CW00347749

Feline Ophthalmology

An Atlas & Text

Keith C Barnett
OBE, MA, PhD, BSc, DVOphthal,
FRCVS, DipECVO,
Principal Scientist and Head, Centre for
Small Animal Studies, Animal Health
Trust, Newmarket, UK

Sheila M Crispin
MA, VetMB, BSc, PhD, DVA,
DVOphthal, MRCVS, DipECVO,
Senior Lecturer in Veterinary
Ophthalmology, School of Veterinary
Science, University of Bristol, UK

W. B. Saunders Company Ltd 24–28 Oval Road
London NW1 7DX

The Curtis Center
Independence Square West
Philadelphia, PA 19106–3399, USA

Harcourt Brace & Company
55 Horner Avenue
Toronto, Ontario M8Z 4X6, Canada

Harcourt Brace & Company, Australia
30–52 Smidmore Street
Marrickville, NSW 2204, Australia

Harcourt Brace & Company, Japan
Ichibancho Central Building, 22–1 Ichibancho
Chiyoda-ku, Tokyo 102, Japan

This book is printed on acid free paper

A catalogue record for this book is available from the British Library

ISBN 0–7020–1662–4

Typeset by J&L Composition Ltd, Filey, North Yorkshire
Colour Separation by Tenon & Polert Colour Scanning Ltd,HK.
Printed in Barcelona by Grafos, S.A., Arte sobre papel

Contents

Contributors

R. DENNIS
MA, VetMB, DVR, MRCVS
Head, Imaging Unit, Centre for Small Animal Studies, Animal Health Trust,
Newmarket, UK

M.C.A. KING
BSc, BVMS, CertVOphthal, MRCVS
Resident in Veterinary Ophthalmology,
University of Bristol, UK

J.R.B. MOULD
BVSc, BA, DVOphthal, MRCVS
Lecturer in Veterinary Ophthalmology,
University of Glasgow, UK

J. SANSOM
BVSc, DVOphthal, MRCVS, DipECVO
Head, Comparative Ophthalmology Unit, Centre for Small Animal Studies, Animal Health Trust,
Newmarket, UK

A.H. SPARKES
BVetMed, PhD, MRCVS
Lecturer in Feline Medicine, School of Veterinary Science,
University of Bristol, UK

Preface

Feline Ophthalmology: An Atlas and Text is intended for veterinary surgeons in small animal practice and for veterinary students in their clinical years. We also hope that veterinary ophthalmologists will find it of value, for one consequence of the immense popularity of cats as household pets is an increasing number of referrals to specialist veterinary ophthalmologists. We believe that the atlas may also appeal to some scientists, breeders and owners interested in the cat as a species.

Many eye problems in the cat are quite different from those found in the dog, or any other animal; corneal sequestrum, for example, appears to be unique to the cat. A number of congenital conditions have been described, but, to date, few of those present from birth, or developing later in life, have been shown to be inherited, quite unlike the situation in the dog. Ocular manifestations of systemic disease are quite common in cats and routine examination may be crucial as an aid to diagnosis. For example, the feline eye appears to be particularly susceptible to the effects of systemic hypertension, a common problem in older cats which can be diagnosed with confidence by examination of the ocular fundus. The diagnosis of neurometabolic storage diseases in kittens is rendered easier if the characteristic cellular accumulations can be visualized directly in the cornea or retina. Deficiencies of taurine and thiamine can change the appearance of the ocular fundus; those alterations associated with taurine deficiency are usually considered pathognomonic. Most commonly, however, it's the diagnosis of infectious disease that is aided by ophthalmic examination; causal agents include viruses such as feline herpesvirus, feline infectious peritonitis virus, feline leukaemia virus and the feline immunodeficiency virus, parasites such as *Toxoplasma gondii* and, in non-temperate climates, a range of yeasts and fungi. Neoplasia in cats is generally more aggressive than that of other domestic mammals and the eye and adnexa may be primarily or secondarily involved; diagnosis and differential diagnosis are challenging as neoplastic infiltration can mimic inflammatory disease.

The format we have followed consists of an initial chapter on methods of examination, followed by a chapter on post-natal development of the eye and one on the recognition and basic management of ocular emergencies, then follows a description of the eye and its diseases in the usual format of separate chapters on the different anatomical parts of the eye. Included in each chapter is a selection of references, which are not intended to be comprehensive and usually include original reports, sometimes of unusual or rare conditions, together with recent references and review articles. At the end of the book we have supplied a Further Reading list of texts that supplement the references supplied with each chapter. We believe it is the illustrations that are the strength of this book and, as such, have paid particular attention to cross-referencing between figures. In writing, our priorities have been to describe the clinical signs and to assist in diagnosis and differential diagnosis, but we have also included notes on management and, when relevant, provided limited details of surgical procedures. Appendices on equipment, congenital anomalies, hereditary eye diseases, neoplasia and systemic diseases have been used to summarize the information found in the main body of the text.

We trust that this *Atlas and Text* will be enjoyable to consult and of help in the accurate diagnosis and successful treatment of the many interesting eye diseases in this fascinating species.

ACKNOWLEDGEMENTS

We are most grateful to a number of colleagues for the loan of illustrations, which have all been individually acknowledged in the text. We particularly acknowledge John Mould for all the beautiful gross and histological figures and Ruth Dennis for her ultrasound measurements of the developing eye and for the diagnostic imaging photographs. We are most indebted to Jane Sansom, Andrew Sparkes and Martyn King for their considerable contributions to the sections on hypertension (Jane Sansom) and neuro-ophthalmology (Andrew Sparkes and Martin King). We readily acknowledge John Conibear and Tracy Townsend of the Photographic Unit, School of Veterinary Science, University of Bristol and Penelope Rothoff-Rook of the Animal Health Trust for her invaluable work in cataloguing transparencies and tracing case histories.

Finally, may we thank most sincerely our colleagues, both past and present, at the Animal Health Trust and Bristol Veterinary School for their interest in this project, for stimulating and valuable discussion and for their encouragement.

1 EXAMINATION OF THE EYE AND ADNEXA

INTRODUCTION

Accurate diagnosis is based on the history and examination. Familiarity with normal appearance (Figs 1.1–1.3) and in the use of ophthalmic diagnostic equipment ensures that examination of the eye (globe) and adnexa (eyelids, lacrimal apparatus, orbit and para-orbital areas) can be undertaken with confidence.

EQUIPMENT

The basic equipment required for examination consists of a pen-light, some form of magnifying device, a condensing lens and a direct ophthalmoscope. A slit lamp biomicroscope is a desirable, but expensive, addition to the basic range. Further details of equipment are given in Appendix 1.

Various disposable items are also needed in order to perform a range of diagnostic tests and these are also listed in Appendix 1.

USE OF INSTRUMENTS

FOCAL ILLUMINATION

A bright pen-light provides a useful light source for examination of the eye and adnexa (Fig. 1.4). In cats it is possible

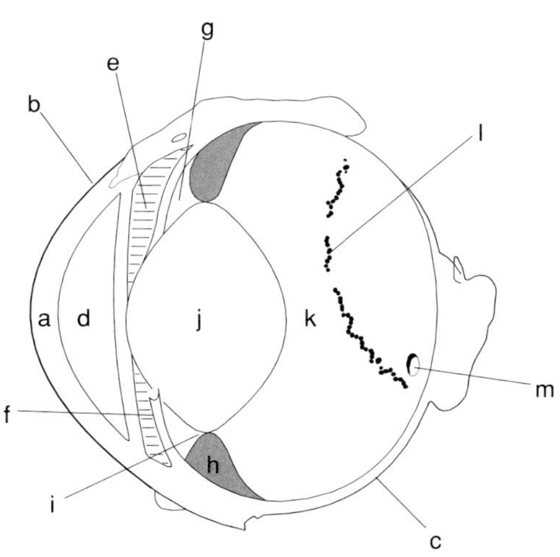

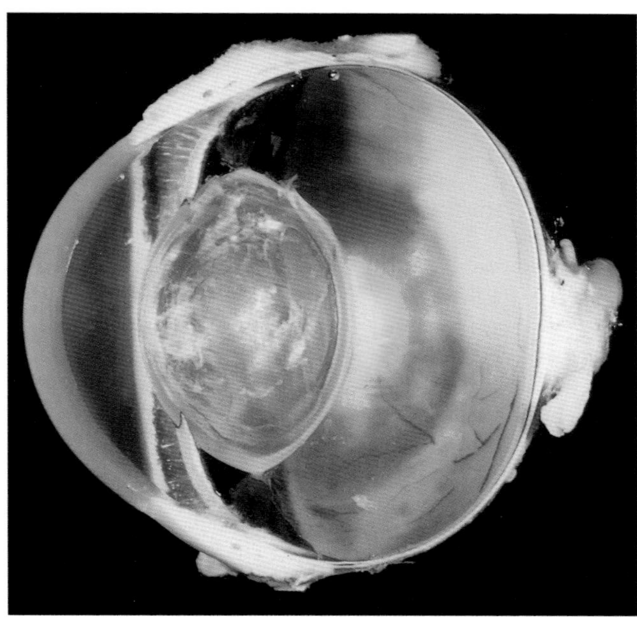

Fig. 1.1 *Gross specimen of feline globe: a, cornea; b, limbus; c, sclera; d, anterior chamber; e, irido-corneal angle; f, iris; g, posterior chamber; h, ciliary body; i, zonule; j, lens; k, vitreous; l, junction between tapetal fundus and nontapetal fundus; m, optic papilla in tapetal fundus.*

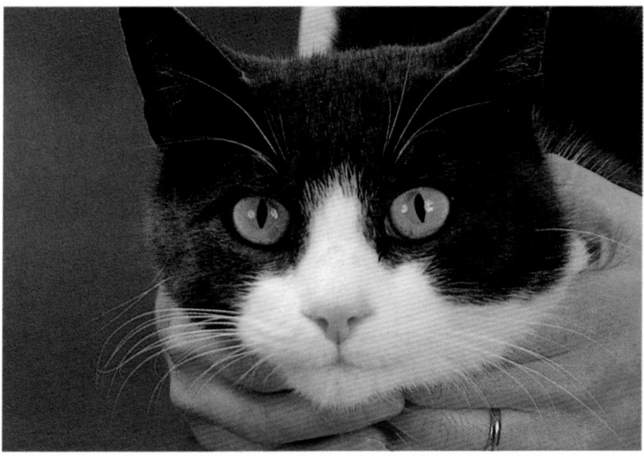

Fig. 1.2 Normal adult cat. Note the symmetry of the face, eyes and pupils.

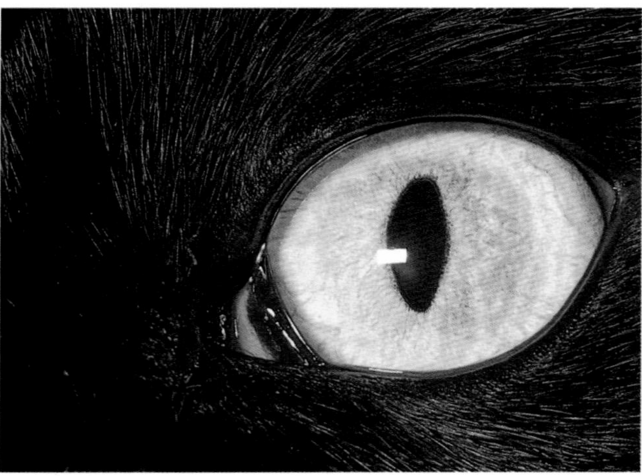

Fig. 1.3 Normal adult cat. The eyelid margins (upper, lower and third eyelid) are clearly defined and heavily pigmented. There is an undisrupted corneal reflex (the camera flash) and the cornea fills almost the whole of the palpebral aperture in this animal with only a small area of bulbar conjunctiva visible laterally (temporally). Note that there is no clear distinction of the pupillary and ciliary zones of the iris (see Chapter 12) and that relative lack of surface iris pigment allows portions of the major arterial circle to be viewed at the iris periphery.

to examine the drainage angle directly using focal illumination (Fig. 1.5) and this technique should be included in this part of the examination. The ease with which the iridocorneal angle can be examined obviates the necessity for routine gonioscopy, but the technique is not difficult to perform when required (Gelatt, 1991).

Magnification

Some form of magnification will be required as a diagnostic aid and this is most readily achieved with a magnifying loupe, an otoscope with speculum removed (Fig. 1.6), a direct ophthalmoscope, or a slit lamp biomicroscope.

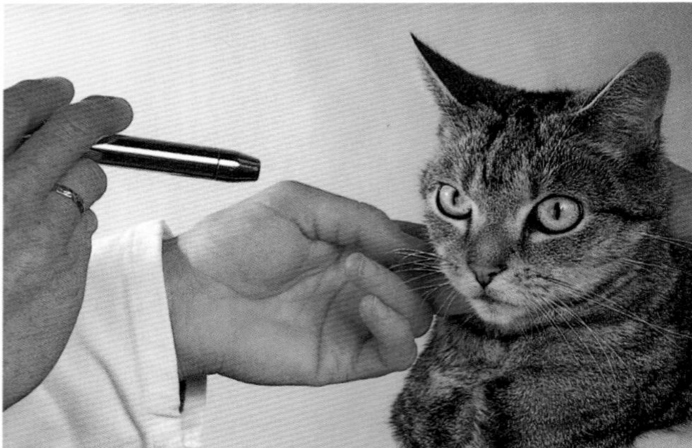

Fig. 1.4 A pen-light being used for examination of the eye and adnexa. This examination should be performed in the dark and the light shone from as many different angles as possible in order to build up a complete picture.

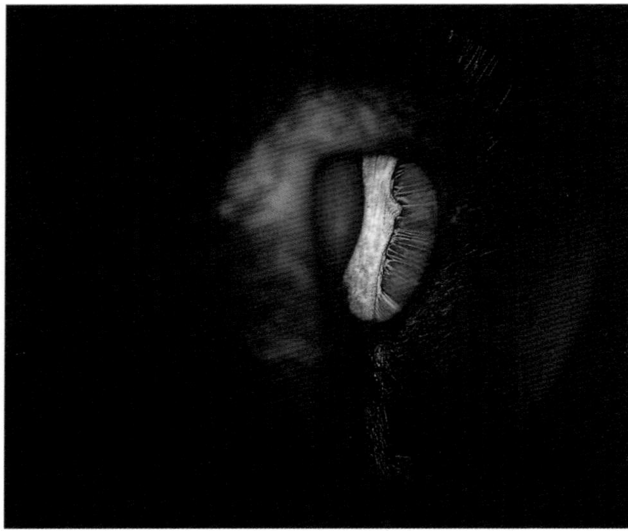

Fig. 1.5 Using a pen-light alone it is possible to examine the iridocorneal angle directly in cats. Note the very wide and deep angle and the clearly defined pectinate fibres which span the cleft between the iris (left) and cornea (right).

Slit lamp biomicroscopy

The slit lamp biomicroscope consists of a light source (diffuse illumination or a slit beam) and a binocular microscope which can be moved in relation to the light source. While primarily a means of providing magnified detail of the adnexa and anterior segment, the posterior segment can also be evaluated if a high dioptre (e.g. +90D) condensing lens is interposed. In cats it is possible to use either a hand-held (Fig. 1.7) or table mounted (Fig. 1.8) slit lamp.

Focal Examination

Gross lesions involving, for example, the eyelids, cornea, anterior chamber, iris, lens or anterior vitreous can be examined with a diffuse beam of light. When the diffuse beam is narrowed to a slit an optical section of, for example, the cornea or lens may be visualized when the beam is directed obliquely.

Retro-illumination

Retro-illumination uses the reflection from the iris, lens or ocular fundus to illuminate the cornea from behind. Minute corneal changes can be detected with this method. The technique is impressive when the fundus reflex is used as the reflecting medium following mydriasis.

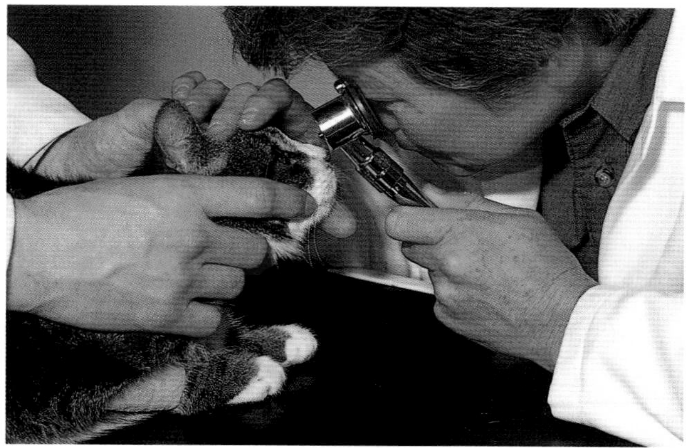

Fig. 1.6 *An otoscope with the speculum removed provides a simple means of combining magnification and illumination. This examination is best performed in the dark.*

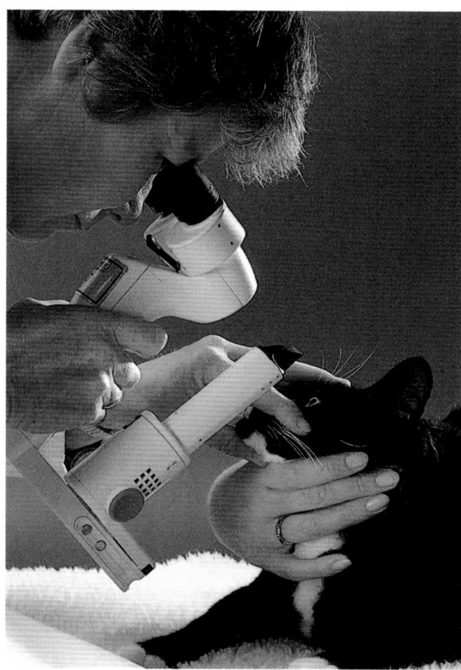

Fig. 1.7 *A portable slit lamp biomicroscope in use. This model (Kowa SL14) is excellent for use in cats. Examination should be performed in the dark.*

Indirect ophthalmoscopy

This technique can be performed most simply using a condensing lens and pen-light (Fig. 1.9). Following mydriasis the lens is held some 2–8 cm from the cat's eye and the fingers of the hand holding the lens should rest lightly on the animal's head. The pen-light is shone through the lens from a distance of 50–80 cm (the distance between the cat's eye and the observer's eye).

Monocular indirect ophthalmoscopy produces an image which is virtual (i.e., viewed indirectly), inverted and magnified, with the magnification depending on the strength of the

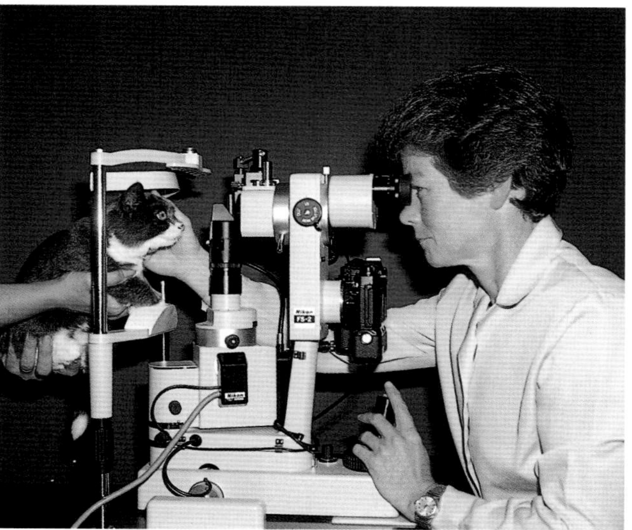

Fig. 1.8 *A table-mounted slit lamp biomicroscope in use. Most cats are tolerant of the procedure. Examination should be performed in the dark.*

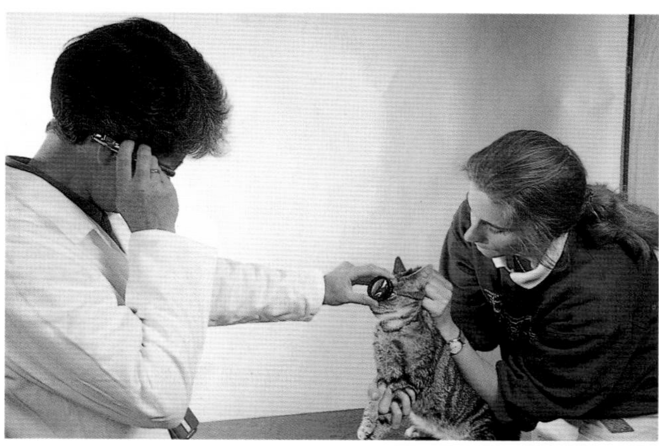

Fig. 1.9 *Monocular indirect ophthalmoscopy being performed with a 28D condensing lens and penlight. Mydriasis is necessary for all types of indirect ophthalmoscopy and the technique must be performed in the dark. A virtual and inverted image should fill the whole of the lens if the technique is carried out correctly.*

lens. More refined and expensive monocular (Fig. 1.10) and binocular (Fig. 1.11) indirect ophthalmoscopes are available commercially.

The advantages of indirect ophthalmoscopy include a wide field of view, a reasonable image, even when when the ocular media are cloudy, and stereopsis, although the last of these can only be obtained when a binocular instrument is used.

Distant direct ophthalmoscopy

Distant direct ophthalmoscopy can be used as a quick screening method prior to more detailed examination (Fig. 1.12), it will provide information about the direction of gaze, pupil size and shape and the presence of any opacities between the observer and the ocular fundus. Any opacities in the path of the fundus reflex (e.g. cataract) appear as silhouettes. The ophthalmoscope is set at 0 and the tapetal or fundus reflex is viewed through the pupil, with the observer at about arm's length from the patient.

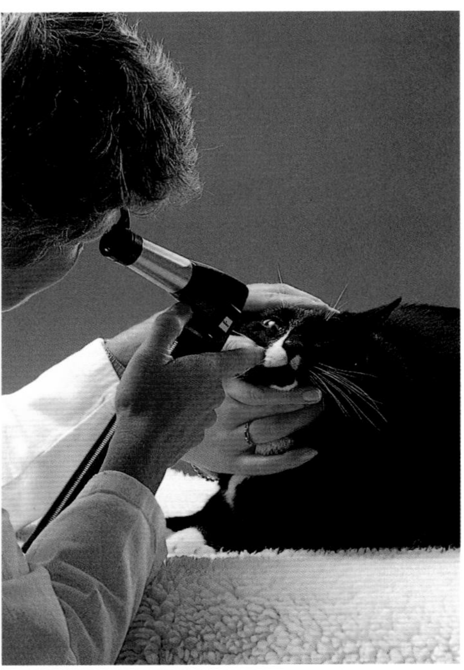

Fig. 1.10 *Monocular indirect ophthalmoscopy using a commercially manufactured instrument. Examination should be performed in the dark following mydriasis.*

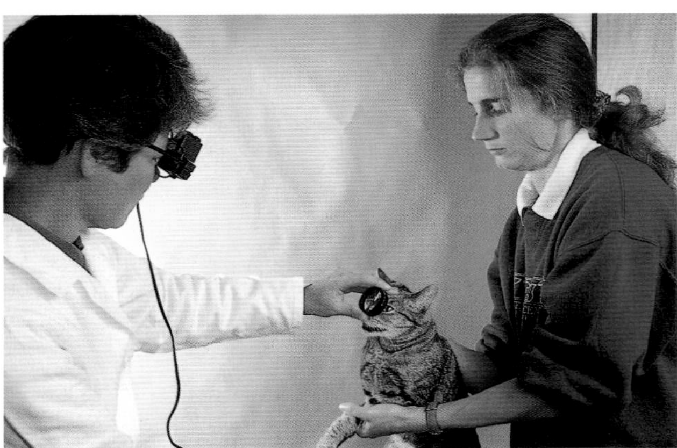

Fig. 1.11 *Binocular indirect ophthalmoscopy using a spectacle indirect ophthalmoscope. Examination should be performed in the dark following mydriasis.*

Close direct ophthalmoscopy

The direct ophthalmoscope consists of an on/off switch with incorporated rheostat, a light source, a beam selector (e.g. large diameter beam, small diameter beam, slit beam and red-free light as an alternative to the normal white light source) and a selection of magnifying (black = +) and reducing (red = −) lenses housed in a lens magazine. The observer looks directly along the beam of light to view the object of interest. Close direct ophthalmoscopy provides an image which is real (i.e. viewed directly), erect and magnified up to 15×.

The direct ophthalmoscope is most commonly used for fundus examination and close direct ophthalmoscopy should be performed with the ophthalmoscope placed as close as possible to the observer's eye and 2 cm from the patient's eye, usually with a setting of 0. Modern halogen bulbs provide very bright illumination, so the examiner should employ the rheostat which is incorporated in the on/off switch, both to ensure that the light intensity is kept at comfortable levels for the patient and to make sure that subtle lesions are not missed because the light is too bright. The instrument should be lined up in the correct position, with the light shining through the pupil, before the examiner looks through the viewing aperture. Fingers of the hand holding the ophthalmoscope can be rested lightly against the cat's head (Figs 1.13 and 1.14).

It is simplest for spectacle wearers to remove their spectacles and set the ophthalmoscope according to the prescription issued for the eye they will use for examination. This allows the instrument to be placed much closer to the observer's eye.

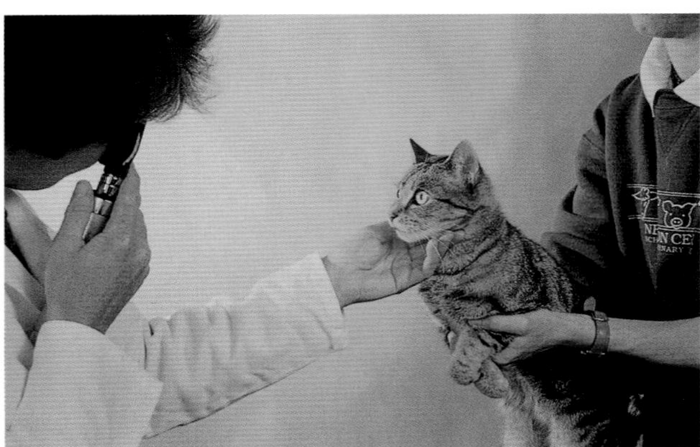

Fig. 1.12 *Distant direct ophthalmoscopy. This technique should be performed in the dark and mydriasis is required.*

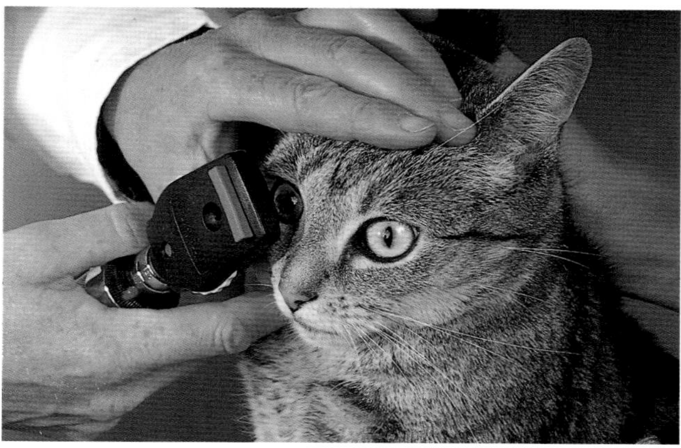

Fig. 1.13 Close direct ophthalmoscopy. The ophthalmoscope is placed in the correct position with the light shining through the pupil before the examiner looks through the viewing aperture. This technique should be performed in the dark and mydriasis is essential for comprehensive examination.

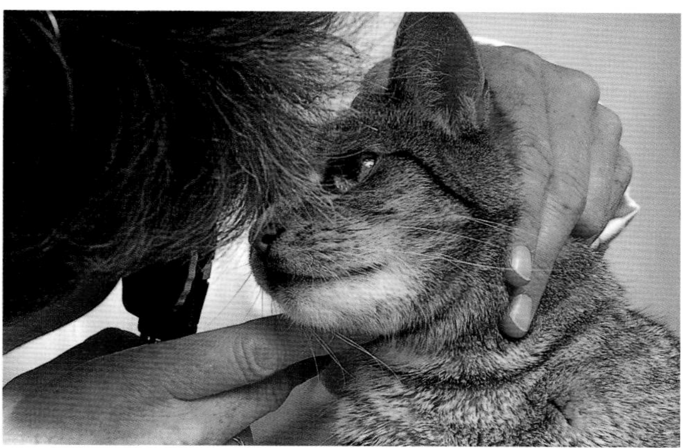

Fig. 1.14 Close direct ophthalmoscopy. The examiner is now viewing the fundus and manipulates the ophthalmoscope to ensure that logical examination of each quadrant is performed. Note how the instrument is steadied against the cat's head by the fingers.

PROTOCOL FOR EXAMINATION OF THE EYE AND ADNEXA

HISTORY

Once the age, breed, sex and vaccination status of the cat has been recorded, information about the present problem and any previous health problems should be obtained. Other relevant enquiries include the management and lifestyle of this cat and any others with which it may come into contact. Details relating to history as an aid to accurate diagnosis are probably more important in the cat than in the dog.

Examination

Examination is usually best undertaken in a quiet room which can be darkened completely and ophthalmic examination follows general and neurological examination (see Chapter 15). Ophthalmic examination is performed in two parts; the first part in daylight or artificial light and the second part in the dark.

Initially, the cat is observed from a distance in order to assess the nature and severity of the ocular problem. If appropriate, the cat should be allowed to move freely about the consulting room; this provides a very crude method of assessing vision (the lighting intensity can be varied).

For detailed examination of the lens, vitreous and fundus, instillation of a mydriatic is essential. This is because, in comparison with the dog, the pupil of normal cats responds briskly and more completely to bright light and the pupil shape changes from round to a narrow vertical slit, resulting in a very limited field of view. Tropicamide 1% is the drug of choice.

In daylight or artificial light The general appearance of the eyes and adnexa is observed and each side compared to ensure that they are symmetrical. The position of the globe in relation to the orbit should be assessed from in front of the patient and from above. The incomplete bony orbital rim should also be inspected both visually and manually.

The lacrimal apparatus is not evaluated in any detail at this stage, although the possibility of abnormalities of production, distribution and drainage may be suspected according to the clinical presentation. The presence and position of the upper and lower lacrimal puncta should be confirmed. The frequency and adequacy of blinking should be noted as an empirical means of assessing distribution of the tear film.

The margins, outer and inner surfaces of the upper and lower eyelids should be examined. There is close apposition of the upper and lower eyelids to the globe, so examination of their inner surface is not always easy. The position of the third eyelid should be observed and its outer surface inspected once the eyelid has been protruded by pressure on the globe through the upper eyelid. The inner surface of the third eyelid is not examined routinely.

The ocular surface is defined as the continuous epithelium which begins at the lid margin, extends onto the back of the upper and lower eyelids, and both surfaces of the third eyelid, into the fornices and onto the globe. Naked-eye examination should indicate whether the appearance of the ocular surface is normal. A pen-light can be used to ensure that the corneal reflex is normal (in this situation the corneal 'reflex' is the light from the pen-light reflected in miniature on the corneal surface without disruption). It may also be appropriate to check corneal sensitivity at this stage, particularly in those situations in which corneal anaesthesia may be part of the clinical presentation (e.g. herpetic keratitis). This can be done in an empirical fashion by touching the cornea with a fine wisp of cotton wool which should elicit a brisk blink in the normal cat. A more elegant and accurate method utilizes an aesthesiometer.

At this point of the examination it is appropriate to apply one drop of 1% tropicamide to each eye if mydriasis is needed as the drug takes approximately 15 minutes to achieve mydriasis.

In the dark Darkness minimizes distracting reflections and is an essential part of ophthalmic examination. A light source and magnification, or a slit lamp biomicroscope, is required. The anterior segment (the internal structures of the globe up to and including the lens) is examined using a light source and magnification, or a slit lamp biomicroscope.

The limbus and cornea are examined first. Most of the limbus is obscured by the eyelids in the normal cat except, sometimes, laterally. The limbal zone is usually clearly defined because of a rim of pigment on the corneal side.

The anterior chamber should be optically clear. A slit beam, rather than a diffuse beam, is used to detect subtle opacities within the aqueous. The depth of the anterior chamber is most easily assessed by use of a slit beam, or by shining a beam of light across the eye from lateral to medial. The anterior chamber is deep and the pectinate ligament of the iridocorneal angle can be observed directly, without a gonioscopy lens.

The iris of most cats is lightly pigmented and the distinction between the pupillary zone (usually darker) and ciliary zone (usually lighter) at the collarette is not always present, so that the iris is of uniform colour. Colour variations may be present between irides and within different sectors of the same iris. Variations of pigmentation produce a range of colours (see Chapter 12). In the least pigmented, genuinely albinotic iris, which is usually pink in colour, the iris is often so thin that it can be transilluminated.

The adult pupil is round when dilated and narrows to a vertical slit on constriction. It is important to observe the size and shape of the pupil, both constricted and dilated, paying particular attention to the pupillary margin, as deviations from normal may indicate posterior synechiae or neurological abnormalities. The pupillary light response is evaluated as part of neurological examination (see Chapter 15).

The whole lens can be examined in detail only when a mydriatic has been used. The light source is used to demonstrate the anterior and posterior lens surfaces by observing the catoptric images which are visualized on the anterior lens capsule (erect) and the posterior lens capsule (inverted). It is easier to establish these boundaries by noting the relative movement of the images in relation to the light source (parallax).

The posterior segment (the internal structures of the globe beyond the lens) is examined next using some or all of a light source, slit lamp biomicroscope, indirect ophthalmoscope and direct ophthalmoscope.

The anterior vitreous is most easily examined with a penlight or slit lamp and should be free of obvious opacities.

Indirect ophthalmoscopy and direct ophthalmoscopy are used to examine the ocular fundus, and, to some extent, the posterior vitreous. Indirect ophthalmoscopy provides low-power examination of a wide area and is particularly useful when the ocular media lack optical clarity. Direct ophthalmoscopy provides a magnified view of a relatively small area (Mould, 1993).

With either type of ophthalmoscopy the optic disc (papilla), which is situated within the tapetal fundus, is located first and its size, shape and colour should be noted. In cats, the optic papilla is usually unmyelinated so that the papilla is round in shape, the optic nerve becoming myelinated posterior to the lamina cribrosa. The retinal vasculature is examined next, paying particular attention to the number and distribution of the retinal vessels. If the choroidal vessels are visible, then they too should be examined. Finally, all four quadrants of the ocular fundus are checked in whichever order the examiner finds most convenient; for example, dorsolateral, dorsomedial, ventromedial and ventrolateral. It is easiest to record any abnormalities using a simple diagram comprising a circle divided into quadrants. Variations, which may or may not be of clinical significance, can only be appreciated if there is an understanding of the normal range of appearances (see Chapters 2 and 14).

Recording

The findings of ophthalmic examination should be recorded by means of annotated diagrams which take only seconds to produce. Photography is also helpful, particularly as a means of charting changes of appearance. Accurate recording should be continued if the cat is examined on more than one occasion.

Diagnostic techniques

Sampling techniques

Swabs and scrapes may be helpful in establishing aetiology (Fig. 1.15) and should be taken from the affected area. Topical local anaesthesia is not necessary when sampling the conjunctiva and eyelid margins, but is essential for corneal samples.

It is important to select the correct culture medium; for example, viral and chlamydial transport medium (VCTM)

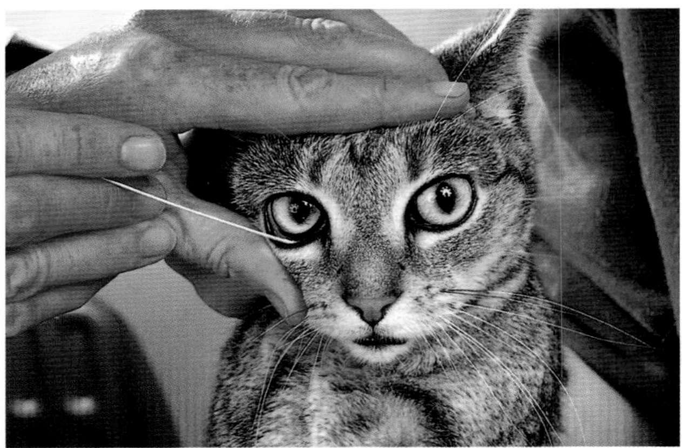

Fig. 1.15 *A conjunctival swab being taken from the lower conjunctival sac.*

is needed for the isolation of chlamydia and viruses, standard bacteriology culture media are inappropriate. If there is any uncertainty about which diagnostic test to perform, it is prudent to contact a diagnostic laboratory before taking the samples. Ocular (conjunctival or corneal) and oropharyngeal swabs will be required as part of the diagnostic work up in most cats which present with ocular surface disease (Fig. 1.16). Dacron or cotton wool swabs have been used traditionally for obtaining superficial cells from sites such as the conjunctiva and cornea but other instruments such as the cytobrush may be superior in terms of the yield, distribution and preservation of cells (Bauer *et al.*, 1996; Willis *et al.*, 1997).

Scrapes are obtained with, for example, a sterile Kimura spatula or the blunt end of a sterile 15# Bard Parker disposable scalpel blade. A smear is made directly onto a clean, dry, glass slide and the preparation is air-dried, fixed in methanol and Gram-stained, or may be submitted to a histopathologist for staining and interpretation.

Impression smears are useful as a means of sampling abnormalities of the eyelid margin or ocular surface. A clean dry glass slide is pressed gently, but firmly, against the abnormal area and the preparation is air-dried and fixed in methanol. As these smears can be difficult to interpret, they are best submitted to a reliable histopathologist. A minimum of two slides should be sent.

Biopsies may be taken from the eyelids and conjunctiva following topical anaesthesia (e.g. proxymetacaine hydrochloride). One drop of local anaesthetic is applied to the eye and shortly afterwards a cotton-wool tip soaked in local anaesthetic is held against the area which is to be sampled for approximately 1 minute. More extensive surgery is best performed under general anaesthesia, with topical anaesthesia as a useful adjunct. A biopsy needle (fine needle aspiration biopsy) or surgical excision is used to obtain the sample, which is transferred immediately into fixative. The amount of fixative should be at least 10 times the volume of the specimen. Neutral buffered formaldehyde can be used for routine light microscopy and immunohistochemistry. Glutaraldehyde (2.5% in 0.1M cacodylate buffer) should be used for electron microscopy.

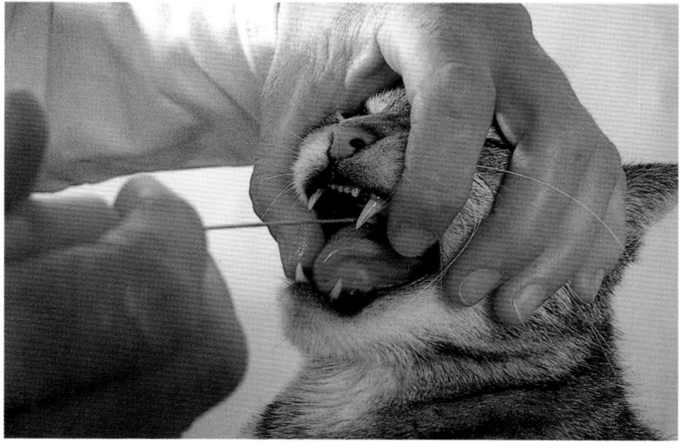

Fig. 1.16 *An oropharyngeal swab being taken.*

Corneal biopsy is useful on rare occasions (e.g. suspected mycotic keratitis). General anaesthesia is required and the biopsy must include the edge of the stromal infiltrate using a microsurgical scalpel blade or disposable skin biopsy trephine. The biopsy can be pressed directly onto a microscope slide for impression cytology.

Aqueous and vitreous paracentesis are not usually indicated as aids to diagnosis in temperate zones, but may be required to confirm and treat mycotic diseases in tropical and sub-tropical areas.

Topical ophthalmic stains

Fluorescein sodium is an orange dye which changes to green in alkaline conditions (e.g. in contact with the normal pre-ocular tear film). It is mainly used to detect corneal ulceration (Fig. 1.17) and is rapidly absorbed by the exposed hydrophilic stroma (see Chapters 3 and 9), fluorescein does not stain the lipid-rich anterior epithelium or Descemet's membrane. Fluorescein should be applied after other tests (e.g. Schirmer tear test, scrapes and swabs for culture and sensitivity) have been performed, as the dye can interfere with certain diagnostic tests (da Silva Curiel *et al.*, 1991). Impregnated strips or single dose vials may be used and it is usual to place the strip or solution in the lower conjunctival sac and allow the blink to distribute the fluorescein. A small quantity of sterile saline can be used as an ocular irrigant to provide sufficient moisture and to flush excess stain from the ocular surface. Subtle staining can be demonstrated with a blue light source.

Fluorescein can also be used as a means of identifying aqueous leakage (Seidel test) following corneal damage or repair (Fig. 1.18) and is sometimes helpful when checking the patency of the naso-lacrimal drainage apparatus (see below).

Rose Bengal is a red dye used to demonstrate ocular surface and tear film abnormalities. It is not employed as a

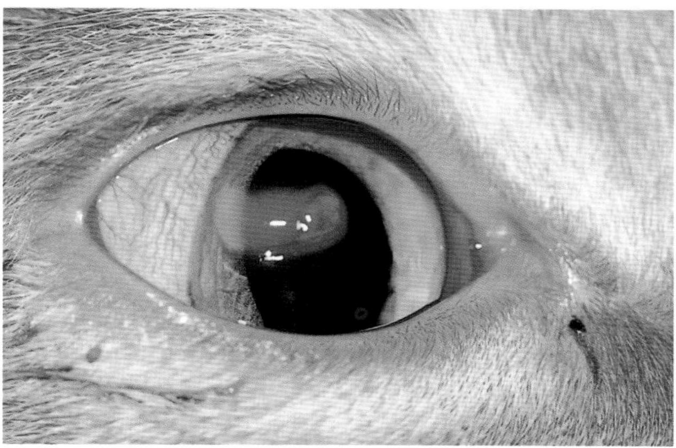

Fig. 1.17 *An 11-month-old Domestic shorthair. A superficial corneal ulcer (the result of a cat scratch) stained with fluorescein. Note the single extra lash in approximately the middle of the lower eyelid which was an incidental finding. See also Fig. 3.25 after the loose flap of superficial cornea has been removed.*

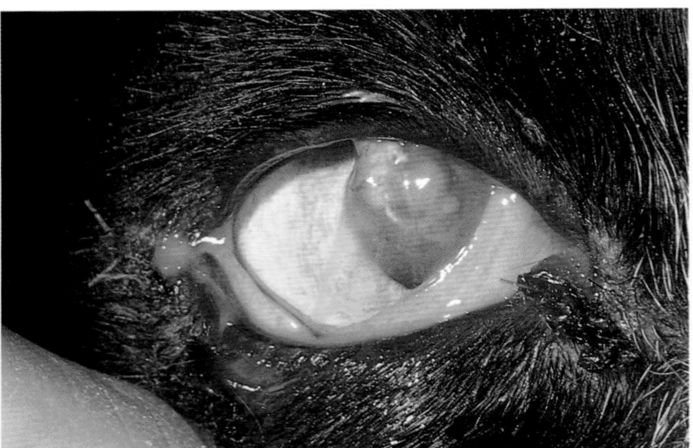

Fig. 1.18 *Seidel test. Aqueous is leaking through a corneal perforation, despite the presence of a conjunctival pedicle graft. The clear aqueous is obvious at approximately '7 o'clock' with fluorescein to each side.*

routine stain because it is irritant to the eye and can interfere with the isolation of pathogens from corneal and conjunctival scrapes (see Chapter 9).

Schirmer tear test

The Schirmer I tear test is the method most commonly employed to test aqueous tear film production. The test should be performed on the conscious, unsedated cat so as to avoid falsely low readings; even so the values are likely to be noticeably lower than those obtained in dogs. Topical local anaesthetic solution is not used for a Schirmer I tear test (STT I) so that it is stimulated (reflex) tear production which is being assessed. Mean values of approximately 12 mm (± 5)/min are obtained in normal cats. Schirmer II testing (STT II) checks basal secretion and is performed after the application of topical local anaesthetic; mean values of approximately 10 mm (± 5)/min are obtained with this technique. With both tests the range of values is wide; in one series of 76 cats the range for Schirmer II tear tests was 1–33 mm and the test results for cats of less than 12 months of age were significantly lower than those obtained for cats of more than 12 months (Waters, 1994). In general, values of less than 8 mm/min should be regarded with suspicion, especially if there is an abnormal ocular appearance or disparity in the STT values between the two eyes. Repeated values of less than 5 mm, together with other clinical signs (see Chapter 7), are indicative of a lack of aqueous component production, manifest clinically as keratoconjunctivitis sicca.

The test is performed using commercially available test strips which are up to 60 mm long, with a notch 5 mm from the tip. The strip is bent at the notched region while still within the packing so as to avoid contaminating the tip with grease from the fingers, the tip is placed just within the conjunctival sac (Fig. 1.19). The strip is removed after 1 min and the value, in millimetres, is read immediately as measured from the notch.

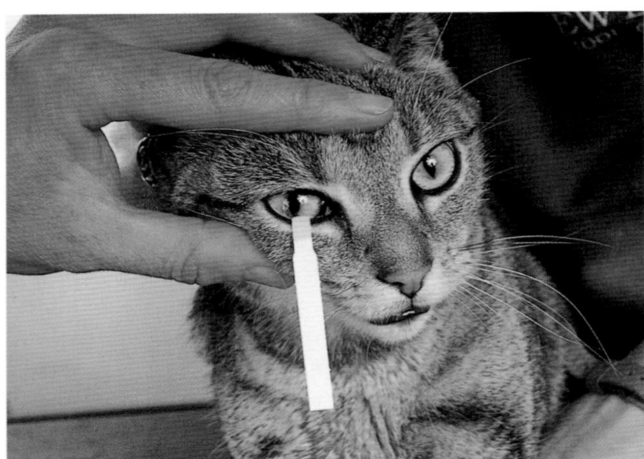

Fig. 1.19 *A Schirmer tear test strip being used to check tear production.*

Investigation of nasolacrimal drainage

The upper and lower lacrimal puncta are small openings located near the eyelid margins approximately 2 mm from the medial canthus. They can be examined directly, but less easily than in the dog, if the medial margins of the eyelids are everted slightly. The excretory portion of the lacrimal system consists of the lacrimal puncta, canaliculi, a rudimentary lacrimal sac and the nasolacrimal duct. The duct passes through the lacrimal bone along the medial surface of the maxilla to the nasal cavity.

Initial examination consists of visual inspection of the lacrimal puncta. Their presence, size and position should be checked, low power magnification may be useful.

Patency of the lacrimal system can be tested using fluorescein drops instilled into the lower conjunctival sac, which may appear at the ipselateral nostril within 1–10 min of application in approximately 50% of normal cats (Fig. 1.20). In the other 50% of normal cats fluorescein fails to appear. A positive result is therefore significant, whereas a negative result does not necessarily mean that the duct is

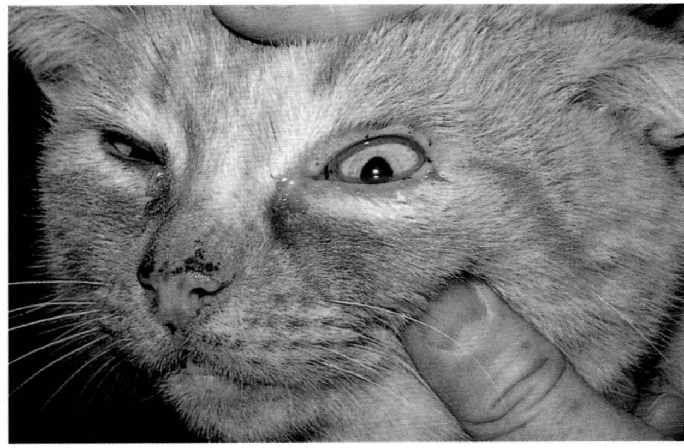

Fig. 1.20 *Fluorescein emerging from the ipselateral nostril after application to the left eye.*

blocked, indeed the fluorescein can sometimes be seen at the back of the throat. Both sides should be tested but with sufficient time between tests to avoid misinterpretation. If samples are required for culture and sensitivity, checking patency with fluorescein is usually omitted.

When samples are required for culture and sensitivity they can be obtained by irrigation with sterile water following cannulation or catheterization of the upper punctum and canaliculus; a range of nasolacrimal cannulae are available (Fig. 1.21). It is better to perform all investigative and treatment techniques under general anaesthesia to reduce the risk of damage to the drainage apparatus. The pharynx should be packed with moist, soft, gauze bandage and the patient positioned with a head-down tilt in order to prevent inadvertent inhalation of the irrigating fluids.

To confirm that drainage is normal, or to re-establish drainage in uncomplicated cases, a set protocol should be followed. Digital pressure is applied over the region of the lacrimal sac to occlude the entrance to the nasolacrimal duct and sterile water or saline is injected via a 25 gauge lacrimal cannula in the upper punctum and canaliculus. Silver lacrimal cannulae are the most satisfactory as they are less traumatic than plastic cannulae and can be reused after sterilization. The liquid is injected with only moderate force and should appear at the lower punctum almost immediately. Once this happens the lower punctum and canaliculus is occluded by digital pressure and fluid should then pass along the nasolacrimal duct and appear at the ipselateral nares a short time after injection. Samples can be collected for culture (aerobic and anaerobic) as they drip from the nares.

If it is impossible to establish patency using irrigation a fine catheter or monofilament nylon may be passed through the drainage system via one of the puncta. The end of the catheter or nylon must be smooth and rounded to avoid iatrogenic damage.

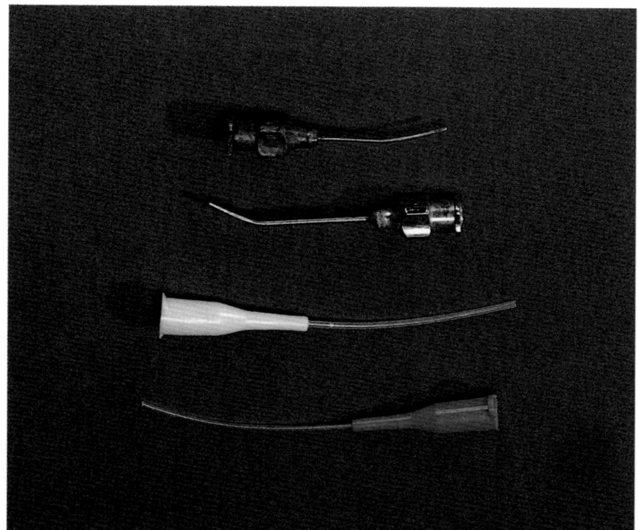

Fig. 1.21 *A range of metal and plastic nasolacrimal cannulae.*

Dacryocystorhinography is a technique whereby an iodine-based contrast agent may be used to delineate the nasolacrimal drainage system. After plain radiographs (usually lateral and open mouth views) have been taken, the upper or lower punctum and canaliculus is cannulated and 2–3 ml of contrast agent is injected as further radiographs are taken.

Tonometry

Tonometry is the measurement of intraocular pressure. The MacKay–Marg electronic applanation tonometer is the most accurate indirect device for use in cats; portable tonometers, such as the ProTon and Tono-Pen (or Tono-Pen XL), are reasonably accurate, although the Tono-Pen has a tendency to underestimate the intraocular pressure. ProTon and Tono-Pen tonometers are still being manufactured, whereas secondhand Mackay Marg tonometers can occasionally be purchased, but are no longer commercially available. Schiøtz indentation tonometry can also be used and is most accurate if used with the human calibration table.

The mean normal intraocular pressure of conscious unsedated cats has been reported as 22.2 ± 5.2 mmHg when measured with the Mackay–Marg tonometer and this correlated with mean readings of 21.6 mmHg obtained with the Schiøtz tonometer and converted into mm of Hg using the human calibration table, the Tono-Pen gave statistically significant lower mean readings of 20.2 mmHg (Miller and Picket, 1992).

Topical local anaesthetic (proxymetacaine hydrochloride) is applied prior to measuring the intraocular pressure; sedation and general anaesthesia should be avoided prior to tonometry as they may affect intraocular pressure.

Diagnostic Imaging

A number of diagnostic imaging methods are available and these are briefly discussed below (see also Chapters 2 and 4).

Radiography can be useful when there are bony changes or radio-opaque foreign bodies, but it is of limited value in aiding diagnosis of soft tissue problems of the eye and orbit.

Ocular ultrasonography (both A-scan and B-scan) is a valuable method for soft tissue imaging in cats and is best performed with a high frequency transducer of between 7.5 and 10 Mz. The technique can be used in conscious cats and general anaesthesia is not usually necessary. Ultrasonography is used in biometric studies, to help with the assessment of cloudy and opaque eyes and for identification of foreign bodies in the eye and orbit. It may also be used to locate intraocular and orbital space occupying lesions, but will not distinguish the tissue of origin and may not always allow differentiation of inflammation and neoplasia.

Computed tomography (CT) will locate and define abnormalities within the eye, orbit and cranium and has been used to evaluate orbital neoplasia in cats (Calia *et al.*, 1994).

Magnetic resonance imaging (MRI) is the best method of imaging currently available and provides superb detail of the eye, orbit and intracranial structures. The excellent spatial and soft tissue resolution allows space-occupying lesions to be delineated accurately – so necessary in surgical planning (Ramsey *et al.*, 1994). Magnetic resonance imaging is available in a number of specialist centres.

References

Bauer GA, Speiss BM, Lutz H (1996) Exfoliative cytology of conjunctiva and cornea in domestic animals: A comparison of four collecting techniques. *Veterinary and Comparative Ophthalmology* **6**: 181–186.

Calia CM, Kirschner SE, Baer KE, Stefanacci JD (1994) The use of computed tomography scan for the evaluation of orbital disease in cats and dogs. *Veterinary and Comparative Ophthalmology* **4**: 24–30.

Gelatt KN (1991) Ophthalmic examination and diagnostic procedures. In: Gelatt, KN (ed.), *Veterinary Ophthalmology*, 2nd edn, p. 195–235. Lea and Febiger, Philadelphia.

Miller PE, Pickett JP (1992) Comparison of human and canine tonometry conversion tables in clinically normal cats. *Journal of the American Veterinary Medical Association* **201**: 1017–1020.

Mould JRB (1993) The right ophthalmoscope for you? *In Practice* **15**: 2, 73–76.

Ramsey DT, Gerding PA, Losonsky JM, Kuriashkin IV, Clarkson RD (1994) Comparative value of diagnostic imaging techniques in a cat with exophthalmos. *Veterinary and Comparative Ophthalmology* **4**: 198–202.

da Silva Curiel JMA, Nasisse MP, Hook RR, Wilson HW, Collins BK, Mandell CP (1991) Topical fluorescein dye: Effects on immunofluorescent antibody test for feline herpes keratoconjunctivitis. *Progress in Veterinary and Comparative Ophthalmology* **1**: 99–104.

Waters L (1994) The Schirmer II tear test in cats. In: *Clinical Research Abstracts*. British Small Animal Veterinary Association.

Willis M, Bounous DI, Hirsh S, Kaswan R, Stiles J, Martin C, Rakich P, Roberts W (1997) Conjunctival brush cytology: evaluation of a new cytological collection technique in dogs and cats with a comparison to conjunctival scraping. Veterinary and Comparative Ophthalmology 7: 74–81.

2 POST-NATAL DEVELOPMENT OF THE EYE

INTRODUCTION

There would appear to be a paucity of clinical descriptions of the post-natal development of the feline eye. This despite the fact that neonatal ocular conditions are by no means rare in this species and, in addition, a number of congenital conditions have been recorded, including some which are inherited. The following description of the appearance of both ocular and fundus development, together with the accompanying illustrations, has been compiled from a study of several individual kittens and litters.

CLINICAL DESCRIPTION

At birth the eyelids normally are closed (Fig. 2.1), as is the external auditory meatus. There is considerable variation in the time the eyes open, with some kittens having wide open eyes at 5 days but others only showing partial opening, from the medial canthus, at seven days (Fig. 2.2); in others the eyes are still closed at 1 week old. Variation occurs within a litter and even between the two eyes of the same kitten. On opening, as might be expected, there is a mild degree of corneal opacity, caused by oedema, which temporarily prevents scrutiny of the anterior and posterior segments of the eye.

At 7–10 days the pupillary membrane is obvious as fine anastomosing vessels occupying the whole pupil (Fig. 2.3), together with tiny red blood vessels visible on the surface of a grey-blue iris. It is not possible to examine any details of the fundus and the fundus reflex at this time is greyish pink in colour. At 10 days the cornea is clear (Fig. 2.4) and a good, but slow, pupillary light reflex should be present. Remnants of the pupillary membrane are still visible across the pupil and the superficial blood vessels on the anterior surface of the iris are more evident (Fig. 2.5).

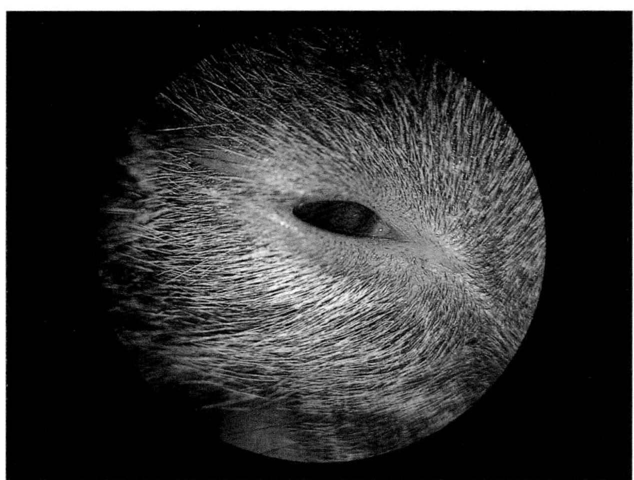

Fig. 2.2 *Eyelids opening from medial canthus (7 days).*

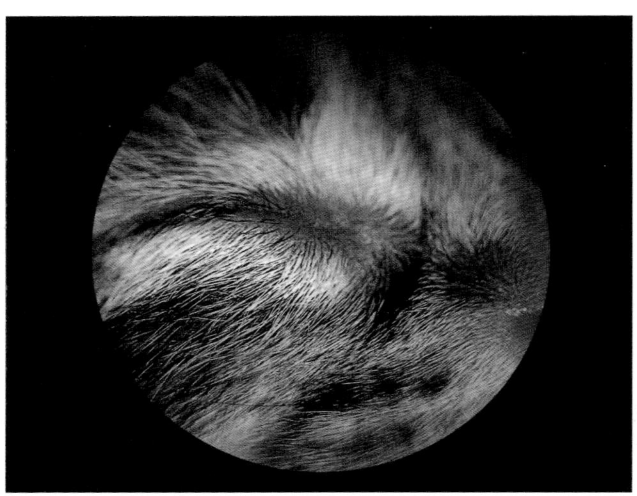

Fig. 2.1 *Eyes closed (1 day).*

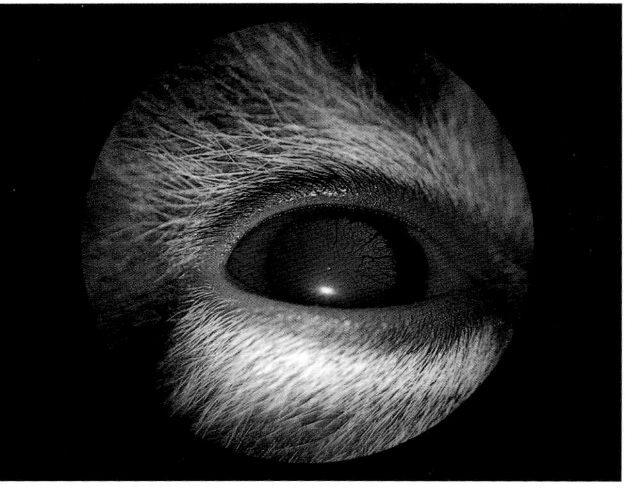

Fig. 2.3 *Pupillary membrane across whole pupil (7 days).*

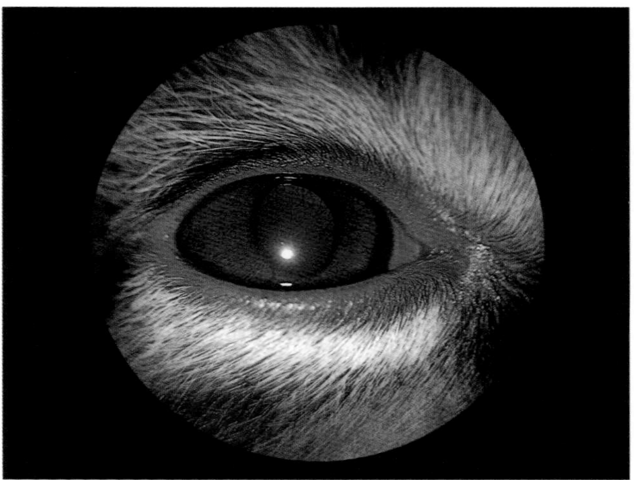

Fig. 2.4 *Clear cornea and note fine blood vessels on iris (10 days).*

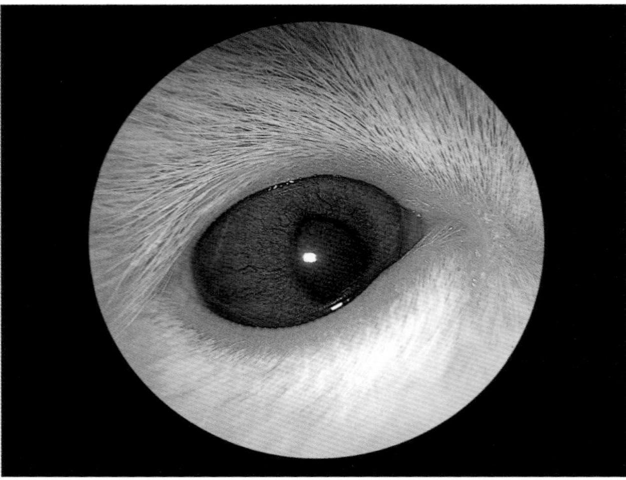

Fig. 2.6 *Change in colour and appearance of blood vessels on iris (14 days).*

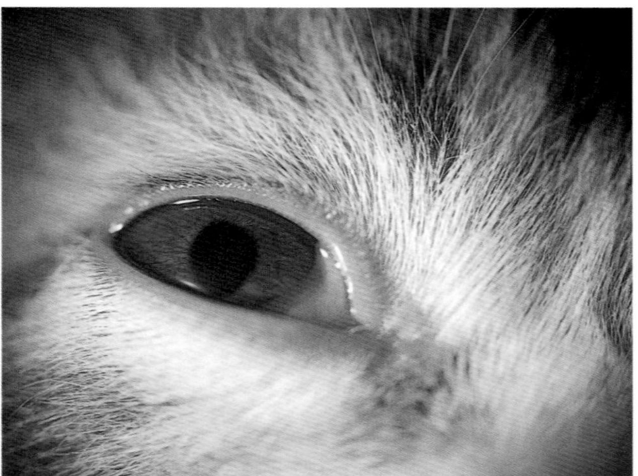

Fig. 2.5 *Blood vessels on iris prominent, pupillary membrane remnants still visible (10 days).*

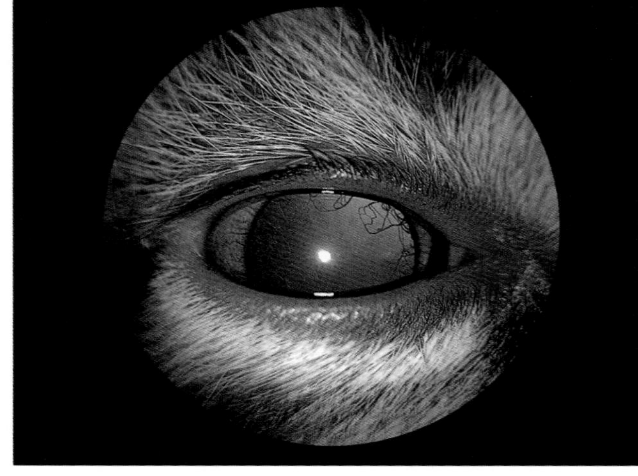

Fig. 2.7 *Breakdown of pupillary membrane but fine vessels still visible from collarette onto lens surface (14 days).*

At 14 days old the blood vessels on the anterior surface of the iris are less obvious and the colour of the iris has lost its intense blue appearance (Fig. 2.6). Further absorption of the pupillary membrane is now evident, although small loops of the anterior tunica vasculosa lentis are visible with blood vessels crossing from the mid iris region (collarette) onto the surface of the lens (Fig. 2.7). Further breakdown of the pupillary membrane occurs (Fig. 2.8) and, with mydriasis, small loops are visible against the lens at the edge of the pupillary aperture. The posterior tunica vasculosa lentis is still complete (Fig. 2.9), together with a hyaloid remnant. The fundus is now visible and a slate grey future tapetal region and a darker nontapetal region (Fig. 2.10) can be distinguished. Faint choroidal blood vessels may be visible in the upper part (Fig. 2.11).

At 3 weeks old the blood vessels which were obvious on the anterior surface of the iris are no longer evident and the appearance is more like that of the adult (Fig. 2.12). With the pupil dilated a few remaining vessels of the posterior vasculosa lentis can be seen (Fig. 2.13) and one or two small loops of the anterior vasculosa lentis may remain. The fundus exhibits the typical lilac colour of the developing tapetum (Fig. 2.14).

The iris at 1 month old shows further change in colour and it is just possible at this age to recognize the almost metallic appearance of the adult iris (Fig. 2.15). Also at one month of age a few remaining fine vessels of the posterior vasculosa lentis are still apparent (Fig. 2.16). The fundus is now distinctly divisible into tapetal and nontapetal parts but the future tapetum is still a lilac-blue colour. The retinal blood vessels (arteries and veins) are now more obvious (Fig. 2.17).

The fundus at 6 weeks (Fig. 2.18; this is the same kitten as in Fig. 2.10) shows the first signs of the adult green

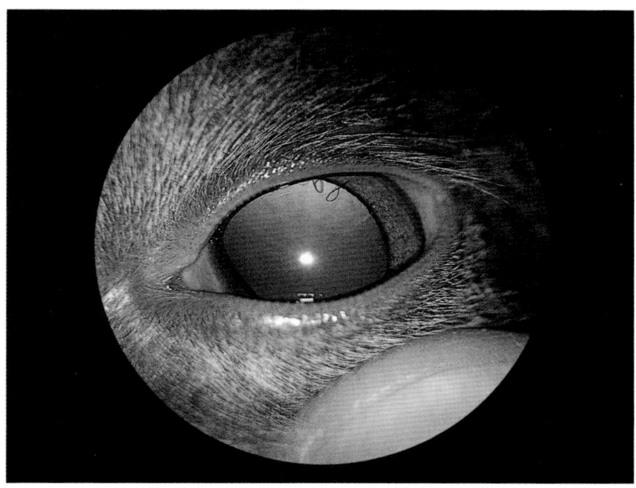

Fig. 2.8 *Further degeneration of pupillary membrane (14 days). Figs 2.7 and 2.8 are of littermates taken on the same day.*

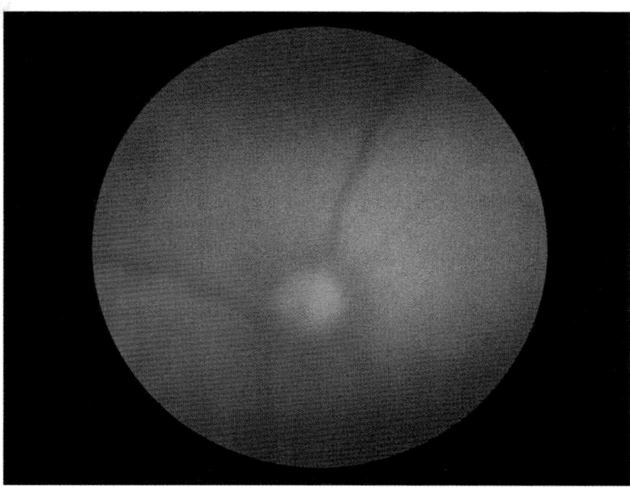

Fig. 2.10 *Fundus showing early differentiation into tapetal and nontapetal parts (14 days).*

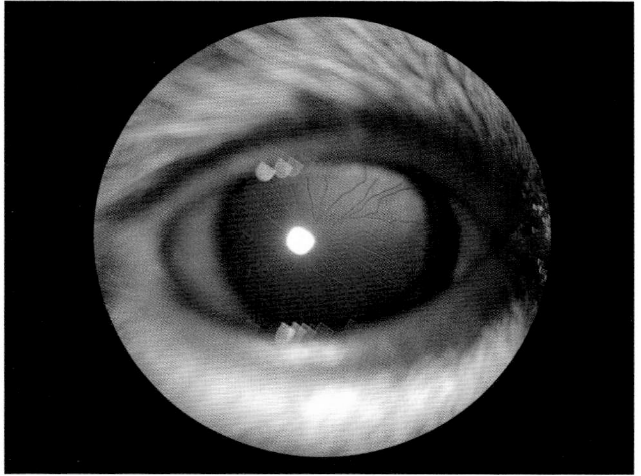

Fig. 2.9 *Posterior tunica vasculosa lentis (14 days).*

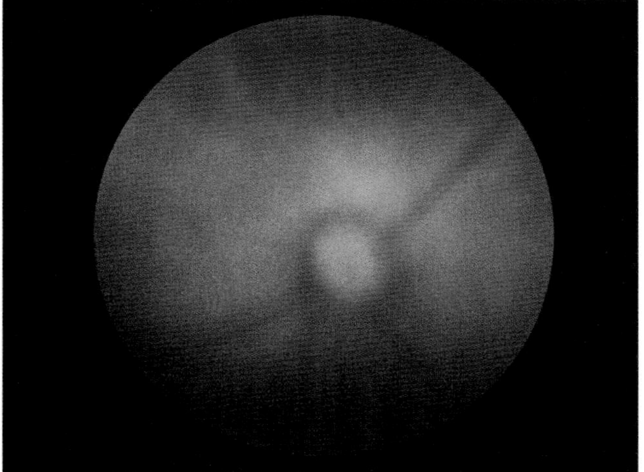

Fig. 2.11 *Another fundus at same age. Note choroidal vessels visible in upper part (14 days).*

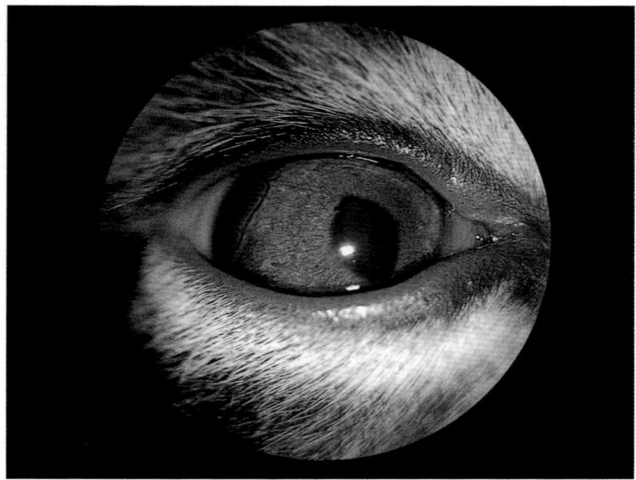

Fig. 2.12 *Further change in appearance of surface of iris (21 days).*

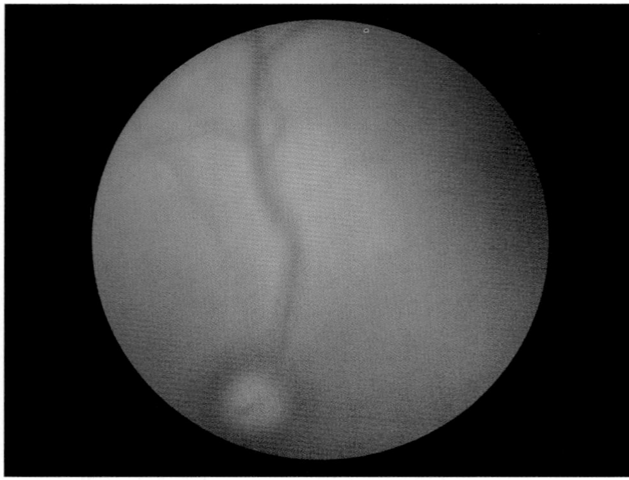

Fig. 2.14 *Fundus showing typical lilac colour of future tapetum (21 days). Note hyaloid remnant superimposed over optic disc.*

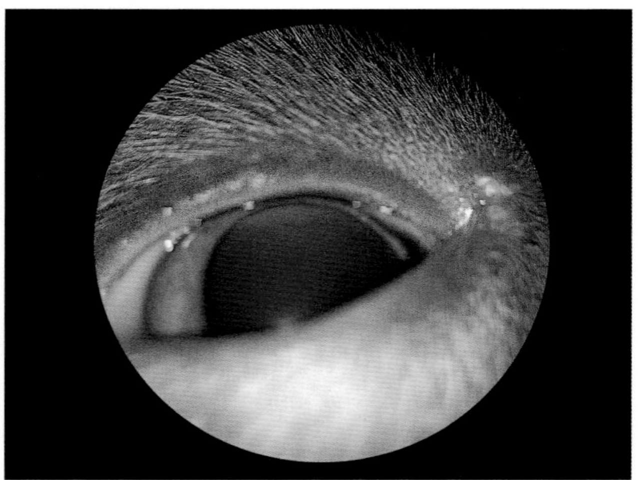

Fig. 2.13 *Few remaining vessels of posterior vasculosa lentis (21 days).*

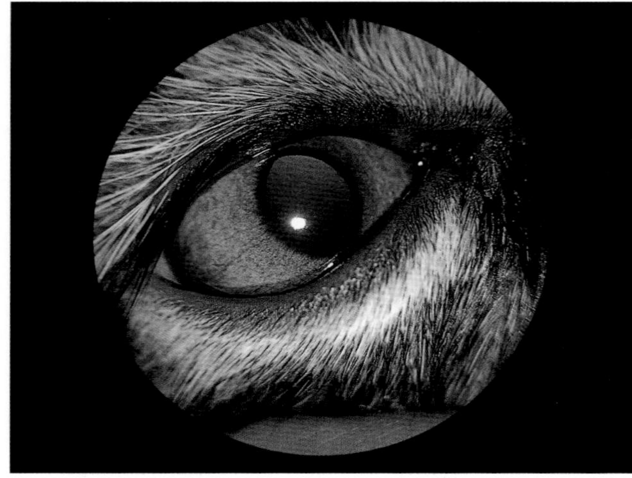

Fig. 2.15 *Developing metallic appearance of adult iris surface (28 days).*

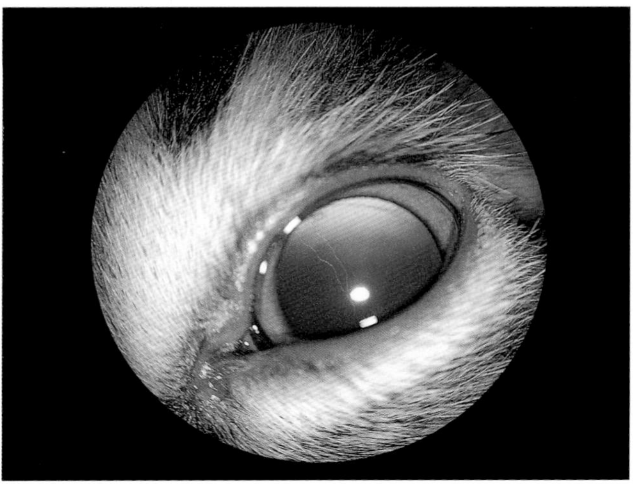

Fig. 2.16 *Few remaining vessels of posterior vasculosa lentis (28 days).*

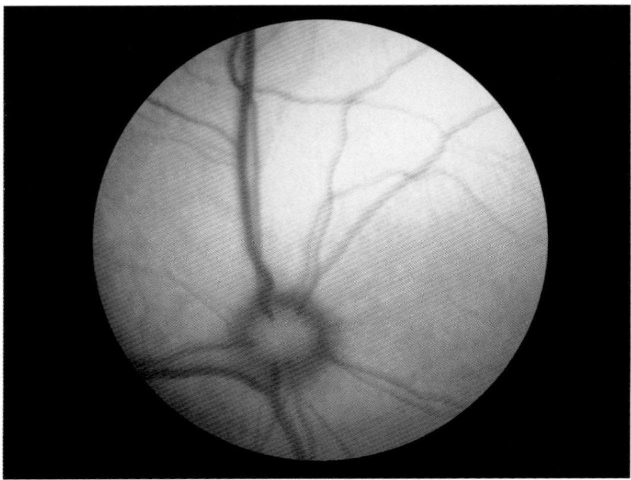

Fig. 2.18 *First signs of adult green tapetum (42 days).*

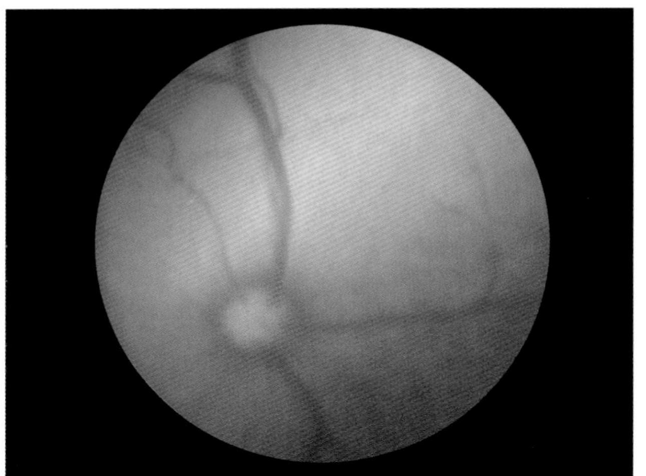

Fig. 2.17 *Fundus showing obvious difference between arteries and veins (28 days).*

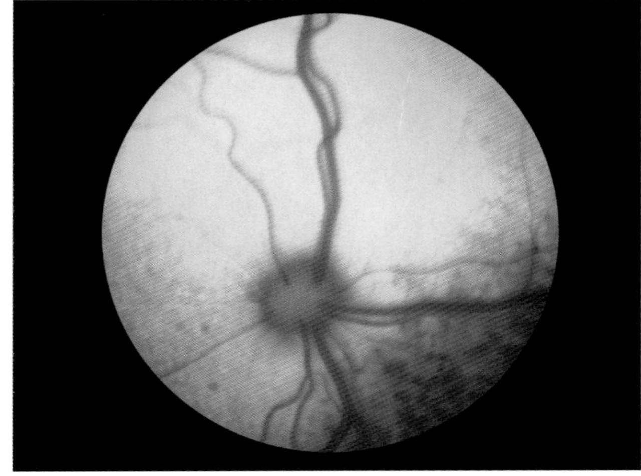

Fig. 2.19 *Development of both tapetal and nontapetal areas (56 days; 8 weeks).*

tapetum. At 8 weeks (Fig. 2.19; this is the same kitten as in Fig. 2.17) the whole tapetal region has taken on this green colour and heavy pigmentation is now evident in the non-tapetal fundus. At this age there is no longer any evidence of the tunica vasculosa lentis and with tapetal development the previously visible choroidal vessels can no longer be seen in the fundus.

By 10 weeks old the tapetal fundus appears yellow-green-blue from its upper part down to the junction with the non-tapetal fundus (Fig. 2.20); at 3 months (Fig. 2.21; this is the same kitten as in Figs 2.10 and 2.18) these colours are more obvious. At 6 months (Fig. 2.22) the fundus appears almost adult and little, if any, changes in appearance of the normal fundus occur after 12 months (Fig. 2.23).

It has been stated that kittens are born with divergent strabismus (Glaze, 1995), apparent after the eyes open, and that normal alignment develops during the second month. However, this phenomenon was not noted in litters studied for this description of postnatal development.

Very occasionally a kitten may be born with the eyes open but in such cases the degree of corneal oedema precludes examination of the rest of the eye (Fig. 2.24).

The post-natal growth of the globe and orbit, as measured by B-mode ultrasonography, is described in Chapter 4.

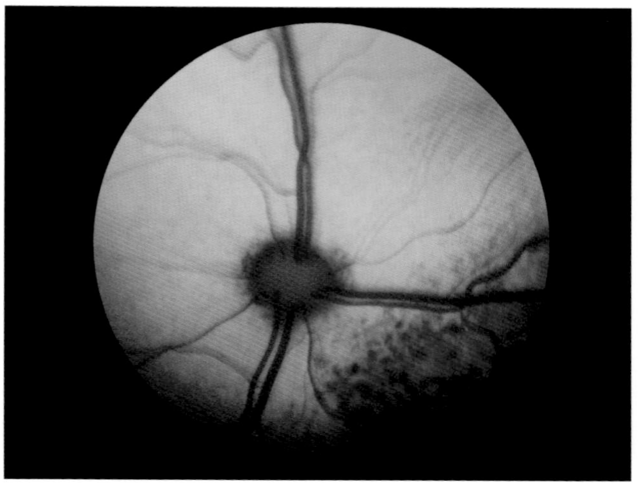

Fig. 2.20 *Yellow-green-blue tapetal region (70 days; 10 weeks).*

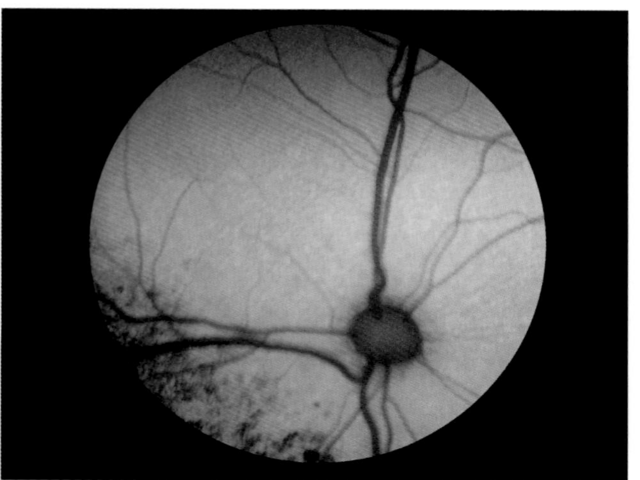

Fig. 2.21 *Further development of fundus (3 months).*

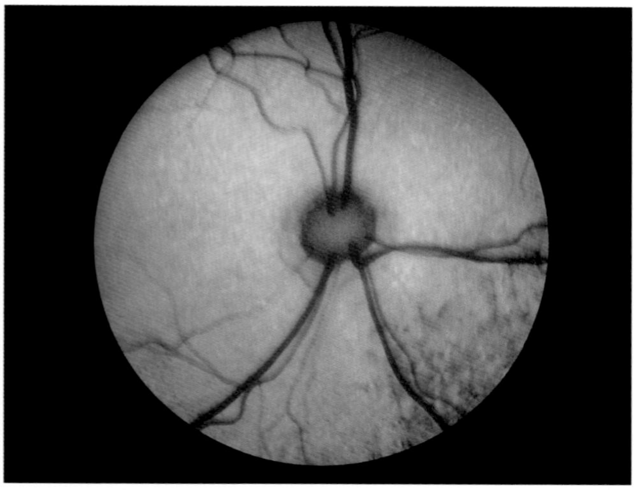

Fig. 2.22 *Further development (6 months).*

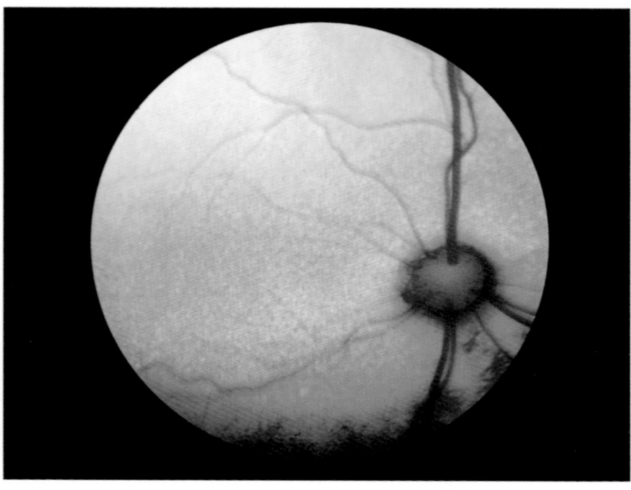

Fig. 2.23 *Adult fundus (1 year).*

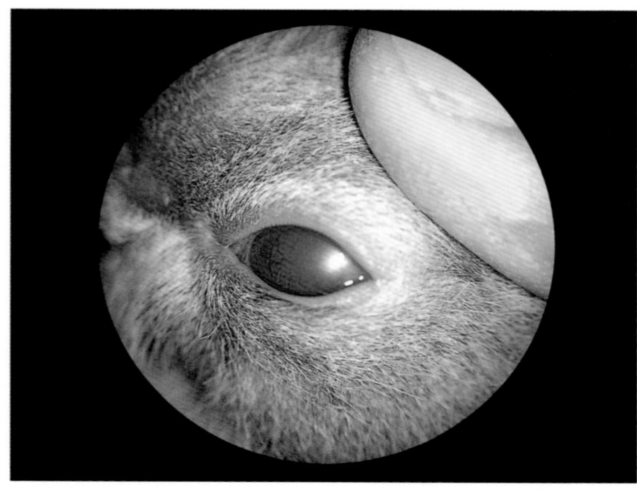

Fig. 2.24 *2-day-old kitten born at full term with eyes open. Note corneal oedema.*

Reference

Glaze MB (1995) In Hoskins, JD (ed.), *Veterinary Pediatrics – Dogs and Cats from Birth to Six Months*, 2nd edn, p. 310. W.B. Saunders Co., Philadelphia.

3 OCULAR EMERGENCIES AND TRAUMA

INTRODUCTION

Ocular emergencies may be defined as situations where prompt intervention is crucial in determining the outcome. Careful patient evaluation will be necessary (Morgan, 1982; Roberts, 1985). If the true extent of the problem cannot be ascertained at the time of the initial examination then it is sensible to seek expert advice without delay.

Traumatic injuries to the eye and adnexa usually require prompt veterinary attention, but it is important to emphasize that when the correct equipment and materials are not available it is better to refer such cases to specialist centres, even though this may delay treatment.

SUDDEN BLINDNESS

Sudden loss of vision (see Chapters 12, 13, 14 and 15) may involve one or both eyes (Fig. 3.1), the pupillary light response (PLR) may be intact or abnormal. There are a great number of possible causes which include trauma, inflammation, neoplasia (Davidson *et al.*, 1991a), vascular accidents, hypertension and hypoxia. Unilateral cases are less likely to be presented unless the owner has actually observed a change of appearance such as anisocoria (see Chapter 15) or intraocular haemorrhage. Sudden loss of vision should be differentiated from gradual loss of vision, since owners often suspect that there has been an acute loss of vision when an affected cat is placed in an unfamiliar environment, but clinical examination reveals long standing pathology.

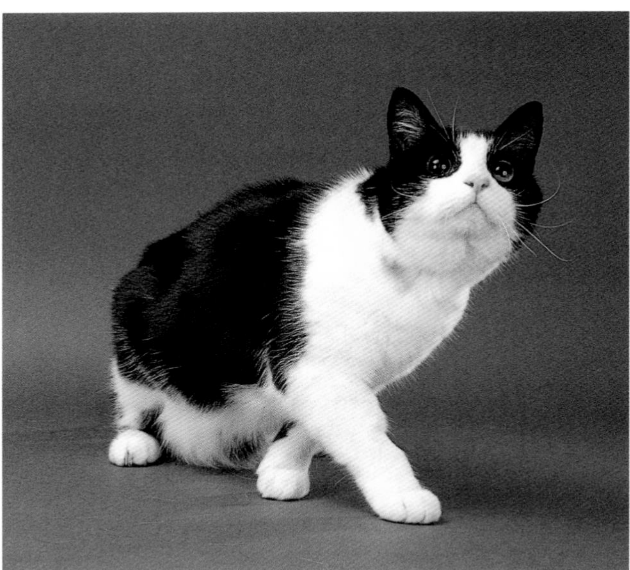

Fig. 3.1 *A 14-year-old Domestic shorthair neutered male presented with sudden loss of vision. The cat was hypertensive and ophthalmic examination revealed bilateral retinal detachment and intraocular haemorrhage. Vision must have been compromised for some time.*

Acute unilateral blindness This is most common following unilateral intraocular haemorrhage, traumatic damage to the eye, including the optic nerve (e.g. traction and avulsion), optic neuritis, retinal detachment and, less commonly, uveitis. It is also possible, but rare, for such cases to be bilateral. The pupil on the affected side is usually widely dilated, but there are exceptions with brain disease and trauma.

Acute bilateral blindness This can follow a head injury and may also be observed as a complication of undetected hypoxia and hypercapnia during or following general anaesthesia, or after cardiac arrest. Affected animals are usually blind but the pupillary light response may be normal, although, again, there are exceptions with brain disease (including trauma). Traumatic brain injury can alter the appearance and reaction of the pupils, as well as affecting vision; the potential clinical presentations are beyond the scope of this book but are reviewed by Griffiths (1987).

Unilateral or bilateral blindness One of the commonest reasons for unilateral or bilateral blindness is systemic hypertension (see Chapter 14). Both primary and secondary types may be associated with retinal detachment and intraocular haemorrhage.

MANAGEMENT

- The underlying cause should be investigated as a matter of urgency, so that rational treament can be given.
- Hypertension is a treatable condition. In those cases which are hypertensive and blind the urgency is to return the blood pressure to normal (aiming for a mean systolic pressure of less than 180 mmHg). Emergency management consists of sodium nitroprusside (Henik, 1997).
- There are other types of blindness which cannot be cured but can certainly be prevented. Surgical removal of the cat's globe can place undue traction on the optic nerve of

the other eye via the optic chiasma and blindness subsequently occurs (see Chapter 14). Careful atraumatic surgery will ensure that this highly undesirable complication is avoided.

- Preventative principles also apply to anaesthetic accidents, especially with regard to proper monitoring during the period of anaesthesia and in the recovery phase until the cat is fully conscious (Clarke and Hall, 1990). The general principles of emergency resuscitation (maintenance of airway, breathing, circulation) apply to problems of this nature in the unconscious animal, as does the necessity for treatment of cerebral oedema (see below). In those unfortunate circumstances where blindness is apparent in the conscious cat following a recognized or unrecognized peri-anaesthetic incident, the most urgent need is to reduce the cerebral oedema that follows hypoxic brain damage by treatment with systemic corticosteroids (e.g. 30 mg/kg methylprednisolone sodium succinate i/v) and diuretics (e.g. 0.25–1.0 g/kg 20% mannitol i/v, initially, followed by frusemide 0.7 mg/kg i/v or i/m 15 min later). A proportion of cases will regain useful or normal vision but others will remain blind.
- The success of treatment for other cases of sudden onset blindness depends upon establishing and eliminating the cause. Optic neuritis and retrobulbar neuritis may be treated symptomatically with oral prednisolone (e.g. 1–2 mg/kg body weight for 5 days with a reducing regime thereafter) while the aetiology is investigated (e.g. viral infection, see Chapters 12 and 14).

Orbital trauma

Both penetrating and blunt injuries (see Chapter 4) can cause orbital trauma (Fig. 3.2). Cats differ from dogs in that they have an internal vascular rete arising from the maxillary artery located in the region of the orbital fissure; haemorrhage may sometimes arise from this site.

Careful physical examination is necessary to determine the extent of the damage, in particular noting pain, swelling, haemorrhage, globe position, loss of symmetry or other facial deformity, epistaxis, crepitus and subcutaneous or orbital emphysema (Wolfer and Grahn, 1995). The last usually indicates involvement of a periorbital sinus. Radiographic examination of the skull is sometimes helpful in confirming fractures of the skull; oblique views are the most helpful. Imaging techniques such as ultrasonography can be of value in trying to establish the extent of the damage and determining whether there is any retained foreign material.

Management

- If orbital haemorrhage is severe the globe will become proptosed and emergency tarsorrhaphy is required both to provide tamponade and to reduce the risk of corneal damage due to exposure keratopathy. After generous lubrication of the globe with a suitable ophthalmic preparation and placing 2–3 horizontal sutures of 4/0 silk, the eyelids should be elevated over the globe so as to avoid direct pressure on the eye itself; lateral canthotomy may also be required. It should be noted that haemorrhage in these cases is so diffuse that it cannot be 'drained' and blunt probing may exacerbate the problem if the maxillary rete is damaged.
- Orbital surgery is needed only if there is gross displacement at the fracture site, sequestration of bony fragments or gross contamination with foreign material.
- A combination of systemic antibiotic, anti-inflammatory and systemic analgesic drugs may be required. A topical ocular lubricant or antibiotic gel is desirable in order to prevent corneal and conjunctival dessication. It may also be necessary to use a therapeutic soft contact lens, third eyelid flap, or temporary tarsorrhaphy for corneal protection.

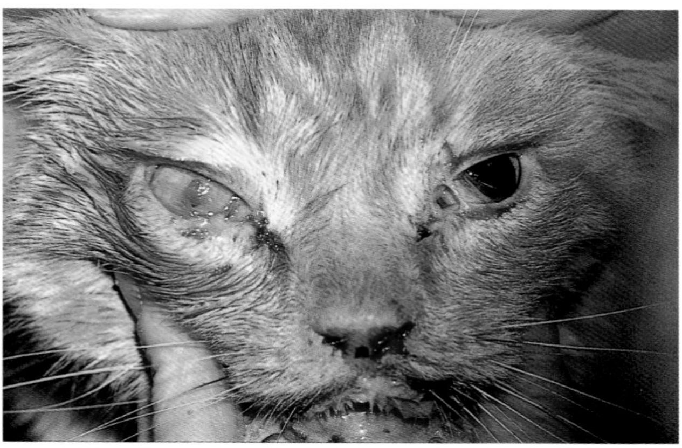

Fig. 3.2 *Domestic shorthair, neutered male approximately 8 years old with extensive head injuries as the result of a road traffic accident. In addition to orbital and ocular damage there were fractures of the mandibular symphysis and maxilla, damage to the hard palate, skin lacerations and epistaxis. There was mild proptosis of the right eye, with pupillary constriction and CN VII damage which had resulted in decreased tear production and exposure keratopathy. In the left eye the pupil was widely dilated; this eye was blind.*

Globe trauma

In almost all breeds of cat the globe is situated in a deep orbit and only the cornea is relatively exposed (see Chapter 4). Traumatic ocular proptosis (Fig. 4.29) is less common in cats than dogs, as might be expected from the anatomy of the feline orbit, and carries an unfavourable prognosis for vision (Gilger *et al.*, 1995). Penetrating injuries are relatively common as a result of fight injuries (see below), whereas blunt ocular trauma is less common but usually more damaging to the globe. Both types of injury may be difficult to assess, especially if gross corneal oedema or intraocular haemorrhage are present (Figs 3.3 and 3.4).

The diagnostic approach is as already described for orbital trauma (see above). Ultrasonography may be useful for assessing the extent of ocular damage (e.g. retinal detachment and splits in the ocular coats). The prognosis for vision is always guarded when extensive intraocular haemorrhage follows either penetrating or blunt injury.

The potential complications of ocular trauma are many and range from loss of the eye to varying effects on vision as, for example, from lens rupture, cataract formation or posterior segment damage (Figs 3.4–3.6) such as retinal oedema, retinal haemorrhage, retinal tears, retinal detachment, full thickness splits in the ocular coats, optic nerve damage and intraocular haemorrhage. Examination of the eye, including the fundus, at the time of the injury may make it easier to determine the prognosis and to explain subsequent complications. However, it is important to emphasize that the eye may appear normal immediately after the injury and sequential examination may be necessary to detect subsequent degenerative changes in the retina, choroid and optic nerve.

Management

- If traumatic proptosis has occurred, the globe should be replaced as outlined above for orbital trauma (see also Chapter 4).
- Blunt injuries are treated symptomatically with a combination of systemic and topical antibiotics, systemic and topical anti-inflammatories and systemic analgesics. Topical mydriatics may also be required because uveitis is a common sequela to blunt injury. If there is a complicating exophthalmos ocular lubrication will also be required

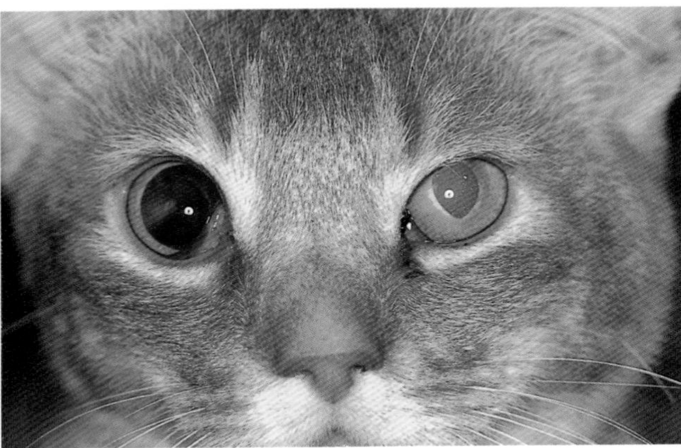

Fig. 3.3 *Young Abyssinian cat injured in a road traffic accident. The pupil of the right eye is dilated and intraocular haemorrhage is apparent within the vitreous. On the basis of ophthalmoscopic examination it would not be possible to establish the extent of intraocular damage. Diagnostic imaging techniques are appropriate and ultrasonography indicated retinal detachment.*

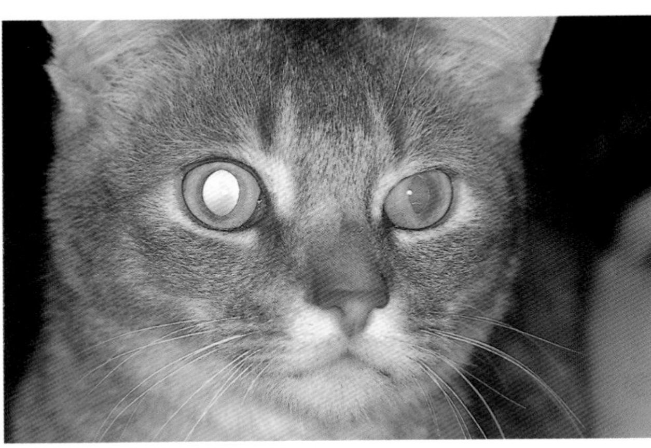

Fig. 3.4 *The same cat as shown in Fig. 3.3 8 months later. The pupil of the right eye remains dilated and retinal detachment is now apparent on ophthalmic examination, the intraocular haemorrhage has resorbed and, although the eye is blind, the cosmetic appearance is perfectly acceptable.*

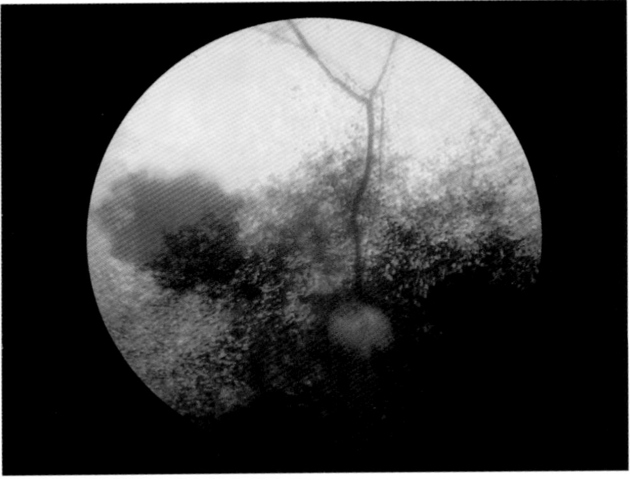

Fig. 3.5 *A 1-year-old Domestic shorthair neutered male with retinal haemorrhage as a consequence of trauma.*

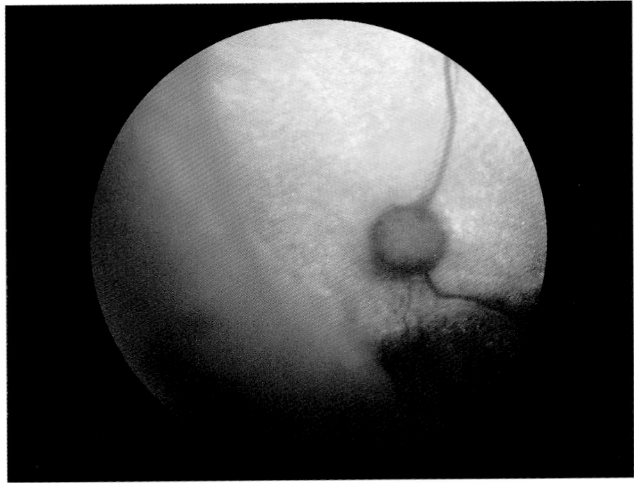

Fig. 3.6 *A 1-year-old Domestic shorthair neutered female. Giant retinal tear and retinal detachment as a result of blunt ocular trauma. There are also small areas of haemorrhage from retinal vessels in the detached retina and from retinal vessels ventral (inferior) to the optic disc.*

as described above. The treatment of penetrating injuries is dealt with below.
- Removal of intraocular haemorrhage should not be attempted unless viscoelastic materials and facilities for microsurgery, including vitrectomy, are available.

Orbital cellulitis and retrobulbar abscess

Many cats fight with other cats and wounds to the head are not uncommon. Infected bite wounds are probably the commonest reason for the development of orbital cellulitis and retrobulbar abscess (see Chapter 4). There is often a lag phase between the traumatic incident and the acute presentation. Other possibilities, such as fractures, foreign bodies and infections in the region of the teeth, mouth, nose and sinuses should also be considered.

Affected animals may present with some or all of acute onset of diffuse periorbital swelling, conjunctival hyperaemia, chemosis, exophthalmos and prominence of the third eyelid (Figs 4.14–4.17). Attempts to retropulse both globes indicates greater resistance on the affected side. Affected animals are usually anorexic and pyrexic. Haematology may indicate neutrophilia with a left shift. Pain is present and is rendered more prominent if the mouth is opened because the coronoid process of the mandible moves rostrally and compresses the inflamed orbital tissues. With the animal under general anaesthesia, it is sometimes possible to see a fluctuating swelling behind the last upper molar tooth.

Management

- The cause should be established and specific treatment given whenever possible. A 10–14 day course of broad-spectrum systemic antibiotics (e.g. newer generation penicillins) is probably the medical treatment of choice. Draining via a probe passed into the ventral orbit behind the last upper molar tooth is also possible (see Chapter 4; Fig. 4.17).

Endophthalmitis and panophthalmitis

Endophthalmitis (severe intraocular inflammation of the ocular cavities and their immediate adjacent structures, but without extension of inflammation beyond the sclera) and panophthalmitis (severe intraocular inflammation which also involves the ocular coats and Tenon's capsule and, rarely, the orbital tissues themselves) are potential complications of serious infections of the eye and orbit (see Chapter 4). These severe inflammations are commonest as a complication of systemic mycoses and ophthalmia neonatorum and following traumatic injuries inflicted by other cats.

The clinical presentation is usually one of pain, redness, loss of vision, pyrexia, lethargy, an ocular discharge, eyelid, conjunctival and corneal oedema and cloudy or opaque ocular media, such that it is often impossible to view the posterior segment (Fig. 3.7). In panophthalmitis the third eyelid may also become prominent if the orbital tissues are involved.

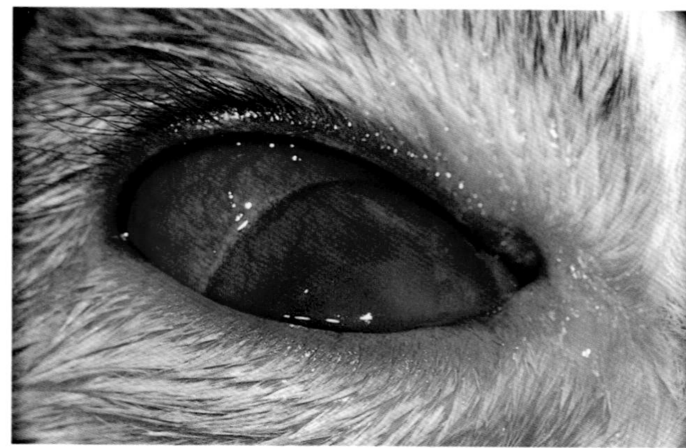

Fig. 3.7 *A 13-year-old Domestic shorthair neutered female with endophthalmitis as a consequence of a penetrating injury (cat scratch) which was not treated.*

Management

- Aqueous and/or vitreous biopsy is indicated in order to obtain material for culture and sensitivity. Smears of the aspirate should be stained and examined to establish, for example, whether Gram-positive or Gram-negative bacteria, yeasts or fungi are involved. Material must also be submitted for culture and sensitivity.
- Treatment is started as soon as the problem is recognized and requires intensive use of appropriate agents; these are administered via the intravitreal route in endophthalmitis, via the systemic, subconjunctival and intravitreal route in panophthalmitis. Corticosteroids can be used to control the inflammatory response if the organisms are sensitive to antibiotics; they are contraindicated if there is fungal infection.
- If pain, inflammation and infection persist and vision is lost then globe removal (endophthalmitis) or orbital exenteration (panophthalmitis) under antibiotic cover is the correct approach.

Foreign bodies

A range of extraocular and intraocular foreign bodies may be encountered in cats. Unfortunately, malicious injuries are relatively common (Fig. 3.8); an airgun pellet, for example, may damage the globe severely and destroy vision before lodging within the orbit. If the ocular inflammation can be controlled and the lens has not been ruptured, enucleation may not be required and there is no need to remove the airgun pellet.

In the majority of cats extraocular and intraocular foreign bodies are unilateral problems of acute onset. If there is a

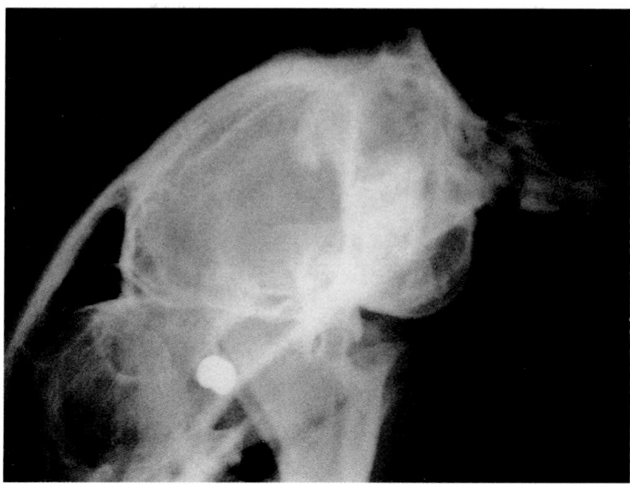

Fig. 3.8 Adult Domestic shorthair. Airgun pellet lodged within the orbit.

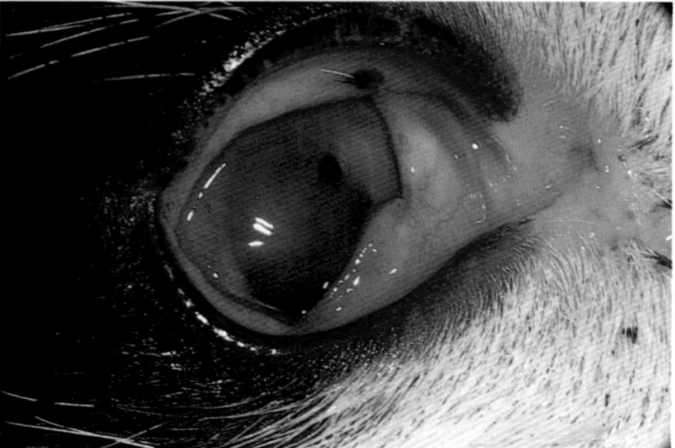

Fig. 3.9 7-year-old Domestic shorthair neutered female. Foreign body (skin and hairs) beneath the upper eyelid, note the deep ulcer that they have caused. The owner reported that the cat had been scratched by another cat a month or so previously and that this scratch had damaged the third eyelid (there is a notch in the free margin as a consequence of this injury). It was assumed that the skin and hairs had been implanted under the upper eyelid at the time of the fight (see Fig. 3.12 for a similar aetiology in another cat). The ulcer healed rapidly after the abnormal region (including the hair follicles) had been excised.

possibility of globe rupture, very gentle handling is essential and, if there is any risk of expulsion of the intraocular contents, detailed examination may be safer under general anaesthesia. The clinical signs are varied; there may be no obvious discomfort or the usual anterior segment triad of pain, blepharospasm and lacrimation. A mucopurulent discharge is more typical of established cases. Because there is a wide range of clinical presentation (e.g. blepharoedema, conjunctival hyperaemia, chemosis, keratoconjunctivitis, ulcerative keratitis, iris prolapse, intraocular haemorrhage) it is important to perform a meticulous examination of the eye and adnexa; this should involve checking beneath the third eyelid, the upper and lower eyelids, the remainder of the ocular surface and the intraocular contents in any situation where there is an acute onset of ocular pain, because a foreign body is not always obvious.

Topical local anaesthesia (several applications) should be employed as a routine aid to examination, general anaesthesia is sometimes also required for complete examination. Imaging techniques may be of value, especially for radio-opaque foreign bodies.

Management

- Foreign bodies may lodge beneath the upper and lower eyelids or third eyelid (Figs 3.9 and 3.10). If the diagnosis is not made promptly, the foreign body may migrate elsewhere and become less accessible. In some cases corneal ulceration develops and, because the ulcer is next to the edge of the affected eyelid and often in line with eyelid movement, the diagnosis should be relatively straightforward. Most foreign bodies in these sites can be removed after several applications of topical anaesthetic solution. However, in longer standing cases, where the foreign body has become embedded, or migrated beyond the fornices, general anaesthesia may be required. A bland ophthalmic ointment should be applied topically once the foreign body has been removed; any accompanying ulceration will heal rapidly.

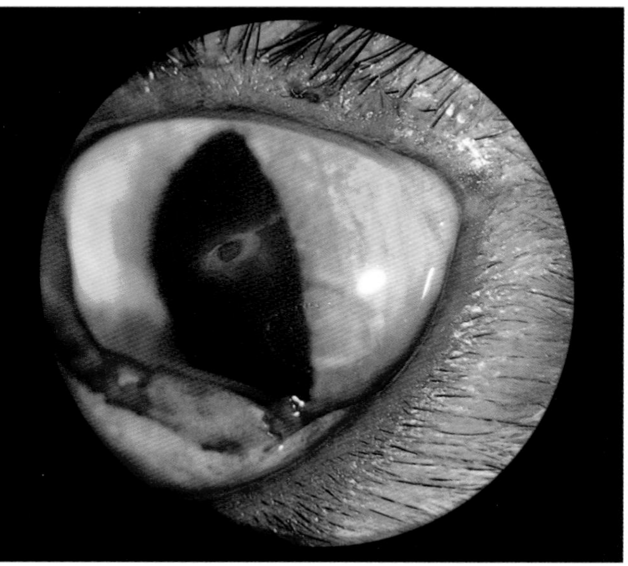

Fig. 3.10 In this young adult cat there is an obvious corneal foreign body in the central (axial) cornea, but ventral to this there is a more subtle oval superficial ulcer close to the free border of the third eyelid. The free border of the third eyelid has a small notch ventrally and part of another foreign body can be seen in the notch. It is the foreign body beneath the third eyelid which is responsible for the corneal ulcer.

- Foreign bodies in the conjunctiva, cornea, limbus and sclera (Figs 3.10–3.14) require removal if they are superficial, or if they are likely to cause, or are causing, irritation. Inert foreign bodies need not be removed unless they migrate and produce irritation. Superficial foreign bodies are easily removed with a foreign body spud, a 25-gauge needle, or by using a pair of fine tissue or mosquito forceps with cotton wool wound tightly round the tips of the jaws (Fig. 3.15). Caution and steady hands are essential for the removal of more deeply placed foreign bodies, to avoid inadvertently pushing them more deeply into the tissues or collapsing the globe. The tip of a protruberant foreign body can be impaled with a fine gauge needle placed at 90° and the object is then removed in the reverse direction to that from which it entered. When the foreign body is more deeply embedded the overlying layers should be incised with a razor-blade fragment or small-gauge scalpel blade to allow access to the foreign body, which can then be undermined and removed with a spud, needle, or fine tissue forceps. Again, if forceps are used it is particularly important to avoid inadvertently pushing the foreign body further into the tissues when the foreign body is grasped.

- Foreign bodies in the anterior chamber, or those which impale the iris (Figs 3.16 and 3.17), can be removed either through the site of original penetration or via a limbal incision with or without a fornix-based conjunctival flap. Arruga's capsule forceps, or similar, are the easiest instru-

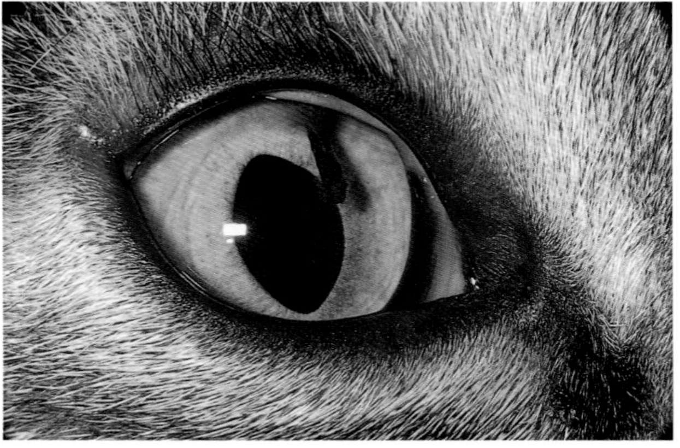

Fig. 3.11 *A 15-month-old Domestic shorthair. There is a foreign body within the anterior chamber of this young cat, but note that there is no sign of corneal penetration and that the eye is 'quiet' and comfortable. The entry site (no longer apparent) was in the dorsal perilimbal region and the foreign body had perforated the iris and come to rest within the anterior chamber impinging on the posterior surface of the cornea. Resorption of the foreign body (presumed organic material) was already occurring when the cat was presented and the remnants are covered by organized fibrous tissue and pigment. Removal was felt to be unjustified in the light of the history and clinical findings and so the cat was simply re-examined at regular intervals while resorption proceeded.*

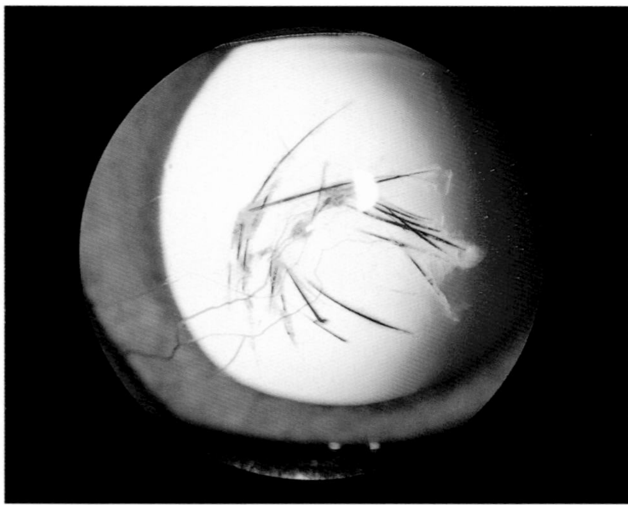

Fig. 3.12 *A 6-year-old Domestic shorthair. Numerous hairs are present within the superficial cornea and there is a mild vascular response, but no discomfort. The hairs had been implanted inadvertently by the cat when it was scratching its ear.*

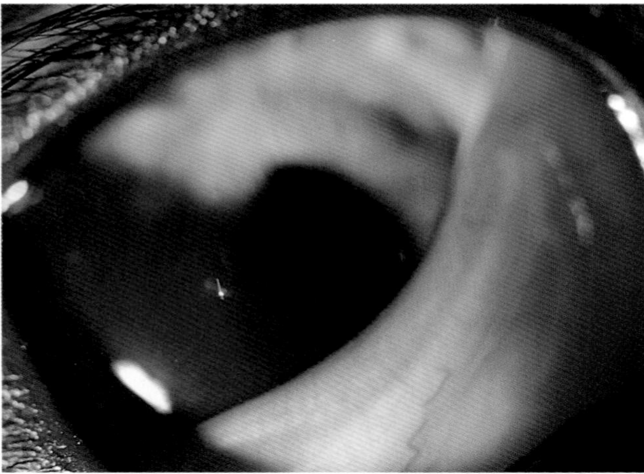

Fig. 3.13 *Adult Domestic shorthair. Several cactus spines were present in this cat's cornea, one is illustrated.*

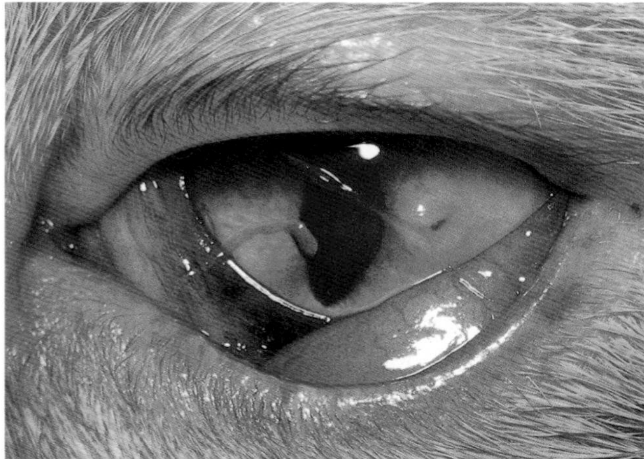

Fig. 3.14 *A 6-year-old Domestic shorthair. Deeper corneal foreign body (thorn). Attempts to grasp the foreign body with forceps have pushed it more deeply into the cornea.*

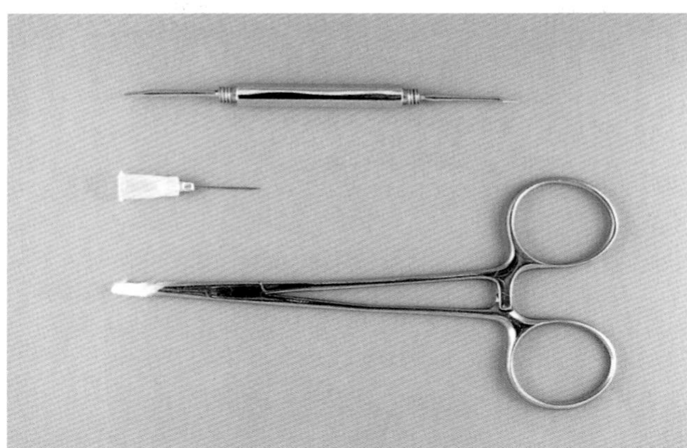

Fig. 3.15 *Equipment for foreign body removal. Mosquito forceps (bottom of figure) with cotton wool wound tightly around the tips are very useful for the removal of superficial foreign bodies as the foreign body becomes enmeshed within the cotton wool. A combined foreign body spud and needle is shown at the top of the figure. The spud is useful for the removal of superficial foreign bodies which are lifted off the cornea by slipping the angled face of the spud beneath them. The needle can be used to impale the foreign body at 90° and then to remove it in exactly the reverse direction to that in which it went in. A microsurgical blade, a small scalpel blade, or the foreign body needle may also be used to undermine deeper foreign bodies prior to removal. A fine gauge hypodermic neeedle can be used in a similar way to the foreign body needle for reasonably superficial foreign bodies. If forceps are used it is safer to apply them at 90° to the foreign body so as to avoid pushing the foreign body further in. Whatever the position of the corneal foreign body, it is wise to ensure that the foreign body is accessible before trying to remove it; this may sometimes mean that corneal dissection is extensive.*

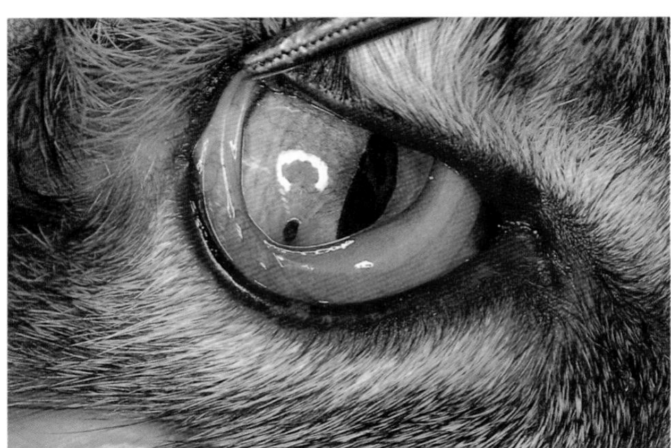

Fig. 3.16 *A 6-year-old Domestic shorthair. A deep foreign body (thorn) has penetrated the cornea and impaled the iris. It was removed without difficulty in the reverse direction to entry using a foreign body needle placed at 90° to the thorn.*

ments with which to manipulate a foreign body in the anterior chamber. Preplaced sutures can make the surgery easier. Viscoelastic material can be used to maintain the anterior chamber. The limbal incision is closed with 8/0–10/0 nylon or polyglactin; the entry wound made by the foreign body does not usually require suturing.

- The inflammatory response to release of lens protein following lens penetration is variable (Figs 3.17–3.19). Cats do not usually develop the severe uveitis which is seen following this type of insult in dogs and horses and

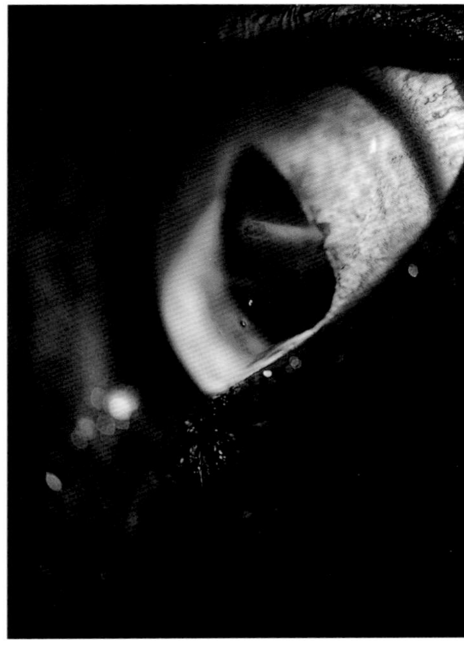

Fig. 3.17 *A thorn has penetrated the cornea, nicked the pupil border and become impaled in the lens of this 2-year-old cat. Removal was effected in similar fashion to that described for Fig. 3.16.*

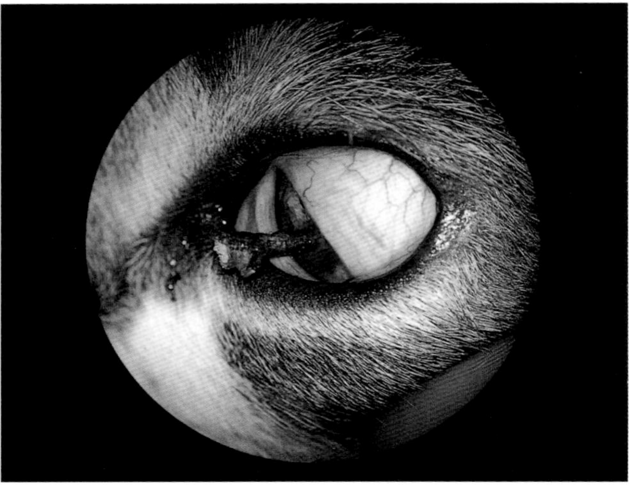

Fig. 3.18 *An 18-month-old Domestic shorthair. A large twig has penetrated the cornea and lens of this young cat.*

symptomatic treatment is usually adequate to control the inflammation if given early enough. The long-term prognosis, however, is guarded because of the putative association between damage to lens epithelium and subsequent development of intraocular sarcoma (Dubielzig *et al.*, 1994).

Eyelid trauma

Eyelid trauma is usually a consequence of fights or road traffic accidents and damage to the upper and lower eyelids (Fig. 3.20) as a result of fighting, is less common than damage to the third eyelid (Fig. 3.21). The damage to the eyelids is usually obvious, but there may be other injuries to the eye, head and body, so careful examination is required.

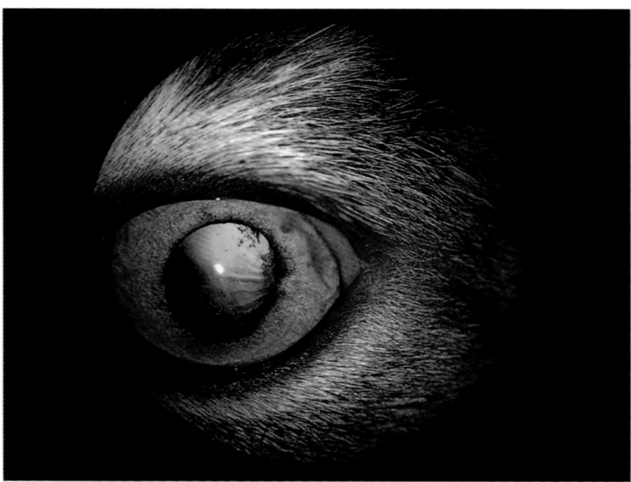

Fig. 3.19 *The same cat as shown in Fig. 3.18 1 week after removal of the foreign body. Although lens protein has escaped from the ruptured lens, the accompanying inflammation was easily controlled. The lens capsule is shrunken with obvious folds in the area of penetration and the site of the original corneal penetration is also obvious.*

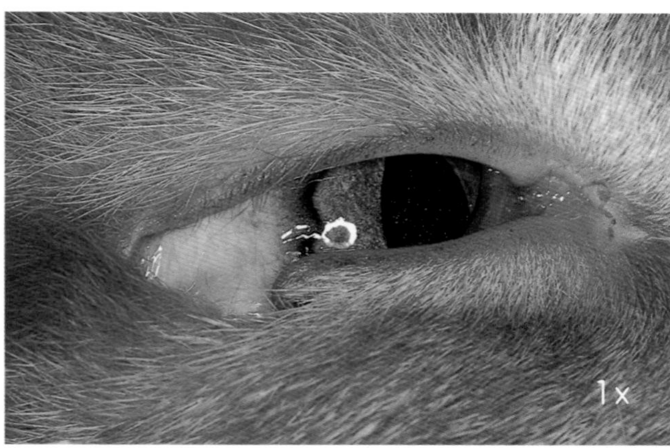

Fig. 3.20 *An adult cat which suffered traumatic injury to the lower eyelid some days previously. Injuries of this type are best dealt with by primary repair, but secondary repair may be imposed if the cat disappears after the injury as this one did. For a recent traumatic injury to the upper eyelid see Fig. 3.32.*

Management

- Upper and lower eyelid contusions are treated conservatively using systemic nonsteroidal anti-inflammatories and topical petrolatum-based antibiotic ointments. Tear replacement therapy should be given if there is a risk of exposure keratopathy.
- Primary repair is the treatment of choice for eyelid lacerations. Potential complications include infection, conjunctivitis, exposure keratopathy, epiphora, and cicatricial ectropion and these are more likely if repair is delayed. Debridement must be minimal because of the close apposition of the normal cat eyelid to the globe. Single or double layer closure is accomplished with 5/0–7/0 absorbable material (e.g. chromic catgut or polyglactin) in a continuous or simple interrupted pattern for the deeper layer and a simple interrupted or figure of eight pattern with 5/0–6/0 absorbable (e.g. polyglactin) or nonabsorbable material (e.g. silk) on a swaged on cutting needle for the skin. The eyelid margin is repaired first and the aim must be for perfect apposition. A 5–7 day course of systemic antibiotics may be necessary if the wound is infected. Nonabsorbable skin sutures are removed 10 days after surgery.
- Trauma near the medial canthus can cause damage to the nasolacrimal puncta, canaliculi and nasolacrimal duct and reconstructive surgery requires microsurgical facilities.
- Traumatic injury to the third eyelid is common in cats. Healing is rapid, unless it is delayed by infection. Superficial lacerations can be left alone or treated with topical antibiotic ointment provided that third eyelid motility is unimpaired. Traumatic avulsion, inadequate mobility and full-thickness lacerations of the third eyelid require

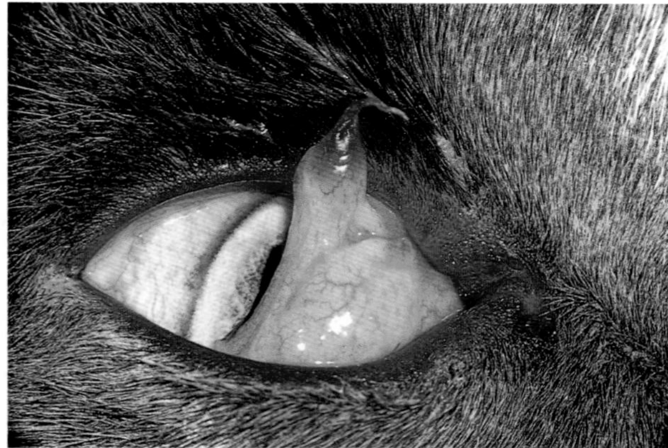

Fig. 3.21 *Avulsion injury to the dorsal aspect of the free border of the third eyelid as the result of a cat scratch in this young cat. Note the conjunctival dessication which is already present within 1 h of the injury. The edge was reattached in this case as third eyelid movement was compromised.*

surgical repair. For avulsion injuries a single simple interrupted suture to reattach the third eyelid may be all that is required, whereas for more extensive trauma a continuous over and over or key pattern buried suture using 5/0–7/0 absorbable material such as polyglactin is ideal. If the cartilage is exposed it should be covered with conjunctiva. The surgery is performed from the outer aspect of the third eyelid and should not penetrate its full thickness, so that there is no possibility of sutures rubbing against the underlying tissues, particularly the cornea. The feline third eyelid is of crucial importance in maintaining ocular health and must be conserved.

Conjunctival trauma

Conjunctival trauma is usually obvious (Fig. 3.22), although chemosis (conjunctival oedema) can obscure the extent of the damage. The possibility of more extensive damage to the globe should always be considered when there is conjunctival trauma, particularly if there appears to be any change in the appearance or arrangement of the intraocular structures, a clear ocular discharge (which may be aqueous) or a decrease of intraocular pressure. Occasionally, eyelid trauma is associated with penetrating injury to the underlying bulbar conjunctiva and sclera and this type of damage can easily be missed.

Management

- No specific treatment, other than protection against dessication, is required in the majority of cases because conjunctiva heals rapidly. Simple excision without suturing may be needed if there is a loose flap of exposed conjunctiva. Buried continuous sutures of absorbable material, as already described for the third eyelid, can be used if there is extensive laceration. Topical antibiotic cover (usually ointment) should be provided for 3–7 days while healing takes place if there is a risk of infection (e.g. cat claw injuries).
- On the rare occasions when there is scleral penetration, prolapsed uveal tissue should be replaced. The scleral wound is closed with simple interrupted sutures of 8/0 nylon or virgin silk and the conjunctiva is closed with interrupted sutures of 6/0 polyglactin. The conjunctival suture line should not overlie the scleral repair.

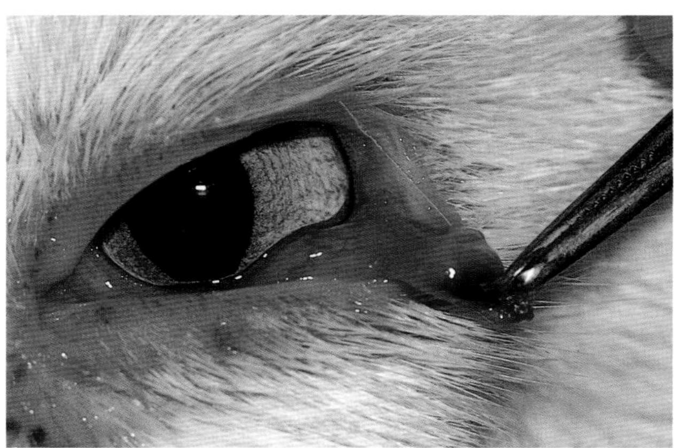

Fig. 3.22 *An 11-month-old Domestic shorthair. Conjunctival trauma as a consequence of a cat claw injury. The traumatized conjunctiva was excised with fine scissors following topical application of local anaesthetic.*

Corneal trauma

Corneal ulceration, laceration, partial thickness and full-thickness injuries are not infrequent in cats (Figs. 3.23–3.35) (see Chapter 9). The clinical presentation is of acute, usually

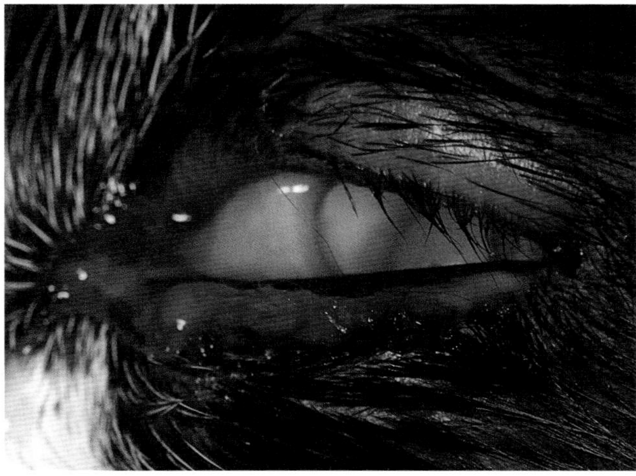

Fig. 3.23 *This adult cat was presented with an acutely painful eye, swollen eyelids and a seromucoid discharge. Careful examination revealed a full thickness penetrating injury 4 mm long at the limbal cornea running parallel to the limbus with underlying damage to the iris, surgical repair was necessary. The history suggested that the injury was the result of a cat fight.*

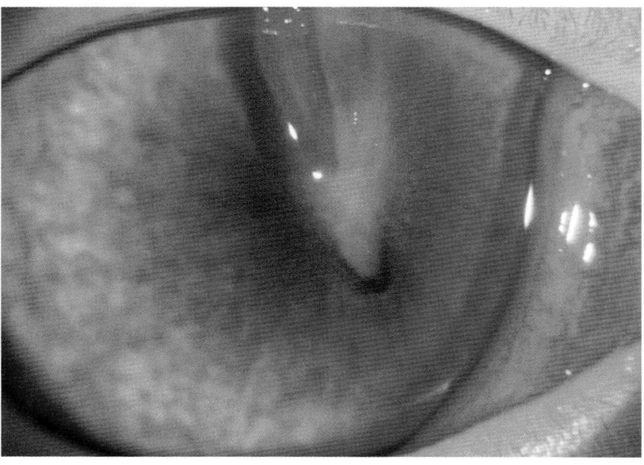

Fig. 3.24 *An 8-month-old Domestic shorthair. Vertical corneal laceration as a consequence of a cat scratch.*

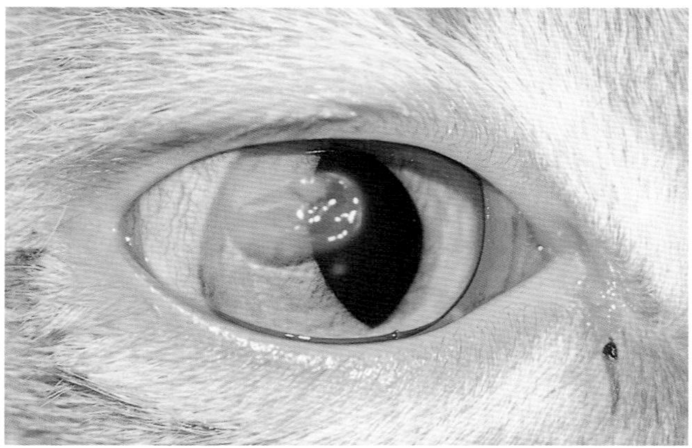

Fig. 3.25 *An 11-month-old Domestic shorthair. Traumatic corneal laceration (cat scratch) after a loose flap of lacerated cornea has been removed following several applications of topical local anaesthetic. The appearance before surgery is illustrated in Fig. 1.17. Note the presence of a single extra lash on the lower eyelid.*

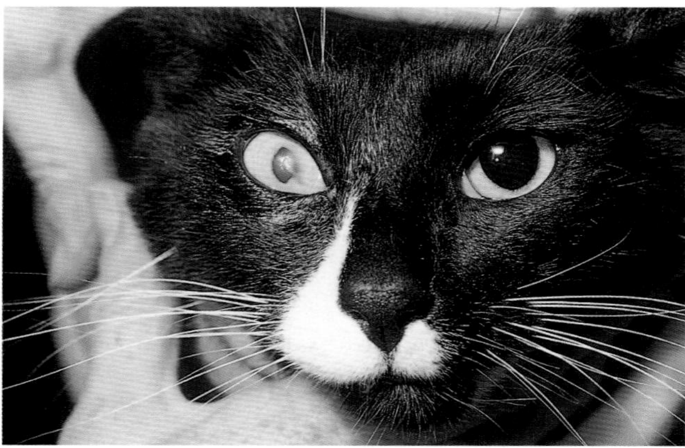

Fig. 3.26 *Domestic shorthair, 4-year-old, neutered male. Traumatic corneal ulceration (cat scratch) involving approximately half the corneal thickness. Note the anisocoria because of uveitis in the affected right eye.*

unilateral, onset of pain, blepharospasm and lacrimation. A transient uveitis mediated by an axon reflex within the trigeminal nerve can follow corneal insult. Aqueous loss or haemorrhage may also be apparent. Corneal injury should always be considered in animals that present with injury to the third eyelid.

Magnification, a bright light and complete darkness are required for detailed examination and a slit beam is also useful. Examination should establish the site of any corneal injury, the position of the iris, the depth of the anterior chamber, if hyphaema is present, the state of the pupil, and whether there appears to be iris and lens damage in addition to corneal damage. Aqueous loss and iris prolapse are common if there has been corneal penetration. Uveitis is usually present, but is not necessarily intense. Lens penetration, with leakage of lens protein (Davidson *et al.*, 1991b) and traumatic lens luxation are less common. Ocular ultrasonography may be of value in assessment when gross corneal oedema and/or hyphaema is present.

Prompt effective treatment gives excellent results in cats provided that the facilities and level of expertise are adequate. A proportion of cats are presented for treatment some time after the injuries have occurred and others have mismanaged injuries. Complications are more likely in such cases (see Chapters 9 and 11) and include excessive corneal scarring, continuing aqueous leakage, uveitis, synechiae, an eccentric, partially mobile or immobile pupil, glaucoma, cataract formation, the development of intraocular sarcoma and blindness (Figs 3.33–3.40).

Management

- Medical therapy consists of either proprietary antibiotic drops or fortified antibiotic solutions. Selection of the appropriate preparation is discussed in Chapter 9.
- A mydriatic cycloplegic (e.g. atropine 1%) is usually indicated when there is deep corneal damage and uveitis. While most cats tolerate atropine ointment better than solution, it is better to select drops rather than ointment if there is any possibility of the ointment becoming trapped in the cornea or entering the anterior chamber during the healing process. Once the pupil has dilated atropine is given only as frequently as is necessary to keep it so.
- Systemic analgesics are indicated if the eye is painful. Topical local anaesthetics are not used beyond the initial diagnostic and treatment stages as they may seriously compromise corneal healing.
- Superficial injuries do not require surgical repair, but wound healing will be enhanced if any loose flaps of corneal epithelium are removed with fine scissors after several applications of topical local anaesthetic.
- It is the extent and the depth of the corneal injury which determines the type of support for corneal wound healing required (Peiffer *et al.*, 1987). Therapeutic soft contact lenses (Schmidt *et al.*, 1977; Morgan *et al.*, 1984) and conjunctival pedicle grafts (Hakanson and Merideth, 1987; Hakanson *et al.*, 1988, Habin, 1995) are the usual means of providing support for healing in those cases in which perforation is likely without some form of corneal support (Figs 3.27–3.30). Third eyelid flaps (see Chapter 5) may be used as an alternative to therapeutic soft contact lenses. Short-term measures to protect the cornea include cyanoacrylate glue (Refojo *et al.*, 1971) and collagen corneal shields.
- It is not always necessary to suture penetrating injuries since if the wound is of small diameter continued aqueous loss is unlikely. If there is no leakage of aqueous from the site of penetration and the anterior chamber has reformed, then medical treatment is all that is required – usually topical antibiotic (e.g. fortified antibiotic solution or proprietary ophthalmic solution) and a mydriatic cycloplegic (atropine 1%). Atropine may be used sparingly once pupil dilation has been achieved but the

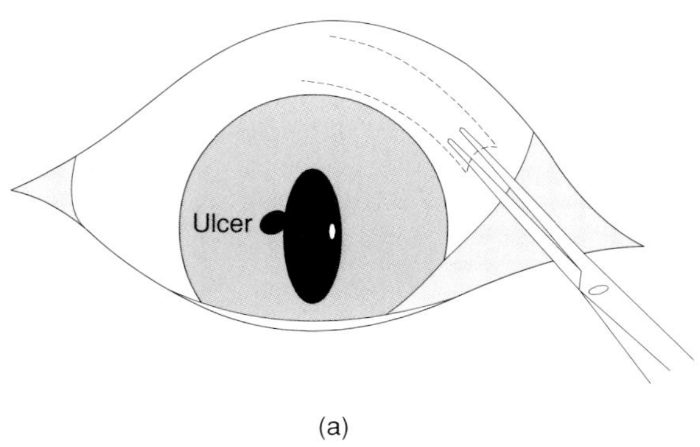

(a)

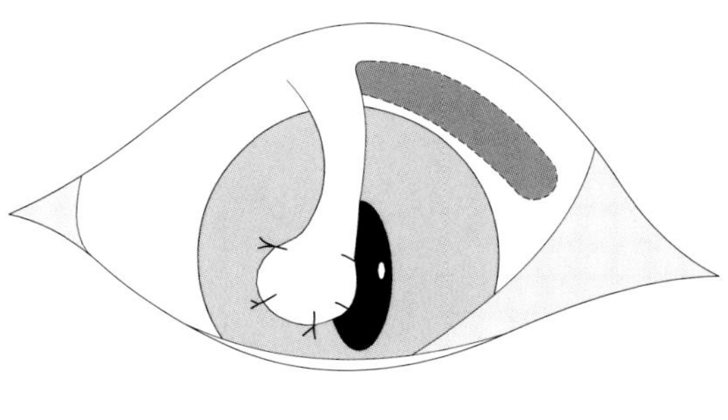

(b)

Fig. 3.27 *Conjunctival pedicle graft. (a) Tenotomy scissors are used for blunt dissection beneath the conjunctiva, parallel with and at least 2 mm from the limbus. The thickness can be varied to suit the depth of the defect to be filled, but the plane of dissection must not vary once the thickness has been selected, to avoid compromising the blood supply. Tenotomy scissors are also used to cut the conjunctiva and shape the graft so that it is slightly broader at the base. The graft is covered with moistened sterile swab while the recipient bed is being prepared. (b) Adequate preparation of the recipient bed is essential. All necrotic tissue must be removed from the area otherwise healing will be delayed and the sutures will not hold. The apex of the graft is sewn in place with simple interrupted sutures of 7/0–8/0 vicryl. The '6 o'clock' suture is the first to be placed and the sutures are passed into the graft, through the wall of the defect and into normal cornea. A continuous pattern may be used in addition to hold the graft firmly in place.*

The paralimbal conjunctival defect is closed with buried continuous sutures of 7/0–8/0 vicryl. The graft can be sectioned with tenotomy scissors once healing is complete. Several applications of topical local anaesthetic will be required prior to the section.

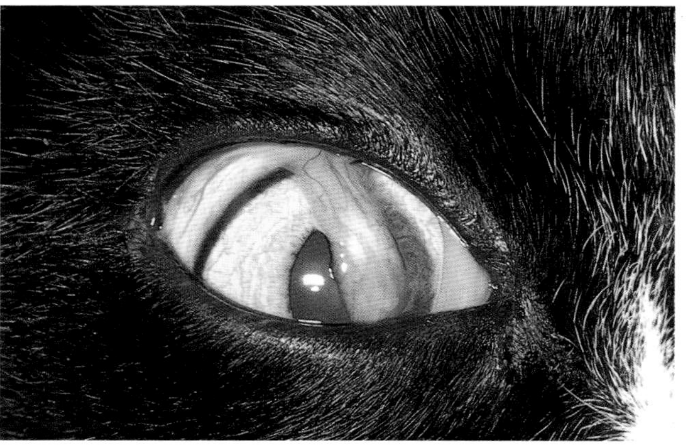

Fig. 3.28 *The same cat as illustrated in Fig. 3.26 approximately 2 months after the original injury with a pedicle graft in place. The graft is about be sectioned under topical local anaesthesia.*

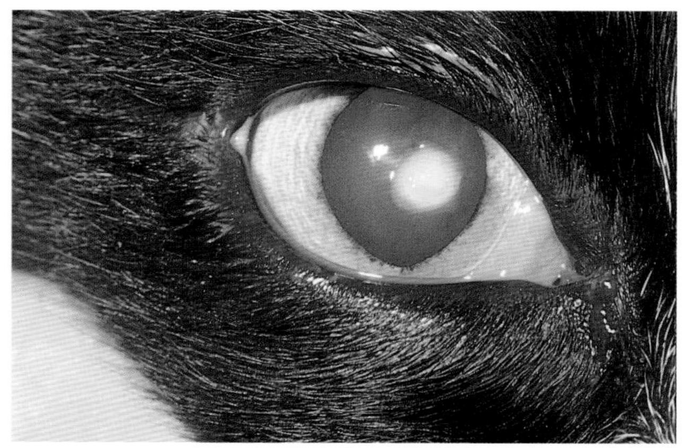

Fig. 3.29 *The same cat as illustrated in Fig. 3.26 approximately 1 week after the pedicle graft has been sectioned.*

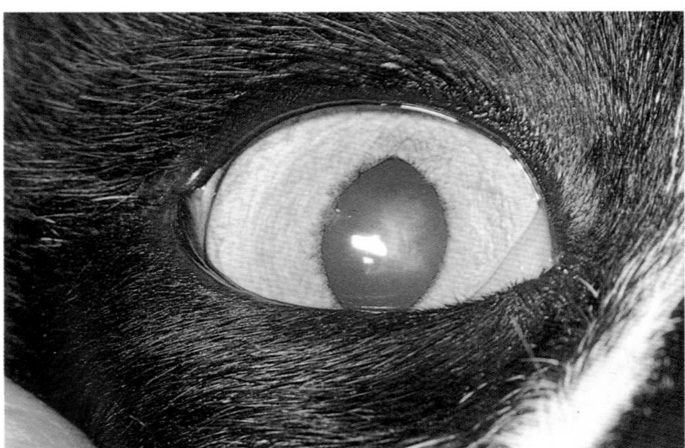

Fig. 3.30 *The same cat as illustrated in Fig. 3.26 6 months after sectioning the pedicle graft. There is little corneal scarring.*

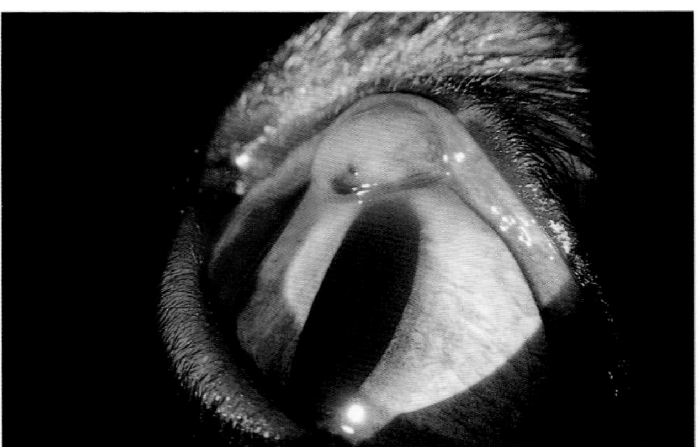

Fig. 3.31 *A 10-month-old Domestic shorthair. Penetrating corneal injury (cat scratch) with iris prolapse and a covering of coagulated aqueous. The anterior chamber is clear and the pupil is distorted because of the iris prolapse. The prognosis is excellent once primary repair has been effected.*

antibiotic should be used initially on an hourly basis until it is clear that healing is proceeding uneventfully.

- Many penetrating corneal injuries require primary reconstructive surgical repair. The wound should be inspected carefully and cleared of foreign debris. Coagulated aqueous invariably covers the corneal wound and this must be removed (Fig. 3.31). Prolapsed iris should be returned to the anterior chamber and it is important to emphasize that abscission of incarcerated iris is rarely, if ever, necessary. Viscoelastic materials will be of value in expelling intraocular haemorrhage and restoring and maintaining normal anatomical relationships within the anterior chamber – high viscosity viscoelastic materials are the best ones to use. Fine suture material (7/0–10/0 monofilament nylon, virgin silk or polyglactin) should be selected and the simple interrupted corneal sutures should penetrate about three-quarters of the corneal thickness and may be preplaced to aid the procedure. Secure watertight closure is essential and it is usual to aspirate the viscoelastic material, because leaks are more difficult to detect with viscoelastics, and to reform the anterior chamber with balanced salt solution and a small bubble of air. Once healing has occurred the sutures can be removed or left, according to their reactivity.
- If the corneal defect is extensive a different suture pattern can be used. A corneal wound of up to 5 mm diameter in

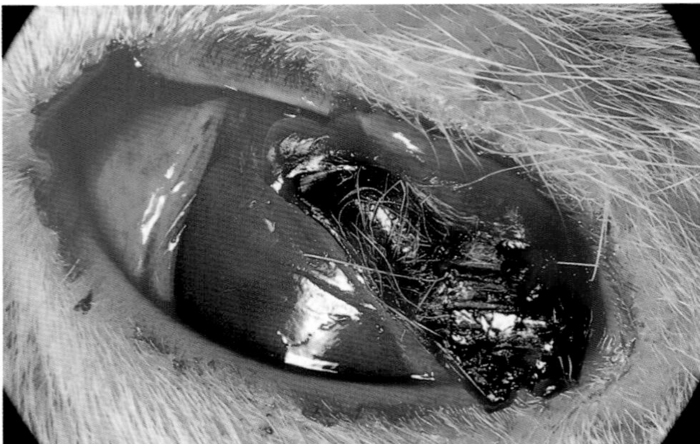

Fig. 3.32 *Adult Domestic shorthair. Full-thickness penetrating corneal injury and upper eyelid trauma (cause unknown, but presumed to be the result of a cat scratch). In addition to damage to the eyelid margin laterally, there is a large and contaminated blood clot at the lips of the corneal wound. Extensive hyphaema is also apparent. The prognosis is obviously guarded as it is impossible to gauge the extent of the damage at this stage. Cases of this type will benefit from specialist assessment and treatment.*

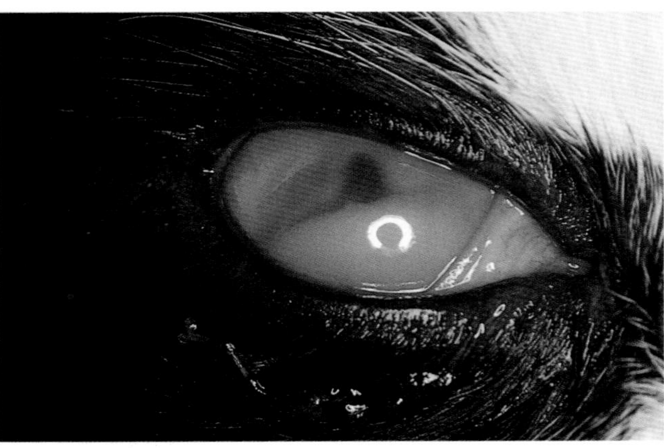

Fig. 3.33 *This 2-year-old cat was scratched by another cat 1 week previously and the owners only sought veterinary help when they noticed the change of appearance produced by marked hypopyon. The eye was painful with anterior uveitis and a fixed, miotic pupil. Pasteurella multocida was obtained in pure culture from a corneal swab at the site of presumed penetration. Note how the hypopyon obscures corneal detail and makes detailed evaluation of the eye impossible. Ultrasound examination indicated that the lens was undamaged and the posterior segment appeared normal.*

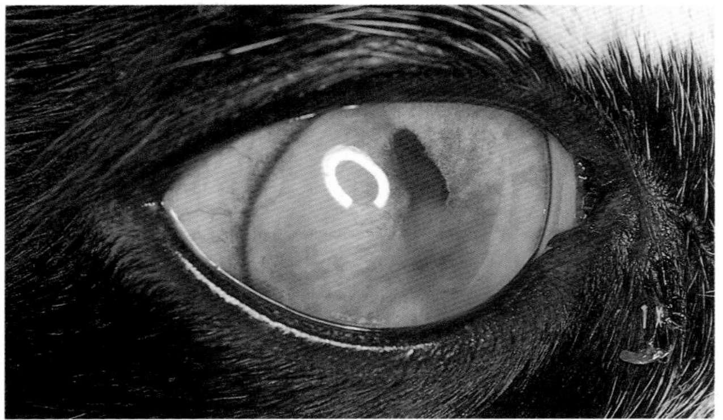

Fig. 3.34 The same cat as in Fig. 3.33 3 weeks later. The site of the corneal penetrating injury is now obvious ventrally in the '6 o'clock' position, the hypopyon has largely resolved, the pupil is still fixed and miotic despite treatment (because of posterior synechiae). The eye is comfortable, but the delay in treatment initially will affect adversely the long-term result.

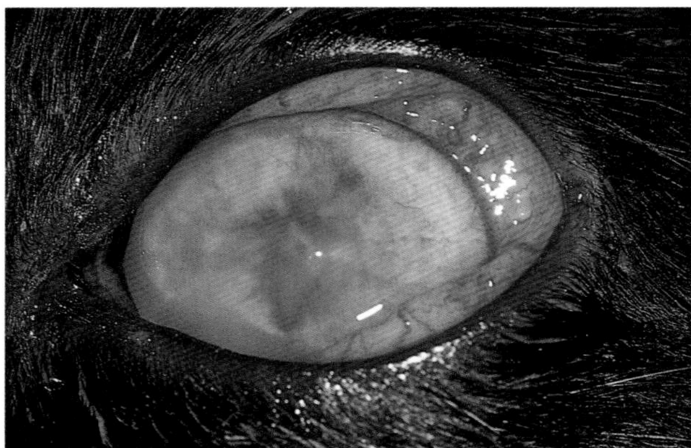

Fig. 3.35 In this adult cat, a penetrating corneal injury (central cornea) has resulted in a severe uveitis and secondary glaucoma (intraocular pressure 70 mmHg). There is chemosis; conjunctival and episcleral congestion; hypopyon; iritis; an irregular, fixed, miotic pupil; extensive posterior synechiae; and the lens capsule is opaque.

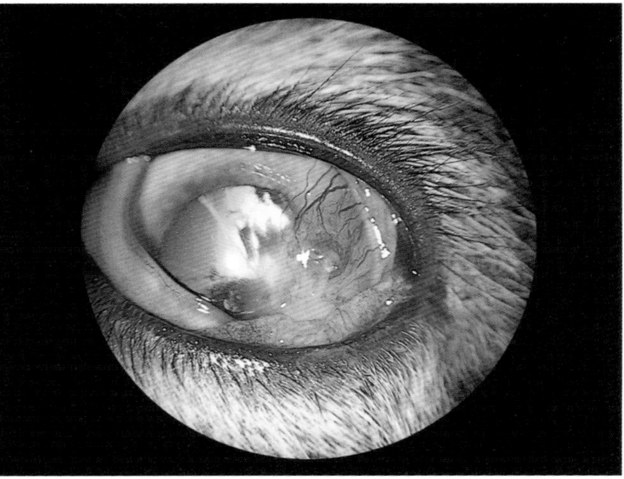

Fig. 3.36 A 4-year-old Domestic shorthair. A full-thickness penetrating injury which was not repaired. The corneal wound has continued to leak aqueous and microsurgical repair is indicated.

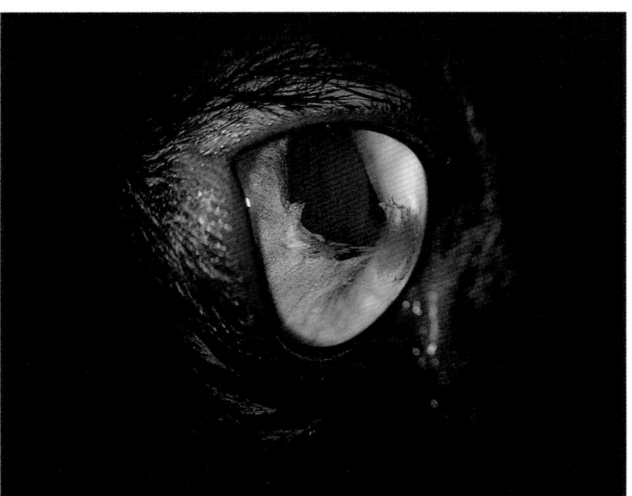

Fig. 3.37 A 5-year-old Burmese cat. Anterior synechiae associated with a previous full thickness corneal penetration. No treatment is required.

its largest dimension can be closed with preplaced horizontal mattress sutures, provided that the wound margins are healthy, but a high degree of astigmatism is inevitable and this technique should not be used if there is excessive tension on the sutures. The same suture pattern can be used to close a descemetocoele, but a thick conjunctival/Tenon's capsule pedicle graft may be a better option. For more complex corneal injuries a number of refined surgical techniques are available (Parshall, 1973; Brightman *et al.*, 1989; Hacker, 1991). Penetrating keratoplasty is also a practical proposition in the cat (Bahn *et al.*, 1982).

- Eye removal is almost never the treatment of choice for acute ocular trauma.

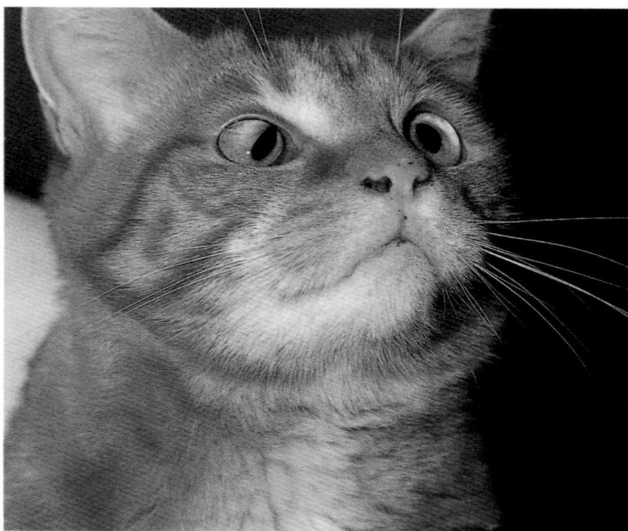

Fig. 3.38 *An 18-month-old Domestic shorthair. Note the eccentric pupil as a consequence of previous penetrating injury at the limbus.*

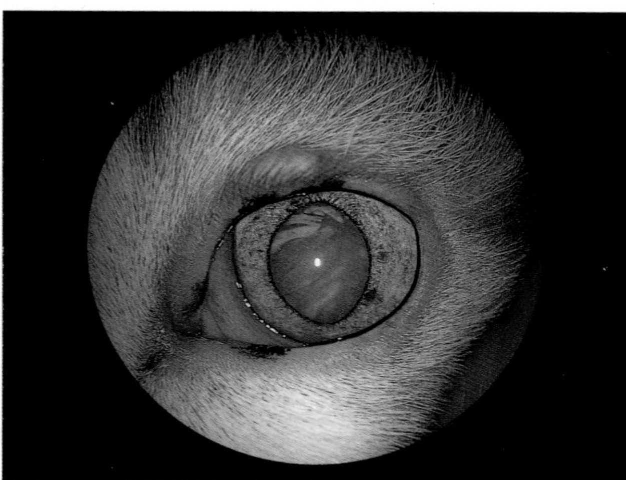

Fig. 3.39 *Adult Domestic shorthair. The swelling of the upper eyelid is caused by scar tissue, a consequence of a cat scratch injury some years previously. The claw also penetrated the globe and post-traumatic cataract developed within a few months of the injury. The cataract subsequently underwent resorption.*

LIQUEFACTIVE STROMAL NECROSIS ('MELTING' ULCERS)

Liquefactive stromal necrosis is rare in cats but may be associated with misuse of topical corticosteroids, feline herpesvirus infection, bacterial pathogens, alkali, necrotic corneal stromal cells and polymorphonuclear inflammatory cells – all of which induce rapid corneal degradation as a result of stromal lysis, necrosis and liquefaction (the so-called 'melting' ulcers). In addition, immunosuppressed animals,

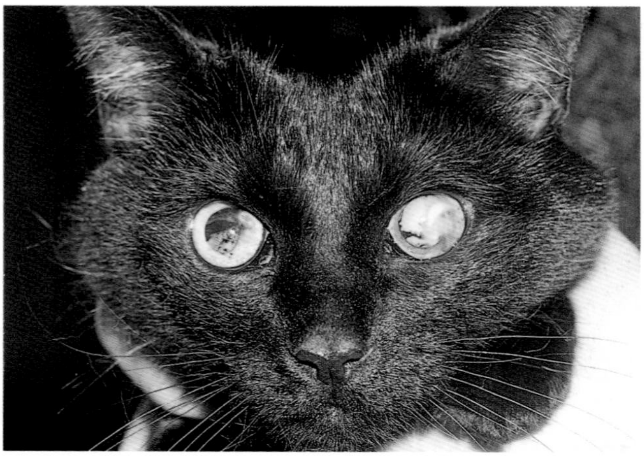

Fig. 3.40 *A 5-year-old Domestic shorthair with bilateral ocular damage following cat claw injuries. Both corneas were perforated and the site of penetration is obvious ('1 o'clock' in the right eye, '5 o'clock' in the left eye), there is also lipid keratopathy in the left eye (a crescent at the axial end of the scar from the penetrating injury) which is illustrated in greater detail in Fig. 9.59. Both lenses have been damaged with a partial cataract on the right and a total cataract on the left. Pigment deposition is also apparent in both pupils and the left iris is darker than the right iris, indicating a more intense uveitis initially.*

for example, those on corticosteroid therapy or infected with the feline leukaemia virus (FeLV), or the feline immunodeficiency virus (FIV) may be more susceptible (Fig. 3.41).

MANAGEMENT

- The principles of treatment are to encourage normal corneal healing, especially epithelialization, and to suppress factors which lead to corneal destruction, such as collagenolysis. Whenever collagenolysis occurs as a feature of corneal disease it is important that specific causes are identified and eliminated. Treatment needs to be early and aggressive if it is to be successful and should be monitored carefully; specialist help may be required.
- Swabs and scrapings should be taken from the affected region of the cornea (to check for feline herpesvirus and bacteria). Ideally, the initial antibiotic treatment is selected according to the results of a Gram stain. The cat should also be checked for toxoplasmosis, FIV and FeLV infection.
- Careful debridement of the necrotic corneal tissue should be performed and an early decision taken with regard to corneal support for healing (e.g. conjunctival pedicle graft) if perforation is considered a possibility.
- Topical medication with a broad spectrum fortified antibiotic solution should be used every hour initially. When the situation is under control a commercial ophthalmic antibiotic solution with a similarly broad spectrum of activity can be substituted. The frequency of application can be reduced when improvement is maintained.

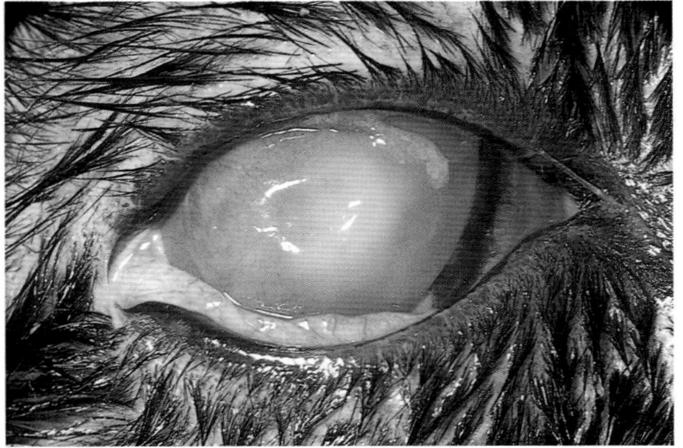

Fig. 3.41 A 9-year-old Domestic shorthair neutered male. Liquefactive stromal necrosis in an FIV positive cat in which the eye had been treated with topical corticosteroids. Note the 'mushy' appearance and opaque nature of the cornea and the presence of hypopyon.

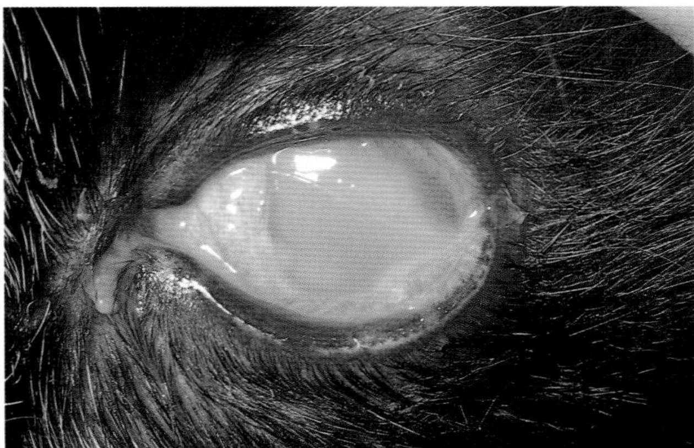

Fig. 3.42 Adult Domestic shorthair with acute keratomalacia as a consequence of accidental splashing from household bleach containing sodium hydroxide (strongly alkaline)

- Fresh autologous serum, topical acetylcysteine and parenteral tetracyclines (e.g. oral doxycycline) have *in vivo* activity against collagenase. Evidence adduced from experimental treatment of alkali burns provides some support for the use of ascorbic acid (e.g. parenterally) and topical 10% sodium citrate (hourly) may also be beneficial.
- Any accompanying uveitis may require symptomatic treatment with a topical mydriatic cycloplegic (atropine 1%).

Chemical injuries to the cornea

Chemical injuries are uncommon. Malicious injuries and accidental exposure to preparations such as bleaches, insecticides, shampoos and surgical skin preparations are possible causes. Alkali has the capacity to penetrate all layers of the eye and strong alkali can irreversibly damage all the tissues with which it comes in contact (Figs 3.42 and 8.16). Acids tend to coagulate and precipitate protein, the damage is therefore more superficial because the coagulated cells on the corneal surface act as a barrier to further penetration.

Diagnosis is based on the history and, ideally, identification of the chemical. An approximate prognosis can be given according to the pH of the conjunctival sac (which is normally on the alkaline side of neutral) and the pH of the chemical responsible; the stronger the pH, the poorer the prognosis. Specialist advice should be sought in complex cases.

Management

- Emergency treatment consists of removal of any particulate matter and flushing the affected area with a continuous gentle stream of cold water for at least 30 min. It may be necessary to anaesthetize the cat to achieve this effect and effective systemic analgesia is important.
- Broad-spectrum topical antibiotic is all that is required for local treatment of superficial damage. More complex cases are managed as described for liquefactive stromal necrosis, but in addition, the intraocular pressure should be monitored. Serious chemical burns may be associated with substantial changes of intraocular pressure (both low and high) and medical therapy will be required for sustained increases.
- In specialist hands, topical corticosteroids may be indicated in the first few days (5–7 days) after injury, to control the inflammatory response, but because they will enhance corneal melting it is essential to monitor the patient every few hours.

Thermal injuries

Thermal injuries are uncommon and usually a consequence of exposure to smoke and heat (Peiffer *et al.*, 1979), although hot liquids may also be implicated. Systemic problems such as hypovolaemic shock and breathing difficulties take precedence over the damage to the eye and adnexa.

Management

- Immediate emergency treatment for the eye and adnexa consists of copious irrigation with cold water. Systemic nonsteroidal anti-inflammatories should also be administered as soon as possible after the incident and for several days afterwards.
- Antibiotic ointment or medicated tulle dressings are ideal as a symptomatic treatment for superficial burns to the skin of the eyelids and it is important to prevent drying as this will help to minimize scarring. Bland topical ophthalmic ointments will be required for damaged conjunctiva in order to reduce the chances of symblepharon formation. Specialist help should be obtained for more serious burns of the eyelids and conjunctiva as early reconstructive surgery may be indicated.
- Thermal injury to the cornea usually presents as corneal oedema and the corneal involvement may be superficial or

deep. The severity of the insult determines the type of treatment. Tear replacement preparations and topical antibiotic solutions will be adequate for uncomplicated cases, but serious injuries will require the type of regime already outlined for liquefactive stromal necrosis.

UVEITIS

Uveitis (see Chapter 12) other than that associated with trauma (Figs 3.32–3.35) is not usually an emergency in cats. Unilateral uveitis is most commonly associated with traumatic injury (discussed earlier) and bilateral uveitis with systemic disease. Blindness is a potential complication of both types, so it is better to regard the investigation and treatment of uveitis cases as deserving urgent attention.

MANAGEMENT

- If the cause of the uveitis is not obvious, blood samples for routine haematology, biochemistry and serology should be taken and urinalysis should also be performed.
- The surgical repair of penetrating injuries, including those with uveal tract involvement, has been outlined earlier.
- A topical mydriatic cycloplegic (1% atropine) is applied to dilate the pupil and relieve ciliary spasm if the pupil is constricted. Once mydriasis has been achieved, atropine is used only as often as is necessary to keep the pupil dilated. It is important to examine the whole eye to establish the extent of the uveitis but complete eye examination may only be possible when anterior segment changes are less florid and the pupil is dilated.
- Broad-spectrum topical fortified antibiotic solutions or commercial antibiotic solutions should be administered when uveitis is a consequence of trauma.
- Iritis and iridocyclitis (anterior uveitis) should be treated with topical anti inflammatory preparations. Choroiditis (posterior uveitis) and optic neuritis will not be affected by topical drug therapy and therefore systemic treatment must be given; both topical and systemic treatment should be given for pars planitis (intermediate uveitis) and panuveitis.
- Topical corticosteroid (prednisolone acetate) should be given if there are no contraindications such as ulceration. Initially, treatment can be applied every hour, an approach which will often bring about a dramatic improvement within a matter of hours. Treatment is then given 2–4 times daily and gradually tailed off some 7 days after the eye has returned to normal.
- Systemic corticosteroid, usually prednisolone, should be used when there is posterior segment inflammation (provided that there are no contraindications). As with topical corticosteroids, a high loading dose should be given initially and then gradually reduced. Abrupt cessation of treatment may produce an acute exacerbation of the clinical signs.

GLAUCOMA

Glaucoma (see Chapter 10) is unusual in cats and the presentation is most typically a chronic one of corneal oedema and globe enlargement, rather than the acute congestive glaucoma so typical in the dog. Possible causes include primary glaucoma and, much more commonly, glaucoma secondary to trauma (Fig. 3.35), haemorrhage, neoplasia and uveitis (see Chapter 12).

Lens luxation, usually secondary to uveitis, is also uncommon in cats and, unlike the situation in dogs, is neither an emergency nor a cause of acute glaucoma.

MANAGEMENT

- Because glaucoma is often secondary to trauma, neoplasia and uveitis the most important aspect of management is to identify and, if possible, treat the underlying cause.
- An osmotic diuretic may be used as a short-lived way of reducing intraocular pressure in an emergency. Intravenous mannitol (1–2 g/kg over 30 min) is the treatment of choice.

REFERENCES

Bahn CF, Meyer RG, MacCallum DK, Lillie JH, Lovett EJ, Sugar A, Martonyi CL (1982) Penetrating keratoplasty in the cat. *Ophthalmology* **89**: 687–699.

Brightman AH, McLaughlin SA, Brogdon JD (1989) Autologous lamellar corneal grafting in dogs. *Journal of the American Veterinary Medical Association* **195**: 469–475.

Clarke KW, Hall LW (1990) A survey of anaesthesia in small animal practice. Association of Veterinary Anaesthetists/British Small Animal Veterinary Association report. *Journal of the Association of Veterinary Anaesthetists* **17**: 4–10.

Davidson MG, Nasisse MP, Breitschwerdt EB (1991a) Acute blindness associated with intracranial tumours in dogs and cats: Eight cases (1984–1989). *Journal of the American Veterinary Medical Association* **199**: 755–758.

Davidson MG, Nasisse MP, Jamieson VE, English RV, Olivero DK (1991b) Traumatic anterior lens capsule disruption. *Journal of the American Animal Hospital Association* **27**: 410–414.

Dubielzig RR, Hawkins KL, Toy KA, Rosebury WS, Mazur M, Jasper TG (1994) Morphological features of feline ocular sarcomas in 10 cats: Light microscopy, ultrastructure, and immunohistochemistry. *Veterinary and Comparative Opthalmology* **4**: 7–12.

Gilger BC, Hamilton HL, Wilkie DA, van der Woerdt A, McLaughlin SA, Whitley RD (1995) Traumatic ocular proptoses in dogs and cats: 84 cases (1980–1993). *Journal of the American Animal Hospital Association* **206**: 8, 1186–1190.

Griffiths IR (1987) Central nervous system trauma. In *Veterinary Neurology*. WB Saunders Co, Philadelphia. Oliver JE, Hoerlein BF, Mayhew IG (eds) pp 303–320.

Habin D (1995) Conjunctival pedical grafts. *In Practice* **17**: 61–65.

Hacker DV (1991) Frozen corneal grafts in dogs and cats: A report on 19 cases. *Journal of the American Animal Hospital Association* **27**: 387–398.

Hakanson NE, Merideth RE (1987) Conjunctival pedicle grafting in the treatment of corneal ulcers in the dog and cat. *Journal of the American Animal Hospital Association* **23**: 641–648.

Hakanson N, Lorimer D, Merideth RE (1988) Further comments on conjunctival pedicle grafting in the treatment of corneal ulcers in the dog and cat. *Journal of the American Animal Hospital Association* **24**: 602–605.

Henik RA (1997) Diagnosis and treatment of feline hypertension. *Compendium on Continuing Education for the Practicing Veterinarian* **19:** 163–179.

Morgan RV (1982) Ocular emergencies. *Compendium on Continuing Education for the Practicing Veterinarian* **4**: 37–45.

Morgan RV, Bachrach A, Ogilvie GK (1984) An evaluation of soft contact lens usage in the dog and cat. *Journal of the American Animal Hospital Association* **20**: 885–888.

Parshall CJ (1973) Lamellar corneal–scleral transposition. *Journal of the American Animal Hospital Association* **9**: 270–277.

Peiffer RL, Williams L, Duncan J (1979) Keratopathy associated with smoke and thermal exposure. *Feline Practice* **7**: 23–36.

Peiffer RL, Nasisse MP, Cook CS, Harling DE (1987) Surgery of the canine and feline orbit, adnexa and globe. Part 6: Surgery of the cornea. *Companion Animal Practice* **1**: 3–13.

Refojo MF, Dohlman CH, Koliopoulos J (1971) Adhesives in ophthalmology: a review. *Survey of Ophthalmology* **15**: 217–236.

Roberts SM (1985) Assessment and management of the ophthalmic emergency. *Compendium on Continuing Education for the Practicing Veterinarian* **7**: 739–754.

Schmidt GM, Blanchard GL, Keller WF (1977) The use of hydrophilic contact lenses in corneal diseases of the dog and cat: a preliminary report. *Journal of Small Animal Practice* **18**: 773–777.

Wolfer J, Grahn B (1995) Orbital emphysema from frontal sinus penetration in a cat. *Canadian Veterinary Journal* **36**: 3, 186–187.

4 GLOBE AND ORBIT

INTRODUCTION

The globe of the cat is relatively larger than the other domestic animals and is almost spherical with a large cornea (Fig. 4.1), occupying a frontal position and giving good binocular vision. The dimensions of the globe are given as 20–22 mm anteroposterior, 19–21 mm vertical, 18–21 mm horizontal.

The globe fits the orbit extremely well (see Fig. 4.3), so that any retrobulbar space-occupying condition rapidly leads to degrees of exophthalmos.

The orbit occupies a considerable part of the total volume of the skull and is large and deep. The orbit is described as open or incomplete, i.e. it is not wholly enclosed but has an incomplete lateral bony orbital rim which is completed by the orbital ligament. The orbit lacks a floor but has an anterior shelf.

Globe development occurs early in embryogenesis from neural and surface ectoderm and mesenchyme. The optic vesicle, which forms from neural ectoderm, invaginates to form the optic cup from which the globe develops.

POSTNATAL GROWTH OF GLOBE AND ORBIT

In an attempt to measure eyeball size and growth in the cat two unrelated litters were studied, six kittens in total (litters of four and two).

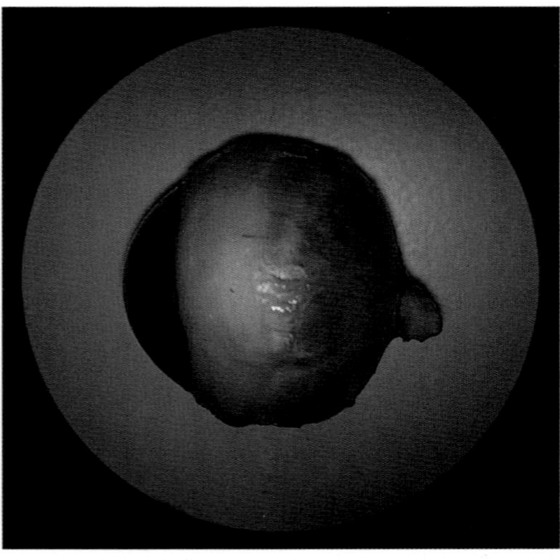

Fig. 4.1 *The globe of the cat. Note spherical shape and large cornea.*

The globes were measured by B-mode ultrasound, both right and left eyes of each kitten. Measurements started at 7 days old when the eyes were first opened and continued at weekly intervals up to 1 month, 2-weekly intervals up to 3 months and 4-weekly intervals up to 9 months and again at 1 year old.

The measurements were the same for both eyes and there was no difference between sexes. Table 4.1 gives the results, in millimetres, averaged for the 12 eyes of all kittens at each age.

Figures 4.2 and 4.3 depict ultrasonograms at 7 days and 9 months old, respectively.

CONGENITAL ANOMALIES

Feline congenital ocular anomalies, including multiple ocular defects, are rare.

Anophthalmos, absence of the globe, has been reported together with absence of the optic nerve (see Chapter 14) and optic tract but is rare. Anophthalmos, and cyclopia (Scott *et al.*, 1975), are included with other congenital abnormalities as teratogenic anomalies following the use of griseofulvin in

Table 4.1 Ultrasound globe measurements of developing kittens.

Age of kitten	Size of globe (mm)
7 days	10.2
14 days	11.1
21 days	11.8
28 days	12.0
5 weeks	12.4
6 weeks	13.1
8 weeks	14.1
10 weeks	14.9
12 weeks	15.9
14 weeks	16.0
5 months	17.1
6 months	17.5
7 months	17.9
8 months	18.2
9 months	18.5
12 months	18.7

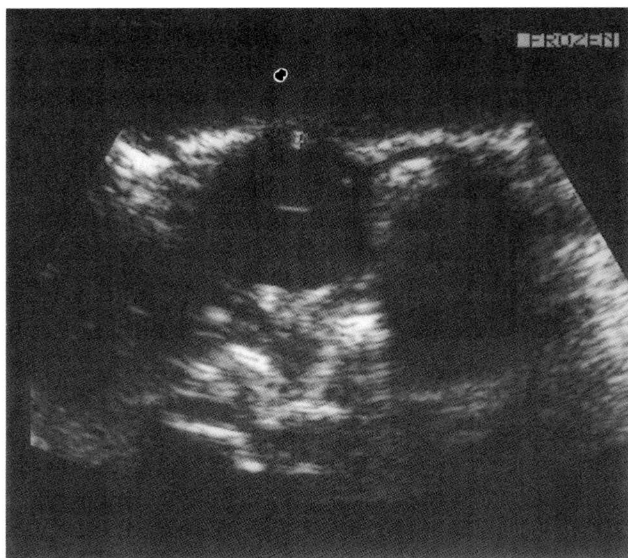

Fig. 4.2 Normal ultrasonogram of the eye of a 7-day-old kitten using the direct corneal contact method. The globe appears anechoic except for short hyperechoic lines representing the front and back of the lens. The cornea is visible as a double echoic line at the top of the image.

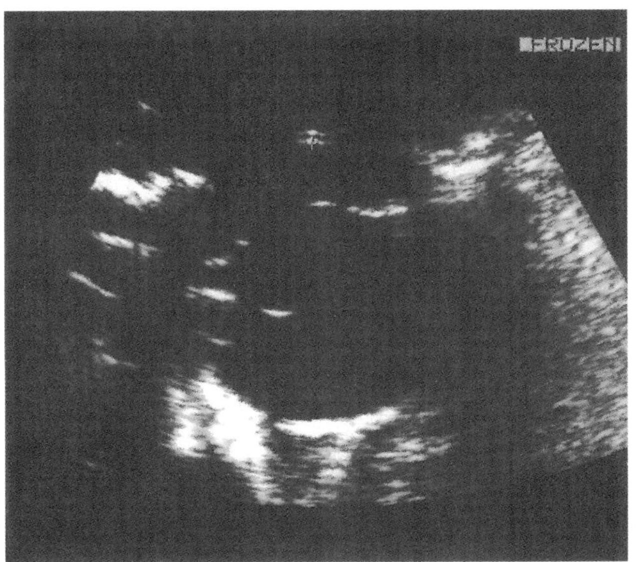

Fig. 4.3 Normal ultrasonogram of the eye of a 9-month-old cat. Description as in Fig. 4.2.

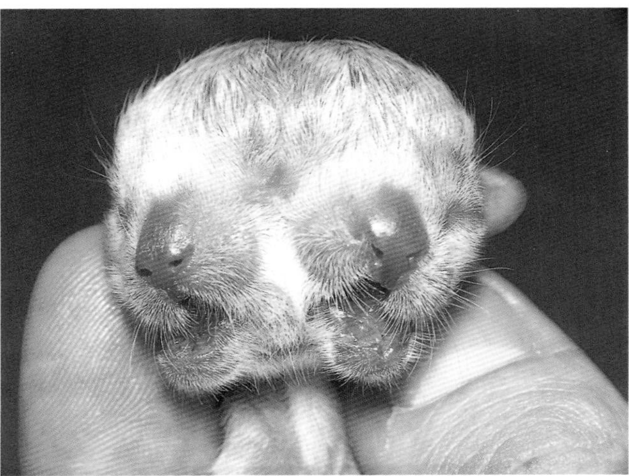

Fig. 4.4 Congenital deformity (no history).

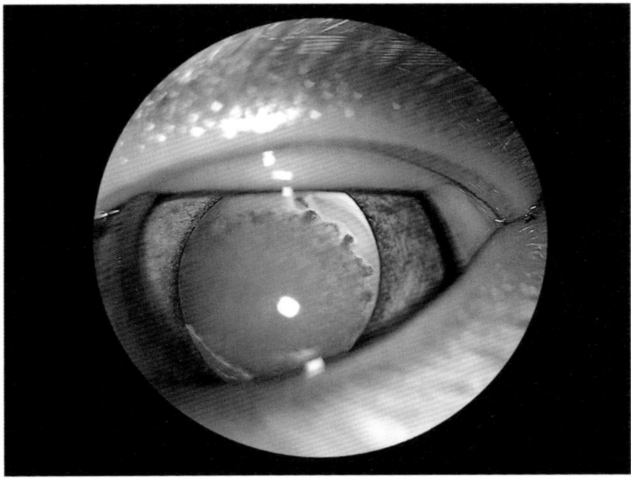

Fig. 4.5 Microphthalmos (mild case). Note prominence of nictitating membrane on the left side and visible sclera on the right side. Also note nuclear cataract, a frequent accompaniment to microphthalmos.

pregnant queens. Other congenital deformities involving the globes and orbits occur rarely, Fig. 4.4 is a single example.

Microphthalmos, a congenitally small eye, is much rarer in the cat than in the dog; with no evidence of either inheritance or breed predisposition, as is the case in the dog. Microphthalmos may be unilateral or bilateral and in severe cases has been recorded in association with a narrow palpebral fissure. Figure 4.5 illustrates a mild case of microphthalmos and, as is often the case, accompanied by other congenital anomalies, in this case nuclear cataract, which is clearly illustrated, and retinal dysplasia. Figure 4.6 depicts a more severe case, again with congenital cataract. Microphthalmos may also be accompanied by degrees of enophthalmos and consequent prominence of the nictitating membrane (Figs 4.7–4.9).

Strabismus (squint), convergent and bilateral, is perhaps the most common feline congenital ocular anomaly (see Fig. 15.20). It occurs particularly in the Siamese and is said to be due to an autosomal recessive gene; the incidence is now much less, due to selective breeding, than was the case years ago (see also Chapter 15).

Nystagmus occurs particularly in the Siamese and not necessarily in association with strabismus. The nystagmus is rapid, oscillatory and intermittent. It has no effect on vision (see also Chapter 15).

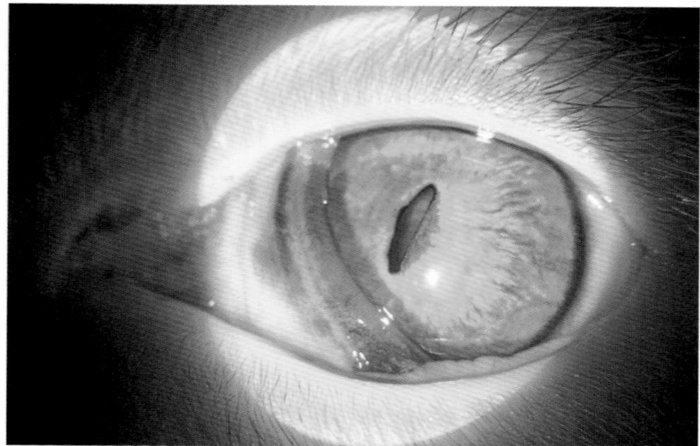

Fig. 4.6 A more severe case of microphthalmos, again with cataract.

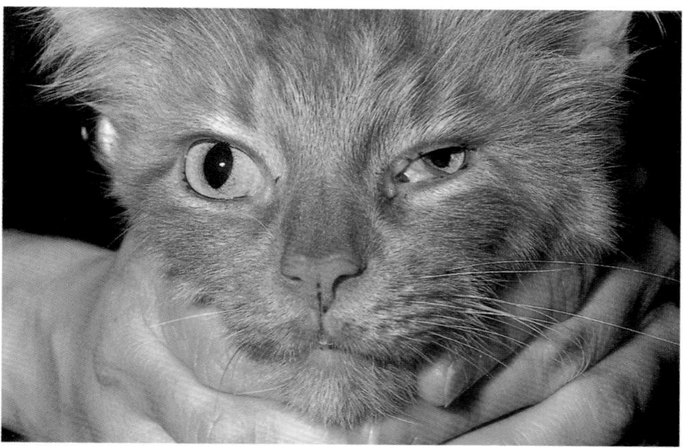

Fig. 4.7 Microphthalmos and multiple congenital anomalies, full face view.

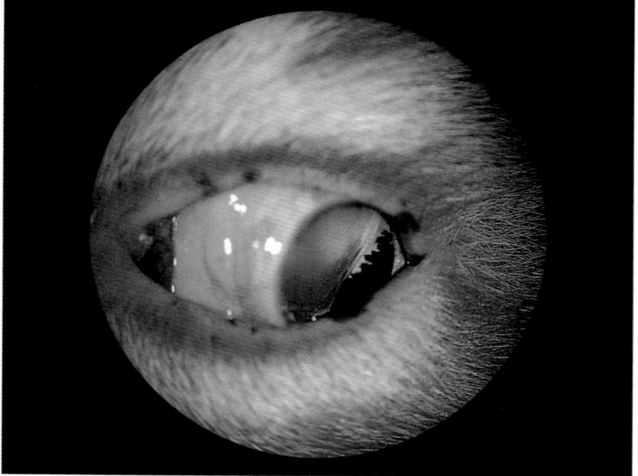

Fig. 4.8 Same case. Note prominence of third eyelid, cataract, lens shape abnormality and irregularity of ciliary processes.

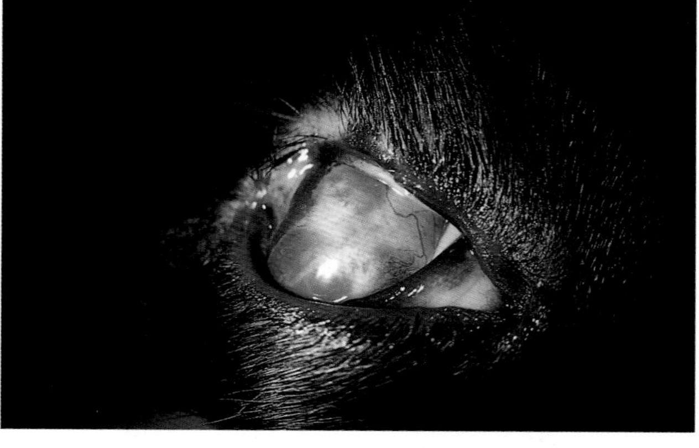

Fig. 4.9 Microphthalmos and enophthalmos with prominence of nictitating membrane. Note also eyelid agenesis in addition to other congenital anomalies.

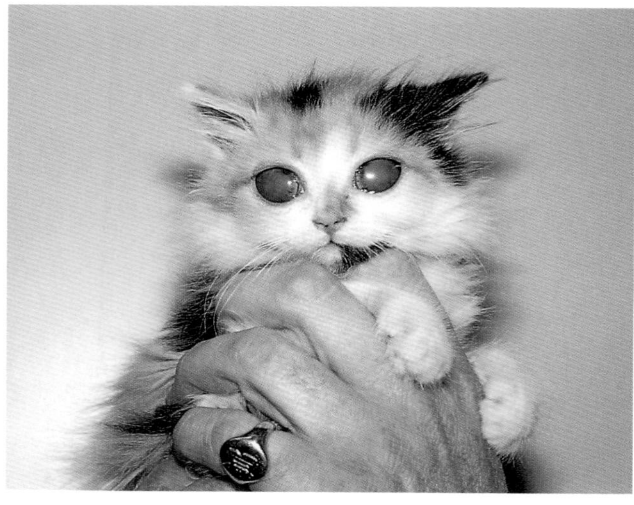

Fig. 4.10 Bilateral buphthalmos in a 9-week-old kitten.

Buphthalmos, the enlarged globe of congenital glaucoma (Fig. 4.10), has been regularly recorded in the kitten (see also Fig. 10.4). The eye is prominent, owing to its increased size, but the nictitating membrane may be retracted. In cases of exophthalmos, in which the eye is also prominent but of normal size, the nictitating membrane is also prominent.

Differential diagnosis of the two conditions is best made by viewing the globe from above; with exophthalmos the globe on the affected side is obviously pushed forwards, whereas this is not so in buphthalmos. Retropulsion of the globe in cases of exophthalmos results in resistance, but not in buphthalmos or hydrophthalmos.

For the management of buphthalmos see hydrophthalmos and glaucoma in Chapter 10.

Ophthalmia neonatorum

Infection within the conjunctival sac prior to opening of the eyelids occurs during birth due to viral infection as the

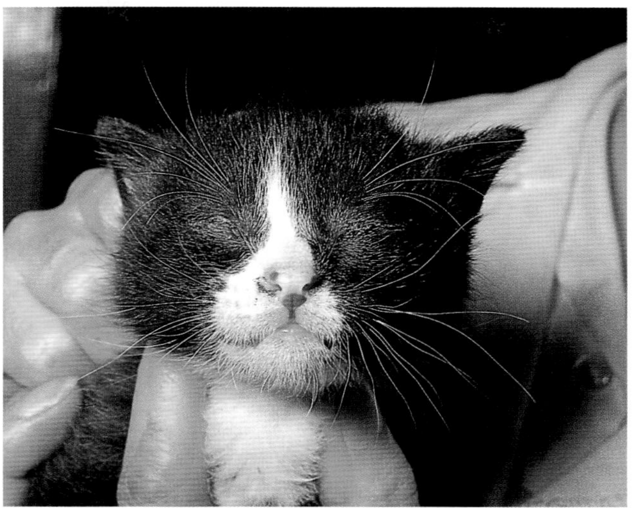

Fig. 4.11 *Ophthalmia neonatorum showing closed lids with swelling behind and oculonasal discharge (see also Fig. 8.8).*

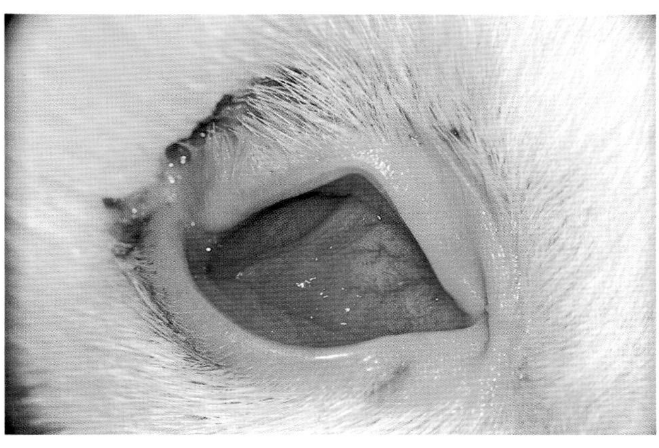

Fig. 4.12 *Phthisis bulbi following penetrating injury. Note enophthalmos and prominence of nictitating membrane.*

kittens pass through the vagina. However, clinical signs may not be apparent until the kitten is several days old and often a number are affected in a litter. The clinical presentation is gross swelling behind closed lids (Fig. 4.11) which do not open at the normal time. Corneal ulceration, which can lead to perforation and endophthalmitis, and subsequent symblepharon may all occur. Treatment is to open the lids with blunt tipped scissors from the medial canthus along their line of fusion. It is important to remove all purulent material by frequent irrigation and ensure that the lids do not seal again. An antibiotic eye ointment should be used and the cornea and conjunctiva kept moist.

Phthisis bulbi

Phthisis bulbi, a shrunken globe, is an acquired condition resulting from serious ocular insult such as trauma (Fig. 4.12), endophthalmitis and (Fig. 4.13) severe uveitis. As with

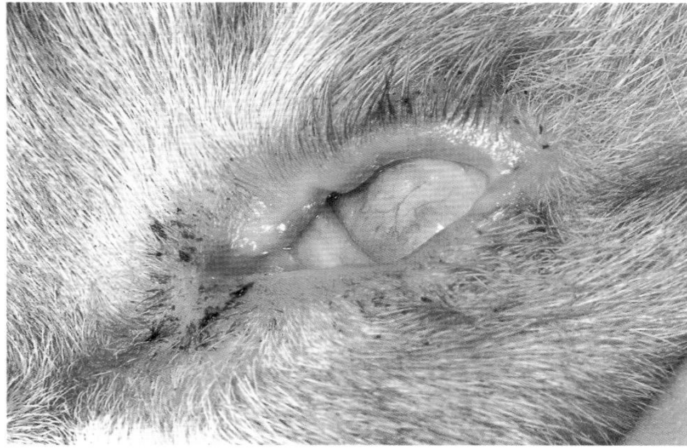

Fig. 4.13 *Phthisis bulbi following severe inflammation (ophthalmia neonatorum).*

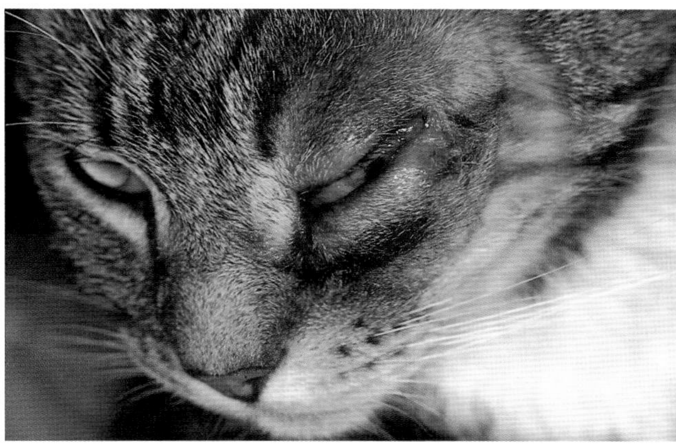

Fig. 4.14 *Orbital cellulitis. Note periorbital swelling and ocular discharge.*

microphthalmos, the small globe is associated with enophthalmos and prominence of the nictitating membrane.

It may be advisable to remove the phthitic globe if excessive discharge is present and persistent.

Exophthalmos

Exophthalmos, abnormal protrusion of the globe, is usually accompanied by prominence of the nictitating membrane and possibly chemosis and strabismus; it is due to some space-occupying lesion. Exophthalmos occurs readily in the cat because of the tight fit of the globe in the orbit. The following conditions all result in degrees of exophthalmos.

Orbital cellulitis

Orbital cellulitis (diffuse inflammation) (Figs 4.14 and 4.15) is not uncommon in the cat and has a varied aetiology, including foreign bodies, which may enter the region via the conjunctiva or the mouth, diseased upper molar teeth, extension from frontal sinusitis, or following fractures or wounds of the region. Other ocular signs in addition to exophthalmos include chemosis, periorbital oedema and sometimes

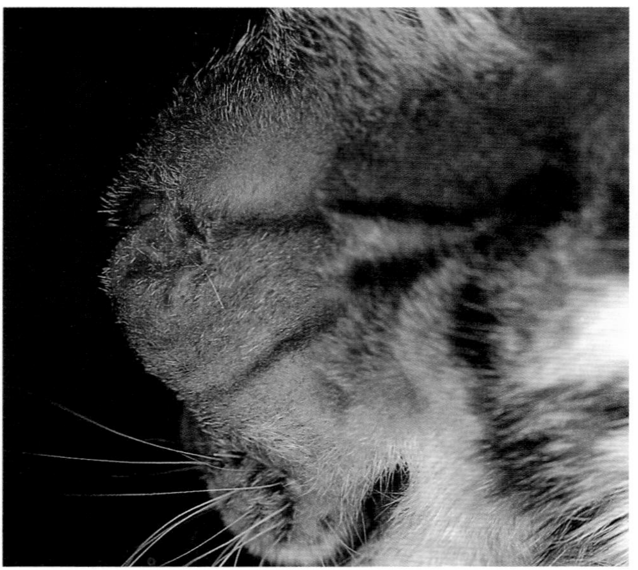

Fig. 4.15 *Orbital cellulitis. Same case as in Fig 4.14.*

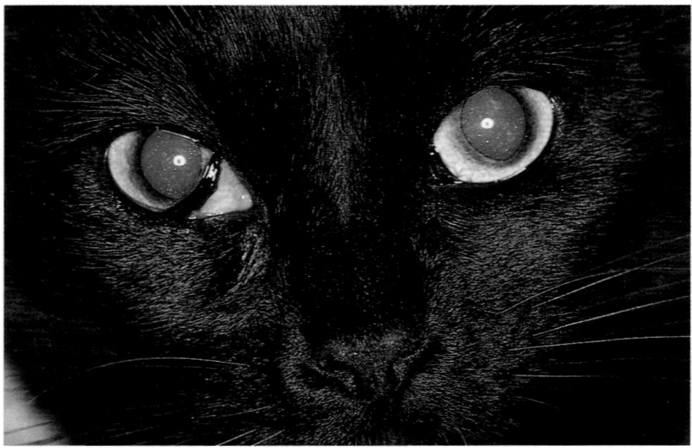

Fig. 4.16 *Retrobulbar abscess. Note minimal discharge and third eyelid prominence.*

pain. Bilateral cellulitis, together with sinusitis and pneumonitis caused by *Penicillium* sp., has been described in a cat (Peiffer *et al.*, 1980). Orbital cellulitis, again bilateral, with optic neuritis and caused by *Pasteurella multocida*, is shown in Fig. 14.75.

Retrobulbar abscess

Retrobulbar abscess (Figs 4.16 and 4.17) is uncommon in the cat but has causes similar to those described under orbital cellulitis, in particular foreign bodies and diseased teeth. Ocular discharge, salivation and pain, particularly on opening the mouth, are more likely than with diffuse inflammation. Defects of the teeth may be obvious but not invariably so and may necessitate detailed dental examination (Ramsey *et al.*, 1996).

The management of orbital cellulitis and/or retrobulbar abscess is similar (see also Chapter 3) and requires a course of broad-spectrum systemic antibiotic. For a retrobulbar abcess it is also possible to establish drainage into the mouth. Under general anaesthesia, with a slight head-down tilt, an endotracheal tube in situ and the pharynx packed with moistened gauze bandage, the mucosa is incised over the space behind the last molar. A fine but blunt pair of artery forceps is introduced through the incision and gently pushed upwards towards the orbit and the jaws of the forceps opened. However, this rarely leads to drainage of obvious purulent material. Swabs for bacterial identification and systemic antibiotic treatment are indicated. It is advisable to extract any fractured molar teeth in the immediate region.

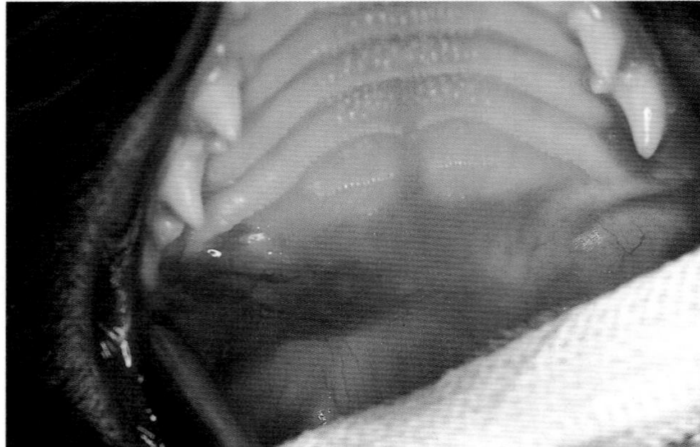

Fig. 4.17 *Retrobulbar abscess. Note drainage established behind last molar tooth.*

Orbital haemorrhage

Orbital haemorrhage is not uncommon following road traffic accidents (head injuries) and bite wounds and may be accompanied by fractures of the orbit and subconjunctival emphysema and haemorrhage. It is important to establish the cause whenever possible and clotting defects should be considered in cases with no obvious evidence of trauma. Exposure keratopathy when present must be treated.

Neoplasia

Orbital neoplasia (Figs 4.18–4.24) is not rare in this species and is frequently malignant. The neoplasia may be primary, arising from any of the orbital structures; secondary, due to extension from adjacent tissue; or metastases from elsewhere. The following tumours have been recorded: lymphosarcoma, squamous cell carcinoma, adenocarcinoma, spindle cell sarcoma, undifferentiated sarcoma, fibrosarcoma, osteosarcoma, rhabdomyosarcoma, osteoma, undifferentiated carcinoma, melanoma, chondroma and haemangiosarcoma. Orbital tumours are usually, but not invariably, unilateral and painless, often slow growing with gradual exophthalmos; they are most common in older cats but have been reported in animals under 1 year old.

Other causes

Exophthalmos caused by a granulomatous inflammatory lesion (Fig 4.25) and, in an aged cat, an eosinophilic infiltrate

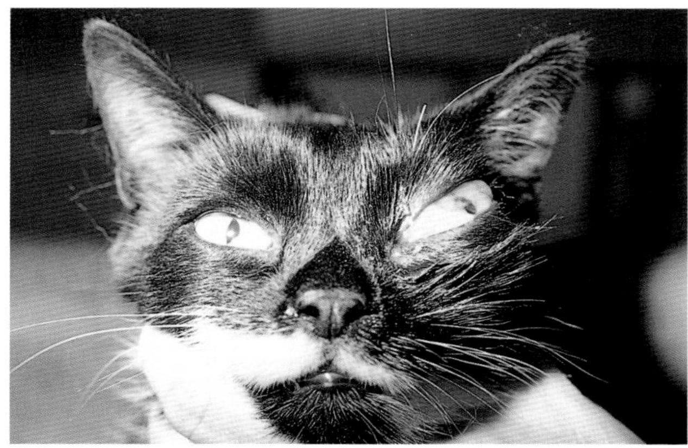

Fig. 4.18 *Retrobulbar tumour. Upward and forward displacement of globe and nictitating membrane. Lymphosarcoma in a 9-year-old Domestic shorthair.*

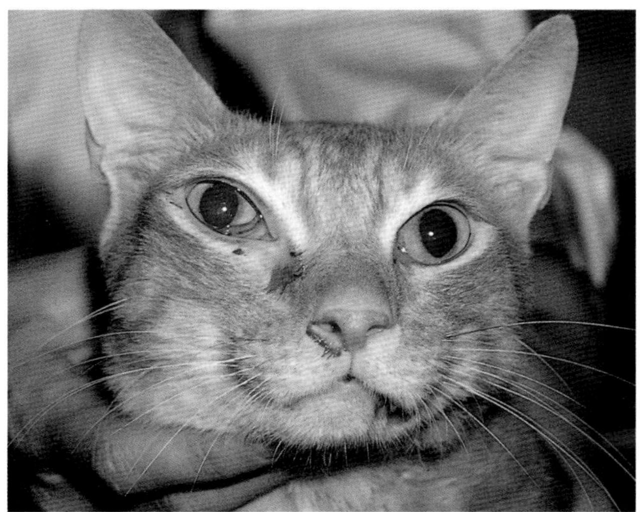

Fig. 4.19 *Exophthalmos and globe deviation caused by nasal adenocarcinoma with orbital extension. Note blood in nostril on affected side.*

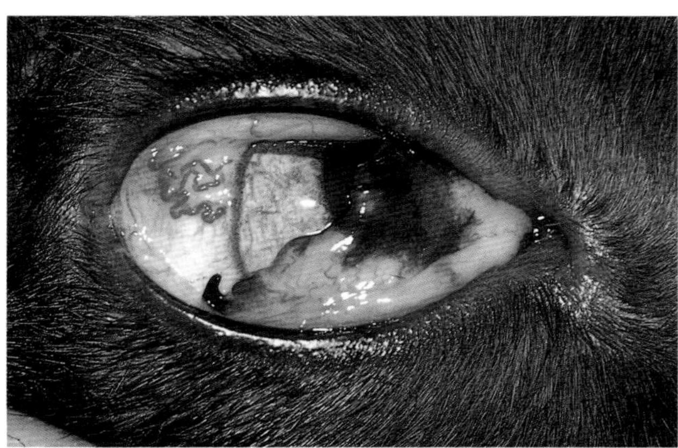

Fig. 4.20 *Exophthalmos caused by nasal tumour with orbital involvement. Note congested superficial blood vessels, chemosis and prominence of nictitating membrane (previous injury to nictitating membrane leaving ragged edge).*

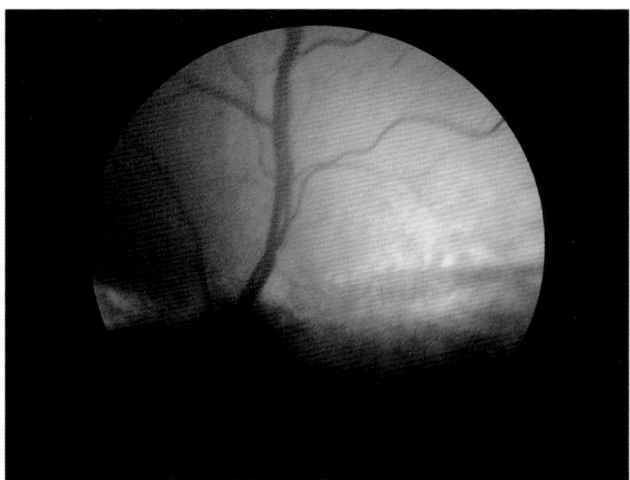

Fig. 4.21 *Fundus photograph showing solid retinal detachment immediately above optic disc (same case as Fig. 4.20).*

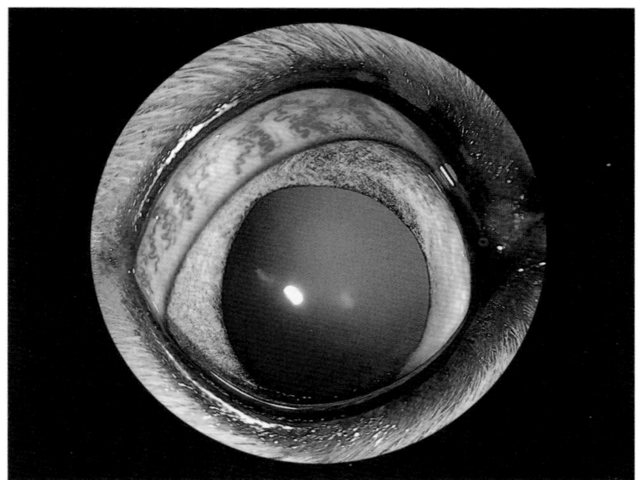

Fig. 4.22 *Multicentric lymphosarcoma including orbital involvement. Note congested superficial blood vessels.*

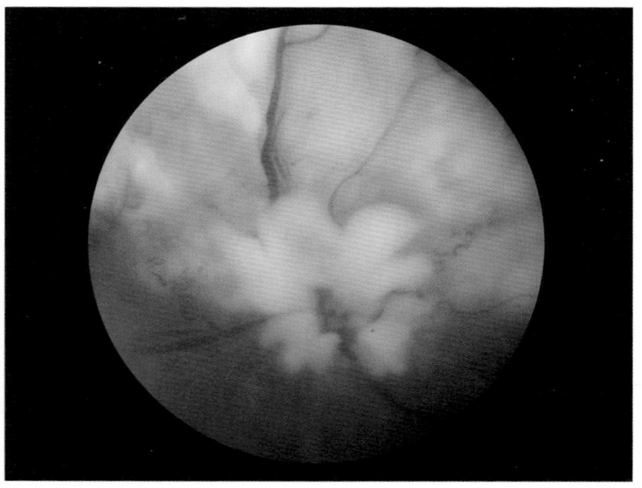

Fig. 4.23 *Same case as Fig. 4.22. Fundus involvement in region of optic disc including retinal detachment and neovascularization.*

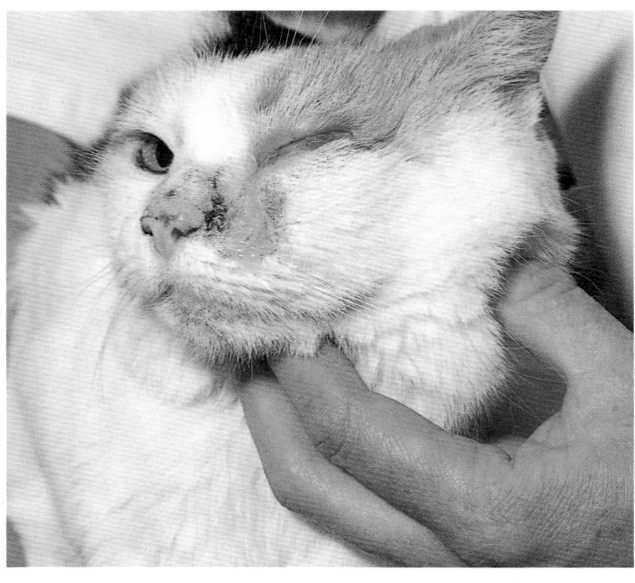

Fig. 4.24 *Orbital lymphosarcoma. Note gross enlargement of local lymph node (between finger and thumb).*

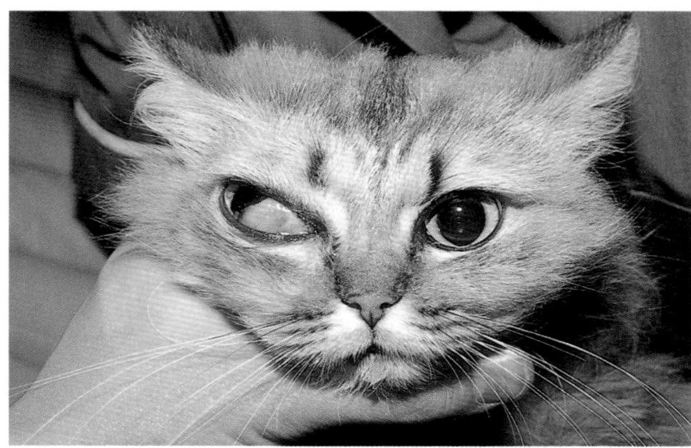

Fig. 4.25 *Exophthalmos due to granulomatous inflammatory lesion (this cat also showed swelling of the hard palate).*

(Dziezyc *et al.*, 1992), have been reported and were both suggestive of retrobulbar neoplasia.

Diagnosis

Further to the clinical signs and procedures described above the differential diagnosis of exophthalmos will be aided considerably by diagnostic imaging techniques. A comparison of these techniques used in a single case of exophthalmos in a cat have been evaluated (Ramsey *et al.*, 1996). Figures 4.26–4.28 depict examples of the use of radiography, which is useful only where bony involvement is suspected, B-mode ultrasonography and magnetic resonance imaging.

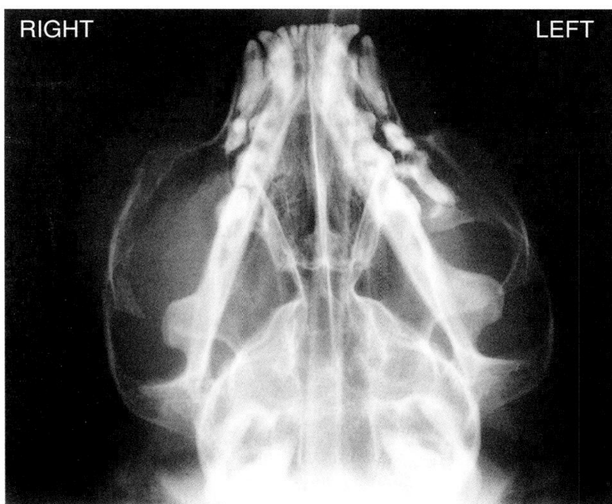

Fig. 4.26 *Dorsoventral skull radiograph of 2-year-old Domestic shorthair with dorsal deviation of the right eye showing extensive osteolysis of the caudal maxilla and rostral zygoma with associated tooth loss. Histopathological diagnosis was ameloblastoma.*

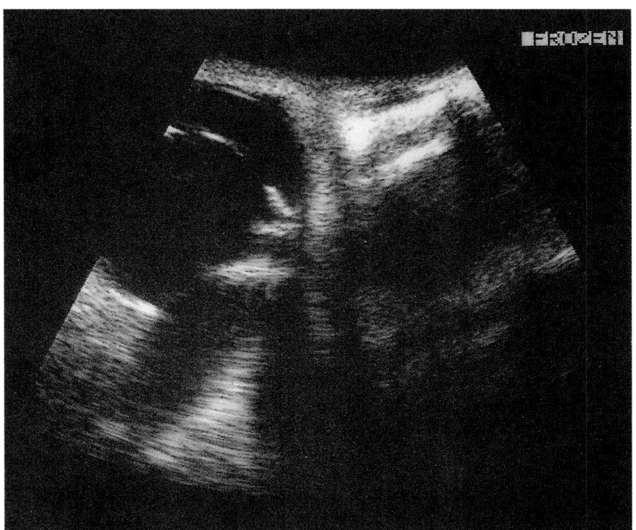

Fig. 4.27 *Ultrasonogram of the eye and orbit of 8-year-old Domestic shorthair with exophthalmos and reduced retropulsion of the globe. A spindle-shaped, hypoechoic mass is visible in the retrobulbar space causing indentation of the back of the globe. Histopathological diagnosis was lymphosarcoma.*

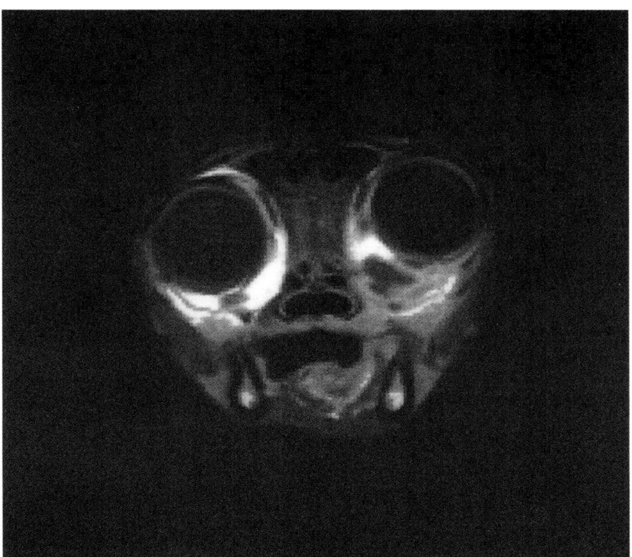

Fig. 4.28 *Transverse T1-weighted MRI scan of the orbital area of 14-year-old Domestic longhair with painful exophthalmos. The normal eye and orbit are visible on the left of the image, the eye appearing hypointense (dark) and orbital fat hyperintense (bright). An extraocular muscle is visible within the fat. On the affected side the globe is displaced and an irregular, thick-walled hypointense lesion is seen in the retrobulbar space. Further scans indicated this to be an abscess, which was subsequently drained. The abscess had mimicked a solid mass on previous ultrasound examination.*

Proptosis

Proptosis (Fig. 4.29), or prolapse, is the forward displacement of the globe from the orbit and between the eyelids which prevent its return to the orbit. Proptosis or prolapse is always caused by trauma and is uncommon in the cat due to the deep orbit; it occurs only with severe trauma and fractures of the orbit.

Management consists of the immediate replacement of the globe in the orbit and this condition should always be considered a real emergency (see Chapter 3). First aid should include lubrication of the cornea and replacement of the globe may necessitate general anaesthesia and possibly lateral canthotomy. Following replacement, suturing of the third eyelid over the globe or, if this is not possible, three or four mattress sutures in the eyelids, will prevent further prolapse resulting from tissue swelling in the orbit. These sutures should remain for 10–14 days and the cat treated with systemic antibiotics and corticosteroids to reduce inflammation and swelling. However quickly the globe has been replaced the prognosis for vision is very guarded.

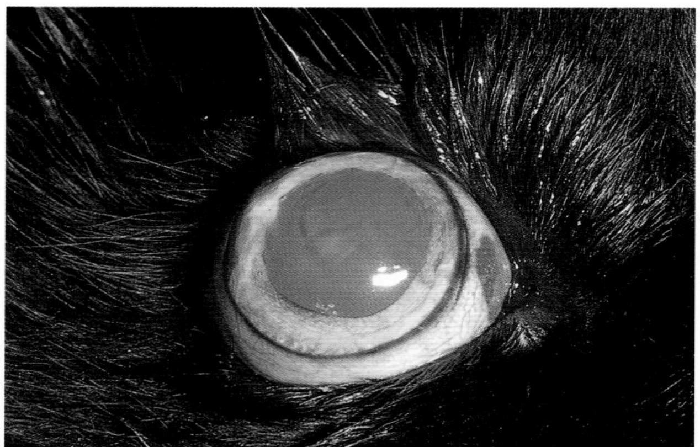

Fig. 4.29 *Proptosis. Note subconjunctival haemorrhage at inner canthus, disappearance of nictitating membrane, inturning of lids behind the globe, visible sclera and mild distortion of corneal surface.*

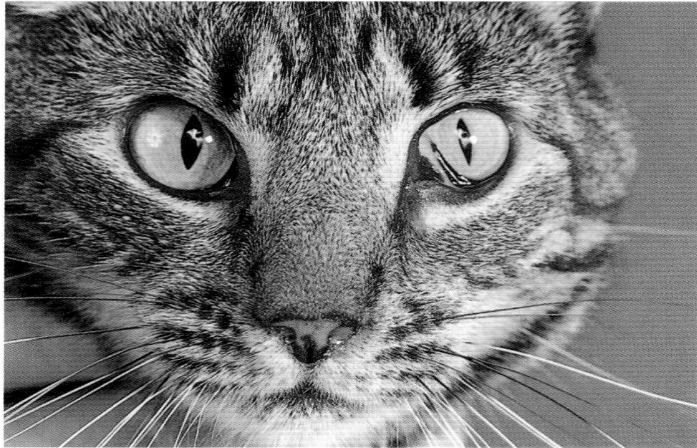

Fig. 4.31 *Enophthalmos with prominence of third eyelid and epiphora on the left side. This was a 3-year-old spayed female Domestic shorthair with nasal squamous cell carcinoma and extension into orbit.*

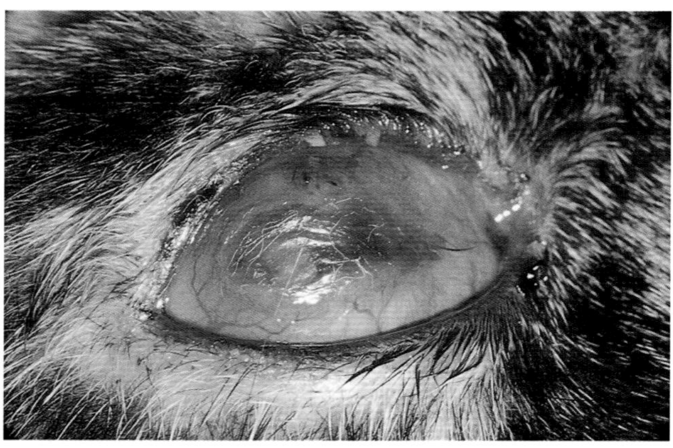

Fig. 4.30 *Hydrophthalmos. Note exposure keratopathy owing to size of globe.*

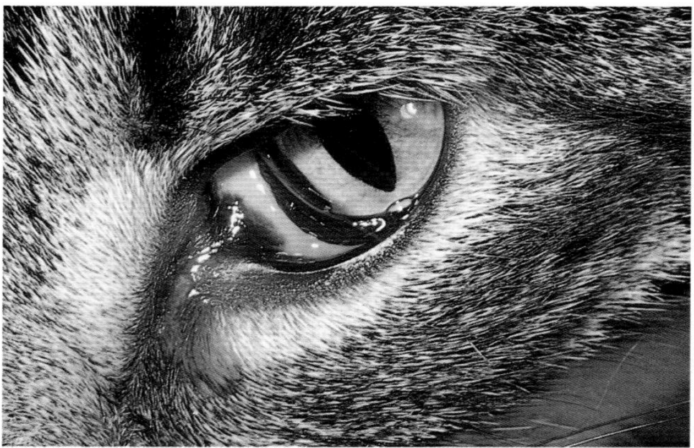

Fig. 4.32 *Same case as Fig 4.31. Close-up of eye showing enophthalmos.*

Hydrophthalmos

Hydrophthalmos (Fig. 4.30) is increased size of globe due to increased intraocular pressure (see also Chapter 10 and Figs 10.17–10.19). Hydrophthalmos implies irreversible blindness caused by retinal and optic atrophy and although, particularly in the cat, the enlarged globe may appear nonpainful the animal may well be more comfortable following removal of a useless eye. Because of the propensity in this species for the development of intraocular sarcomas (see below) removal of the globe is the treatment of choice.

Enophthalmos

Enopthalmos (Figs 4.31 and 4.32), recession of the globe into the orbit, occurs in a number of conditions:

(1) Severe ocular pain.
(2) In cases of microphthalmos (Figs 4.5 and 4.9).
(3) With phthisis bulbi (Fig. 4.12).
(4) Rarely in cases of orbital tumour and depending upon the site of the tumour (Figs 4.31 and 4.32), exophthalmos being the much more common sign.
(5) As part of Horner's syndrome (see Figures 15.8 and 15.9; see also Chapters 6 and 15).

Post-traumatic sarcomas

In recent years a number of reports have been published of intraocular sarcomas in the cat following trauma, infection or surgery (Figs 4.33 and 4.34) (Dubielzig 1984; 1994; Peiffer *et al.*, 1988; Hakanson *et al.*, 1990; Dubielzig *et al.*, 1994). These reports have all been in older cats, with the intraocular sarcoma occurring several months to several years after the initial insult. There has been little or no evidence of pain and since the eye is usually opaque tumour development may go unnoticed. The sarcomas develop within the globe but extraocular extension, usually via the optic canal, does occur. It is thought that the neoplastic cells are derived from

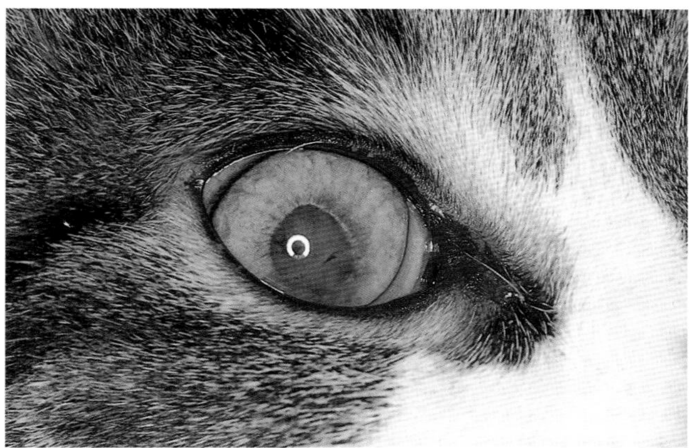

Fig. 4.33 Intraocular sarcoma in a 9-year-old cat following perforating injury two years earlier.

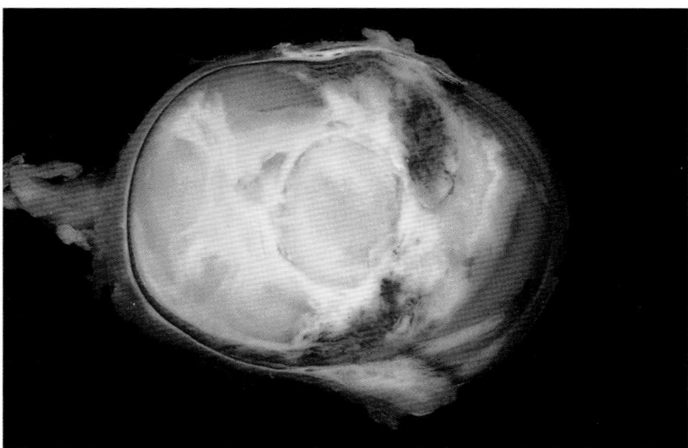

Fig. 4.34 Intraocular sarcoma following trauma in a 14-year-old cat (courtesy J. R. B. Mould).

released lens epithelial cells. These sarcomas have developed in phthitic eyes and are a sound indication for enucleation of both hydrophthalmic and phthitic eyes in the cat.

REFERENCES

Dubielzig RR (1984) Ocular sarcoma following trauma in three cats. *Journal of the American Veterinary Medical Association* **184**: 578–581.

Dubielzig RR, Hawkins KL, Toy KA, Rosebury WS, Mazur M and Jasper TG (1994) Morphologic features of feline ocular sarcomas in 10 cats: light microscopy, ultrastructure, immunohistochemistry. *Veterinary and Comparative Ophthalmology* **4**: 7–12.

Dziezyc J, Barton CL and Santos A (1992) Exophthalmia in a cat caused by an eosinophilic infiltrate. *Progress in Veterinary and Comparative Ophthalmology* **2**: 91–93.

Hakanson N, Shively JN, Reed RE, Merideth RE (1990) Intraocular spindle cell sarcoma following ocular trauma in a cat: case report and literature review. *Journal of the American Animal Hospital Association* **26**: 63–66.

Peiffer RL, Belkin PV and Janke BH (1980) Orbital cellulitis, sinusitis and pneumonitis caused by *Penicillium* sp. in a cat. *Journal of the American Veterinary Medical Association* **176**: 449–451.

Peiffer RL, Monticello T and Bouldin TW (1988) Primary ocular sarcomas in the cat. *Journal of Small Animal Practice* **29**: 105–116.

Ramsey DT, Gerding PA, Losonsky JM, Kuriashkin IV and Clarkson RD (1994) Comparative value of diagnostic imaging techniques in a cat with exophthalmos. *Veterinary and Comparative Ophthalmology* **4**: 198–202.

Ramsey DT, Marretta SM, Hamor RE, Gerding PA, Knight B, Johnson JM and Bagley LH (1996) Ophthalmic Manifestations and Complications of Dental Disease in Dogs and Cats. *Journal of the American Animal Hospital Association* **32**: 215–224.

Scott FW, LaHunta A, Schultz RD, Bistner SI and Riis RC (1975) *Teratology* **11**: 79–86.

5 Upper and lower eyelids

Introduction

The upper and lower eyelids should lie in close apposition to the cornea and within the palpebral fissure there is very little exposed conjunctiva (Figs 1.2–1.3), except for a small portion of third eyelid conjunctiva at the medial canthus and, sometimes, a small area of bulbar conjunctiva laterally. Measurements of the length of the palpebral fissure in adult cats (Stades *et al.*, 1992) indicated a mean length of 27.8 ± 2.7 mm, with a longer mean length of 28.7 ± 2.9 mm in the Persian cat. The eyelid margins are usually pigmented, especially when there is dark skin or fur around the eyes. Some cats have small pigmented patches on the eyelid margins which grow slightly larger with age and some pale-coloured cats completely lack pigment; there is a great deal of variation between eyes and between breeds. The upper and lower lacrimal puncta may be distinguished on the inside of the eyelids in the medial canthus region.

Adult cats blink infrequently, a complete blink takes place about once every 5 min and incomplete blinks are rare. As in humans, the upper eyelid is more mobile than the lower.

The eyelids consist of two laminae which are separated anatomically by a layer of fascia, the orbital septum. The anterior lamina consists of skin and orbicularis muscle, the posterior lamina consists of tarsal plate, those structures which act as eyelid retractors and the conjunctival layer (Fig. 5.1). Eyelid retractors comprise smooth muscle fibres (with sympathetic innervation) and, in the upper eyelid, the levator palpebrae superioris (innervated by the oculomotor nerve: CN III). There is a generous blood supply to both eyelids.

Fine hairs cover the skin and many of the hair follicles are closely associated with glandular tissue. Thicker hairs act as rudimentary eyelashes (cilia) on the upper eyelid, but the eyelid margins of both the upper and lower eyelids are normally devoid of hairs. The thin orbicularis oculi muscle (innervated by the facial nerve: CN VII) encircles the palpebral opening and is closely attached to the overlying skin.

The openings of the well-developed meibomian (tarsal) glands, which number 25–35 for each eyelid (more on the upper than lower eyelid) are obvious in a shallow groove on the inner aspect of the eyelid margin and the extent of the glands is apparent beneath the palpebral conjunctiva; those of the upper eyelid are better developed than those of the lower eyelid. The meibomian glands lie within the fibrous connective tissue known as the tarsal 'plate'; a misnomer given the nonrigid structure of the perimeibomian connective tissue and the quantity of glandular tisue present. Any rigidity the eyelid does possess is largely determined by the complex way in which the connective tissue is arranged, especially at the eyelid margin and to a lesser extent within the substance of the eyelid.

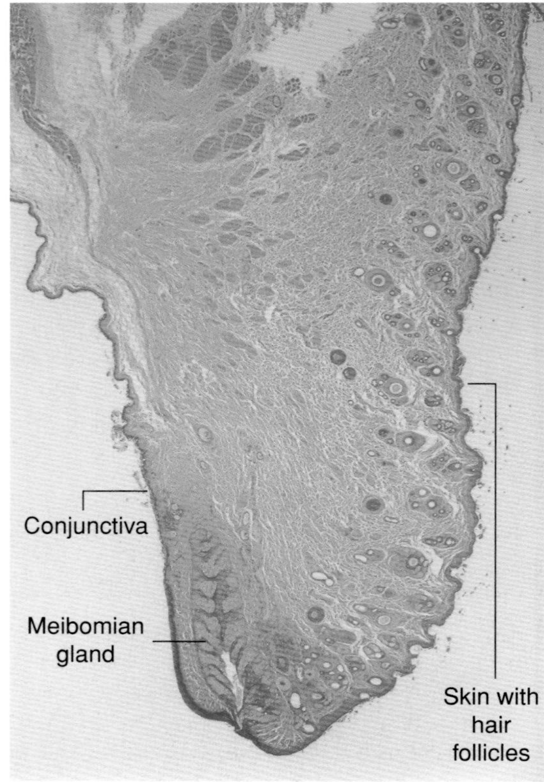

Fig. 5.1 Histological section through the feline uper eyelid. The conjunctival portion is on the left and the skin portion on the right.

The eyelids of neonatal kittens remain fused for some time after birth (usually 4–12 days). On rare occasions kittens are born with the eyelids open and it is not unusual for one eye to open before the other.

Disorders of the upper and lower eyelids

Ankyloblepharon

Congenital ankyloblepharon, in which the upper and lower eyelids are joined by a thick membrane, has been reported in Persians.

Occasionally, infection (usually FHV-1) behind the closed eyelids results in ophthalmia neonatorum (see Chapters 4 and 8), so that the eyelids remain fused beyond the normal time (Fig. 4.11). There is usually swelling behind the closed eyelids and, in early cases, a clear ocular discharge oozes from the region of the medial canthus. The ocular discharge in untreated cases soon becomes mucopurulent and secondary bacterial infection is common (Fig. 5.2).

Ophthalmia neonatorum is a condition which must be recognized and treated if vision-threatening complications are to be avoided (Fig. 5.3); for management see Chapter 4.

Cats which have had previous ophthalmia neonatorum, especially those that were untreated, may present with complex eyelid defects when they are older and the management of each case requires careful assessment. Complications of ophthalmia neonatorum include corneal ulceration, ocular perforation, endophthalmitis, panophthalmitis (see Chapter 3), inadequate tear production and drainage (see Chapter 7) and symblepharon (see Chapter 8).

Agenesis and coloboma

Complete (agenesis) or partial (coloboma) absence of all the eyelid layers, or some of the eyelid layers may affect one or both eyes (Figs 5.4–5.8); it is the commonest congenital eyelid abnormality of cats, both domesticated and wild (Bellhorn *et al.*, 1971). The region most frequently affected is the lateral part of the upper eyelid, but occasionally the medial and lateral canthus is involved. Rarely, the centre of the eyelid is involved. Multiple ocular colobomas in the Snow Leopard were first recorded by Wahlberg (1978) and there have been subsequent reports including Barnett (1981) and Gripenberg *et al.* (1985). No specific aetiology has been established, although a number of possibilities, including teratogenicity, environmental influences and genetic predisposition have been suggested. Ocular manifestations range from single defects (eyelid coloboma) (Fig. 5.9) to multiple ocular defects (eyelid colobomas, microphthalmos, cataract, retinal dysplasia, choroidal and optic nerve colobomas). Similar multiple congenital ocular anomalies have been reported in domestic shorthair kittens (Martin *et al.*, 1997). A genetic predisposition to incomplete development of the eyelids at the lateral and medial canthus is suspected in certain lines of Burmese cats (Fig. 5.10) and epibulbar dermoids may also be part of the developmental defect in this breed (Koch, 1979). Gross eyelid defects can also be a complication

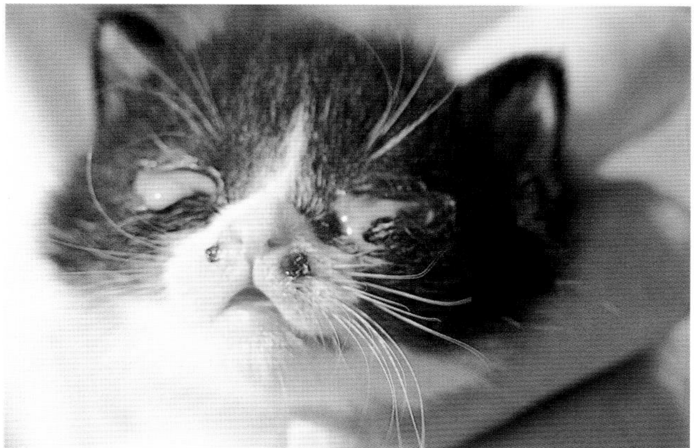

Fig. 5.2 *Ophthalmia neonatorum in a 10-day-old kitten with severe secondary bacterial infection. Note the nasal discharge. (Courtesy of A. L. Lange).*

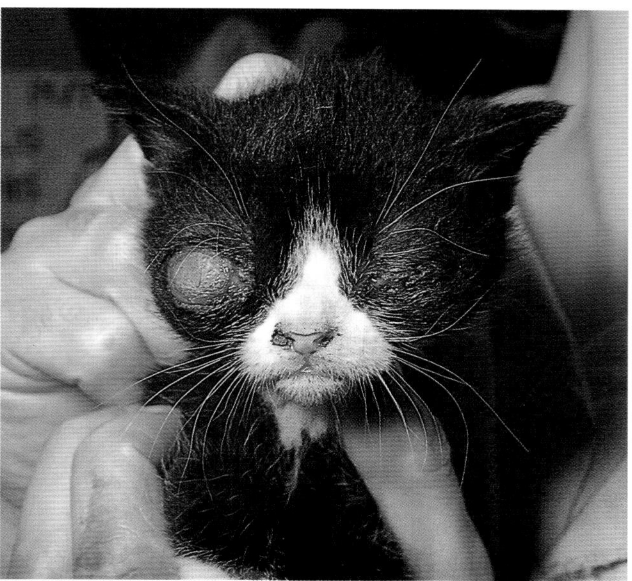

Fig. 5.3 *Ophthalmia neonatorum in a kitten approximately 3 weeks old. Endophthalmitis is present on the right and there is an ocular discharge and swelling behind the eyelids on the left. Note the nasal discharge.*

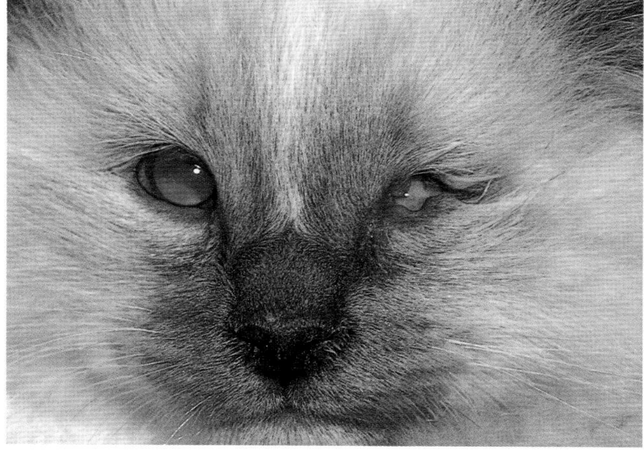

Fig. 5.4 *Multiple ocular anomalies in a Birman kitten.*

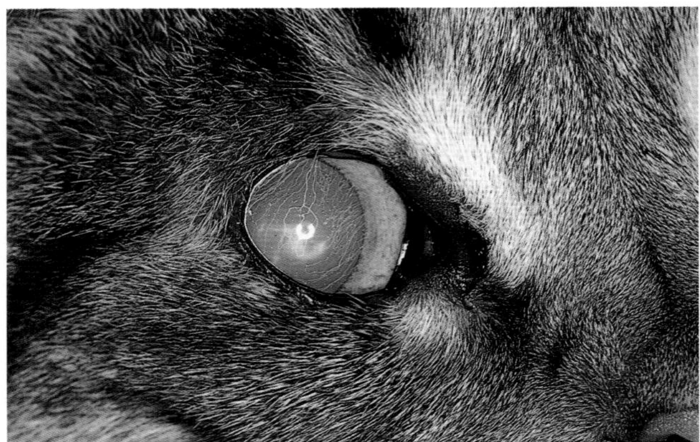

Fig. 5.5 *Eyelid coloboma affecting all but the medial aspect of the upper eyelid margin in a Domestic shorthair. There is an accompanying mild vascular keratitis, largely a result of trichiasis (from skin hairs).*

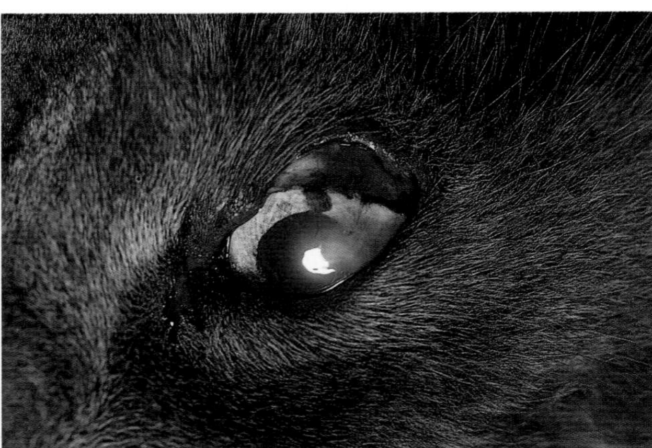

Fig. 5.6 *An extensive upper eyelid coloboma affecting about two-thirds of the length and much of the depth of the upper eyelid in a Domestic shorthair. The exposed bulbar conjunctiva is pigmented and there is also an exposure keratopathy.*

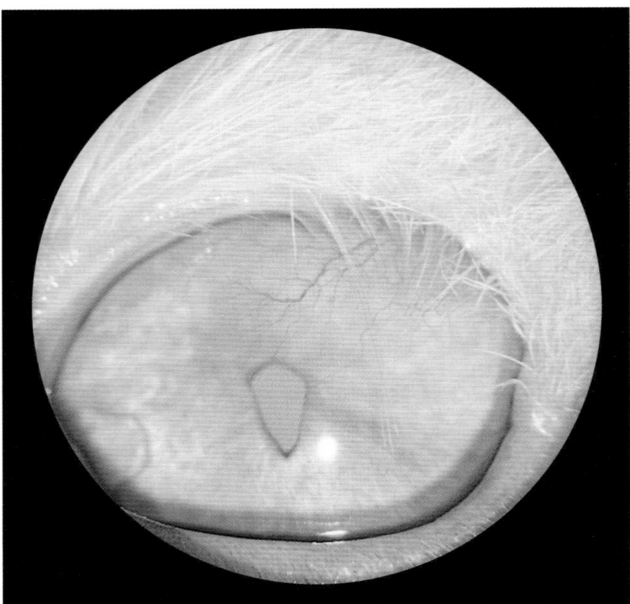

Fig. 5.7 *Lateral eyelid coloboma with trichiasis in a 6-month-old Colourpoint. The coloboma is affecting the lateral aspect of the upper eyelid, the canthus and a small portion of the lower eyelid. There is also an atypical coloboma of the iris at '12 o'clock'. The other eye was also affected.*

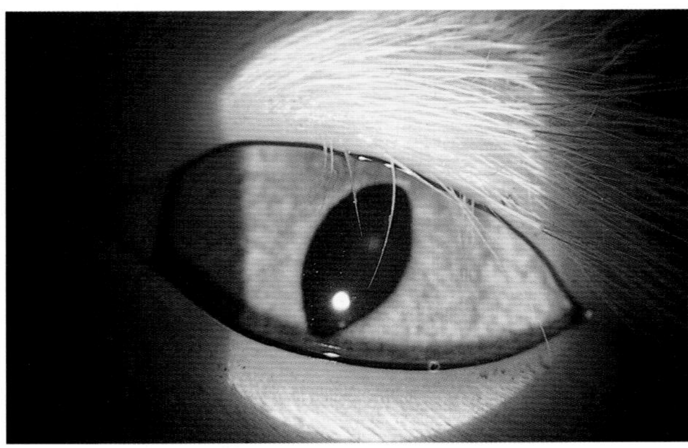

Fig. 5.8 *A 2-year-old Domestic shorthair with coloboma affecting the middle portion of the upper eyelid. Note the trichiasis from the skin hairs. No meibomian glands were apparent in the affected region and a similar colobomatous defect was present in the other eye.*

of prenatal and perinatal infections, in which case the whole litter is affected to varying degrees and ocular defects such as symblepharon (see Chapter 8) are likely to be present.

The extent of the eyelid defect in affected cats determines the severity of the clinical signs. In conjunction with the lack of eyelid margin there may be no obvious meibomian glands in the affected area. The effects on the cornea range from minimal to marked exposure keratopathy and, sometimes, direct corneal trauma because of irritation from contiguous hairs (a form of trichiasis, in that it is skin hairs rather than eyelashes which contact the cornea). It is important to check for any other ocular or adnexal abnormalities in affected animals.

Treatment consists of cleaning and ocular lubrication for minimally affected cases; a similar conservative approach may also be adopted until more severely affected animals are old enough for surgery. Repair may be effected by a number of techniques, depending upon the extent and site of the defect (Peiffer *et al.*, 1987a, b; Collin, 1989; Dziezyc and Millichamp, 1989; Mustardé, 1991). Given the anatomy of the upper eyelid, its greater mobility and the effects of gravity, it is inevitable that surgery of the upper eyelid is more challenging than surgery of the lower eyelid. While detailed reconstructive eyelid techniques are beyond the scope of this book, it is worth emphasizing that successful eyelid surgery aims to retain or construct eyelid margins, to provide conjunctival lining and to preserve functional eyelid movement.

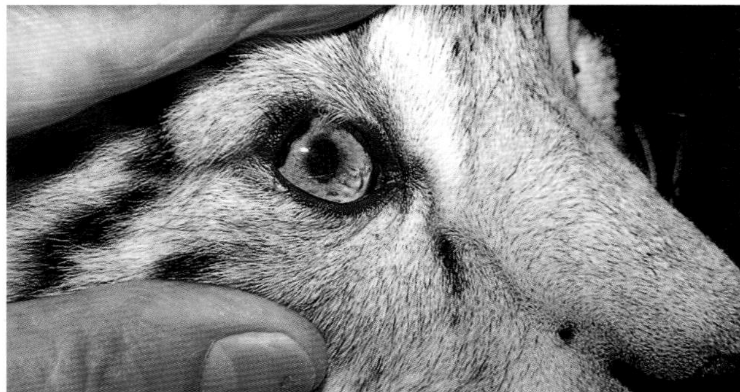

Fig. 5.9 *Snow Leopard with a colobomatous defect of the middle portion of the upper eyelid. The left eyelid was similarly affected.*

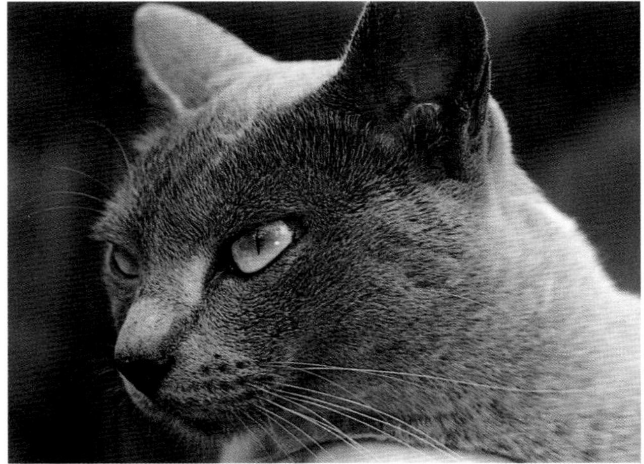

Fig. 5.10 *Adult Burmese with incomplete development of the eyelids at the lateral canthus. (Courtesy of A. L. Lange).*

In simple terms, this means that primary closure is the treatment of choice when it can be undertaken without producing eyelid distortion and that for more extensive repairs eyelid tissue from the same eyelid or the other eyelid should be used whenever possible. For small colobomatous defects (up to one-quarter of the margin) simple one or two layered closure is often all that is required following very limited freshening of the edges of the defect and creation of an elongated pentagon. For larger defects (up to one-third of the margin) a releasing technique at the lateral canthus may be required. For even larger defects (more than one-third of the margin) more complex surgery is required and the technique employed should aim to provide a minimum of an inner mucus-secreting layer and an outer skin-covering layer. Many surgical techniques have been described for extensive lesions, but a high proportion make no attempt to preserve eyelid margin and thus create long-term problems because normal skin hairs contact the cornea and produce chronic corneal damage – a particular problem with extensive surgery of the upper eyelid. A full-thickness 'switch-flap' technique avoids these problems by rotating an attached sector of the full thickness of the lower eyelid through 180° to fill a defect in the upper eyelid. The pedicle must be wide enough to ensure that the blood supply is not compromised and the pedicle is usually sectioned some 12–14 days after surgery (Mustardé, 1991).

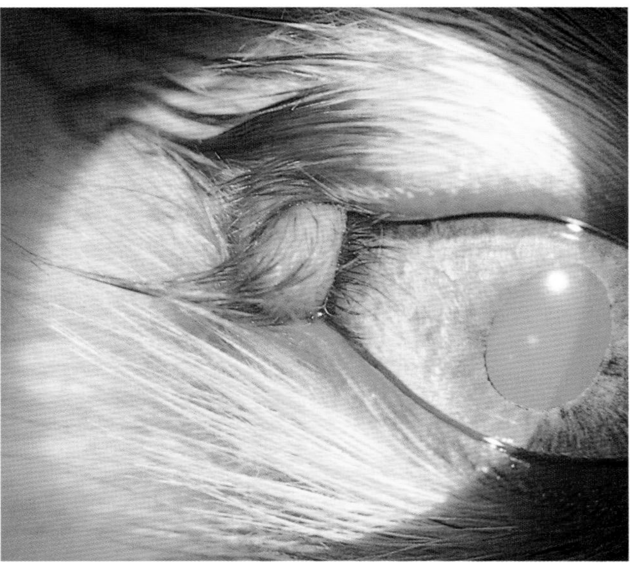

Fig. 5.11 *A 10-week-old Birman kitten. Dermoid (choristoma) at the lateral canthus.*

Symblepharon

See Chapter 8.

Epibulbar dermoid

Epibulbar dermoids or choristomas are congenital malformations containing many of the elements of skin. They may be the result of incomplete fusion of the eyelids, with displacement of skin elements into the dermoid. In cats, they are usually located on the skin (Fig 5.11) or conjunctiva (see Chapter 8) in the region of the lateral canthus, but they may be found at other sites and corneal involvement is also encountered (see Chapter 9). Certain lines of Birman cats show a genetic predisposition (Hendy Ibbs, 1985) and the possible inheritance of eyelid defects and dermoids in the Burmese cat has been mentioned above.

Surgical excision is the treatment of choice for epibulbar dermoids. The incisions should be made in normal surrounding skin and the wound closed with a pliable material such as 6/0 polyglactin or silk, starting nearest the eyelid margin. Silk sutures should be removed after 7–10 days, polyglactin sutures can be left.

Entropion

Entropion is the inturning (inversion) of the whole lid or part of the lid and is an uncommon problem in the cat (Figs 5.12–5.14). It may be classified as anatomical entropion, spastic entropion (a result of anterior segment pain) and cicatricial entropion (a result of scarring/fibrosis).

Anatomical Entropion

Anatomical entropion is most commonly seen in the Persian cat. In this breed it may be present from an early age and usually involves the lower eyelid and particularly the medial aspect of the eyelid initially (Figs 5.12 and 5.13). Entropion may also be seen, unrelated to breed, associated with microphthalmos (see Chapter 4). Anatomical entropion is sometimes a complication of chronic anterior segment pain and, in such cases, the reason for the pain must be addressed in addition to the complicating entropion.

Anatomical entropion is treated most simply using the Hotz–Celsus procedure and the wound is closed with simple interrupted sutures of 6/0 polyglactin or silk (the latter requires removal after 7–10 days). Unyielding materials like monofilament nylon should not be used. Entropion can be a frustrating problem to treat in cats as it may recur. When blepharospasm appears to be a complicating feature of anatomical entropion and a possible reason for repeated surgery it is wise to ensure that there are no other inciting causes such as calicivirus infection.

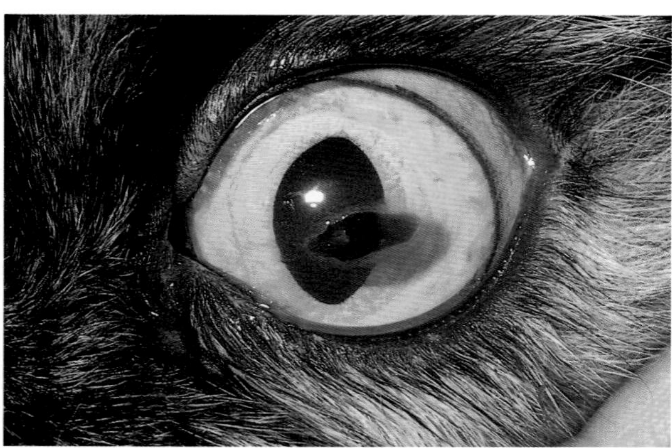

Fig. 5.12 *A 4-year-old Persian. Bilateral lower medial eyelid entropion; the left eye is shown. Careful examination, without manipulation of the eyelids, is required to ascertain the extent of the entropion. In particular, the eyelid margins should be observed directly to ensure both that they are present and that they are correctly aligned. Note the mild epiphora and the presence of a corneal sequestrum which may be associated with chronic low-grade irritation.*

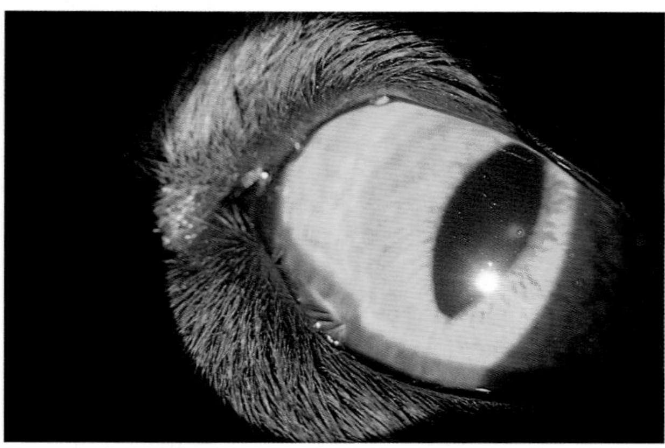

Fig. 5.13 *A 2-year-old Persian. Magnified view of lower medial eyelid entropion. Note the 'trichiasis' (skin hairs).*

Spastic Entropion

If a spastic component is suspected or obvious (see Chapter 9), topical local anaesthesia is an essential part of the investigative procedure and, if the blepharospasm and accompanying entropion resolve following the application of local anaesthetic, then entropion surgery is not required. It is not uncommon for topical anaesthesia to produce only partial resolution and a temporary lateral tarsorrhaphy is sometimes needed while the cause of the anterior segment pain is identified and treated.

Cicatricial Entropion

This is not particularly common in cats (Fig. 5.14). Causes include previous infection, chronic inflammation, trauma, previous surgery and injuries from heat and caustic chemicals. The problem is usually resolved in simple cases by a Y to V plasty which releases the tension on the inverted lid margin. More complicated cases require cosmetic surgery on an individual case basis.

Ectropion

Ectropion is an outward turning of the eyelid. There is a gap between the eyelid and the cornea so that the conjunctiva and cornea are relatively exposed and the tear film is disrupted. Poor eyelid anatomy, for example, the over long palpebral fissure of some Persian cats, will predispose to entropion (see above) and, less commonly, ectropion (Fig. 5.15).

All types of ectropion, other than that caused by insults (e.g. inflammation, trauma, thermal injury, abscesses) and neoplasia, are rare in cats. If eyelid lacerations are not

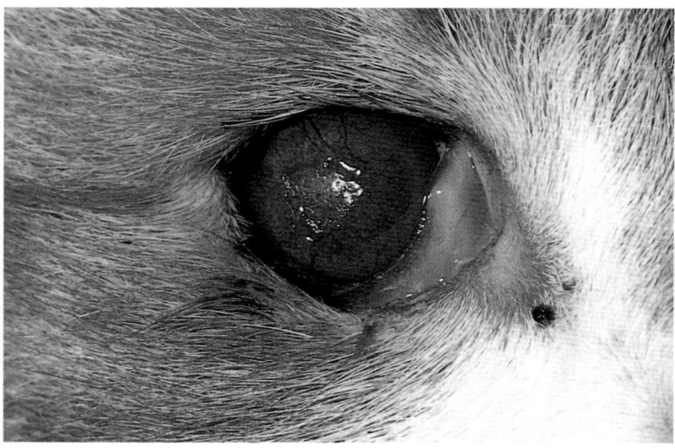

Fig. 5.14 *Domestic shorthair, approximately 2 years old, with complications from previous herpes conjunctivitis. Keratoconjunctivitis sicca and ulcerative keratitis has resulted in a spastic entropion affecting especially the lateral canthus and the lower lateral eyelid of the right eye.*

repaired promptly at the time of the injury, distortion of the eyelid is a likely complication, because of disruption of the eyelid margin and scar contraction. This type of cicatricial ectropion can usually be corrected using simple V to Y plasty. Cases of ectropion associated with symblepharon require individual assessment (Fig. 8.8).

Distichiasis and ectopic cilia

Distichiasis is very rare in the cat compared with the dog. Agenesis and coloboma of the eyelid may be associated with distichia-like hairs on the edge of the abnormal area, where the eyelid margin should be and this anomaly is associated with aberrant eyelid development (Fig. 5.16).

Distichia emerging from the meibomian gland openings, which are so common in dogs, are extremely rare in cats (Figs 5.17 and 5.18). They particularly affect the lower eyelid and may be removed by catholysis if they are causing ocular discomfort or corneal trauma. Their presence usually gives rise to increased lacrimation as the only obvious abnormality, but occasionally corneal damage such as ulceration and sequestrum formation (see Chapter 9) can occur.

There is a single case report of an ectopic cilium, arising from the palpebral conjunctiva at the base of the meibomian glands in the upper eyelid of a Siamese cat, which was treated using nitrous oxide cryotherapy (Hacker, 1989).

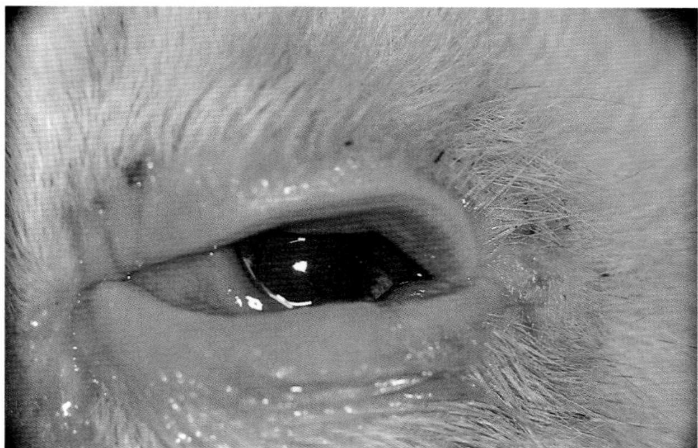

Fig. 5.15 *A 2-year-old Persian cat with ectropion. The over-long palpebral aperture and chronic inflammation from calicivirus conjunctivitis have exacerbated the tendency for the eyelid to turn outwards.*

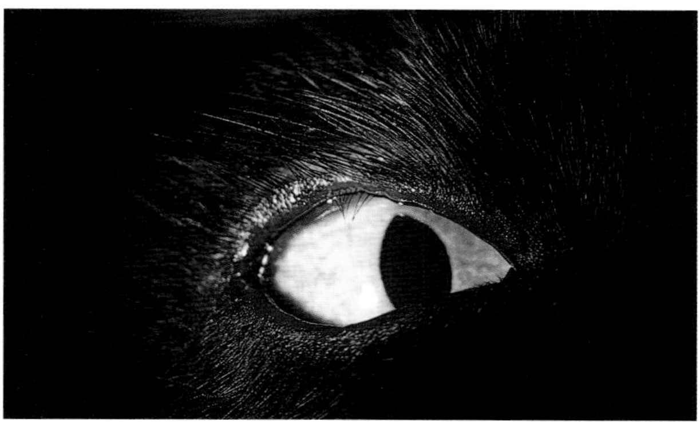

Fig. 5.16 *'Distichiasis' and symblepharon in a 1-year-old Domestic shorthair. As with 'trichiasis', these are not eyelashes, but skin hairs, and probably reflect failure of the upper eyelid margin to differentiate properly (the mildest form of eyelid coloboma). In this case the combination of symblepharon and a mild eyelid margin deformity may be a consequence of earlier infectious conjunctivitis.*

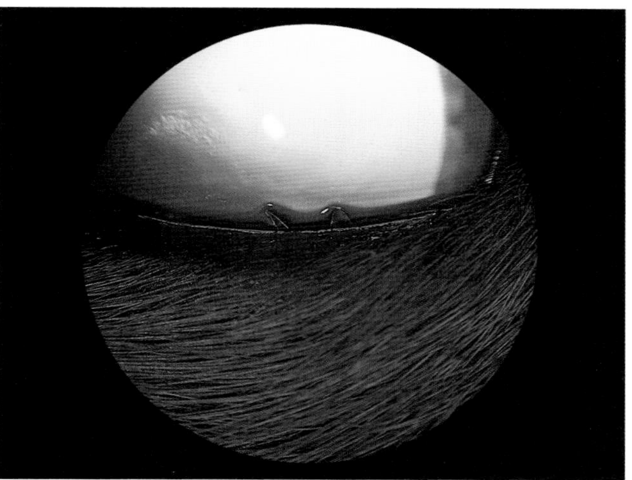

Fig. 5.17 *In this 7-year-old Birman cat the abnormal hairs emerge from the meibomian gland openings of the lower eyelid and can therefore be designated distichia. Note the subtle corneal disruption produced by the distichia.*

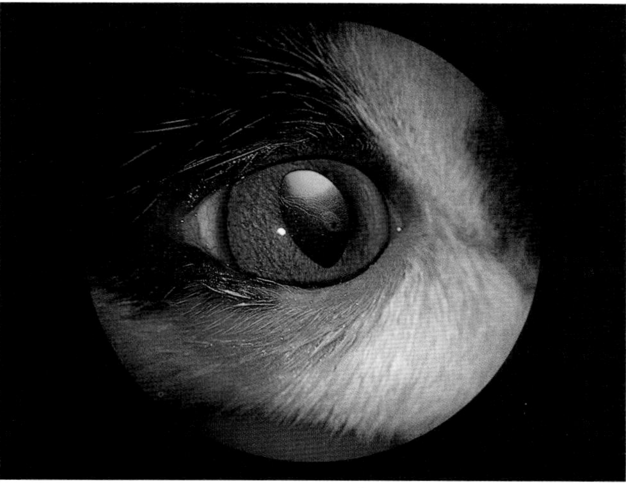

Fig. 5.18 *A 5-month-old Domestic shorthair. In addition to distichiasis affecting the lower eyelid of the right eye, there is a small corneal sequestrum, possibly the result of chronic low grade trauma. A Schirmer I tear test gave readings of 25 mm/min in the right eye and 5 mm/min in the left eye. This cat also had a history of occasional sneezing.*

Dermatoses

Eyelid dermatoses (see Figs 5.19–5.27) may be caused by viral, parasitic, fungal and bacterial infection and immune-mediated problems. The cause is sometimes obscure and it is often advisable to seek advice about diagnosis and management from a veterinary dermatologist. Sampling the lesion (skin scraping, culture and biopsy) is usually the easiest means of confirming the diagnosis.

Viral

Feline pox virus affects kittens and immunocompromised cats most severely and is usually associated with skin lesions, rather than eyelid lesions (Fig. 5.20), although characteristic multiple nodules, papules, crusts and ulcerative plaques may sometimes involve the eyelids. Systemic signs, which include pyrexia, conjunctivitis, an oculonasal discharge and pneumonia, develop in a proportion of cases (Bennett *et al.*, 1990).

There is no specific treatment for pox virus infection in cats and most animals eventually recover. Immunosuppression as a consequence of naturally occurring concurrent disease (e.g. FeLV and FIV infection) or inappropriate treatment (e.g. corticosteroids and megoestrol acetate) will complicate the clinical picture and affected cats may succumb to severe systemic disease.

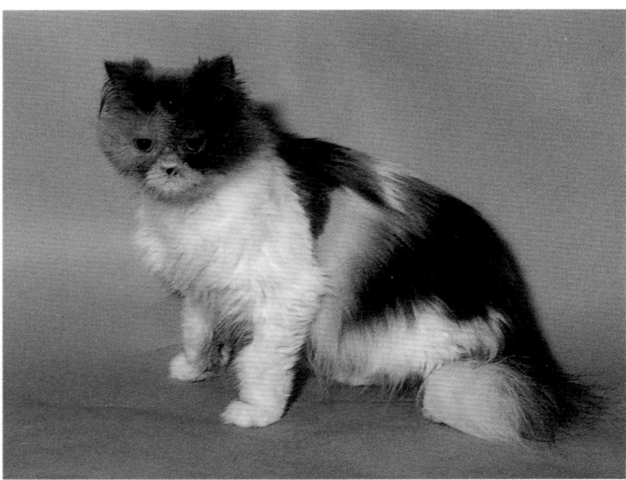

Fig. 5.19 *Chronic blepharitis in a 22-month-old Persian cat. The facial anatomy of this breed predisposes them to eyelid and periocular problems and, in this cat, the situation was exacerbated by a food allergy and self inflicted trauma with secondary bacterial eyelid infection. Note the staining on the front legs where the cat has been rubbing her face.*

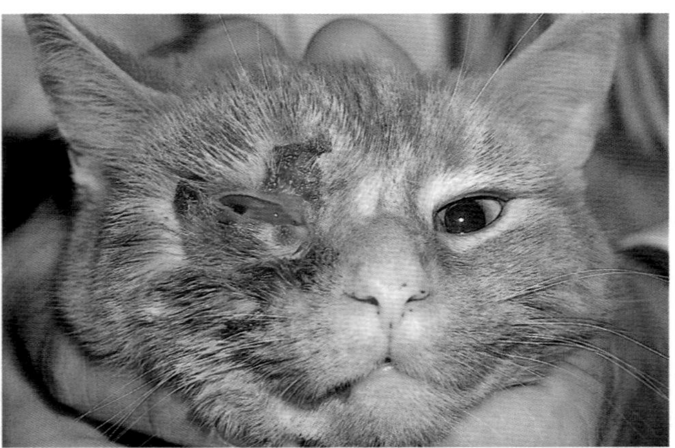

Fig. 5.20 *Cow pox in a 4-year-old Domestic shorthair. The condition resolved with no treatment other than nursing care over the course of approximately 1 month.*

Parasitic

Feline scabies, caused by *Notoedres cati* is rare. The parasite causes an intense pruritis around the head and neck and there is usually some hair loss, with skin thickening and encrustation. Demodicosis is a rare cause of nonpruritic blepharitis in cats (Fig. 5.21) and generalized demodicosis is often associated with a compromised host (as described for pox virus above). Cuterebra larvae are a rare cause of eyelid myiasis.

Fungal

Dermatophytosis with a range of clinical appearances is usually caused by *Microsporum canis,* although, on rare occasions, other dermatophytic fungi may be isolated. Fungal culture should be undertaken to confirm the diagnosis.

Systemic mycotic infections (cryptococcosis, blastomycosis, coccidioidomycosis and histoplasmosis), are rarely seen in the UK unless the animal has been imported from abroad or is severely immunocompromised. Diagnosis is confirmed by histopathology and culture of biopsy specimens. Cryptococcosis is the commonest cause of systemic mycosis (Fig. 5.22). Treatment with 5-fluorocytosine, ketoconazole and itraconazole has met with varying degrees of success.

Bacterial

Infected bite and claw wounds are the commonest reason for suppurative blepharitis. The clinical signs are similar to those

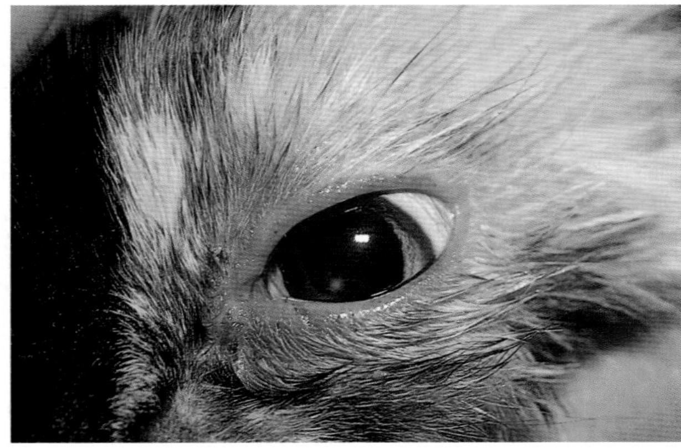

Fig. 5.21 *Demodicosis (bilateral) in a domestic shorthair (courtesy of M.P. Nasisse).*

of an abscess elsewhere, with swelling, heat and pain. Conservative treatment of diffuse suppurative blepharitis combines local therapy using warm compresses with a course of systemic antibiotic. In addition to providing a course of systemic antibiotic, large swellings should be drained and, on occasions, it is better to leave a drain (e.g. Penrose) *in situ*. If no treatment is given, the abscess may burst and discharge via the conjunctiva, or the eyelid skin and extensive swelling may be associated with necrosis and sloughing of the overlying skin. It is wise to perform skull radiography if discharging sinuses are present to verify that there are no additional complications such as fractures or bone sequestration.

Chronic bacterial blepharitis and blepharoconjunctivitis, which are most commonly caused by *Staphylococcus* spp., are occasionally seen in adults (Fig. 5.23). The clinical signs include bilateral discomfort and pruritis with a degree of exudation and ocular discharge. There is usually erythema

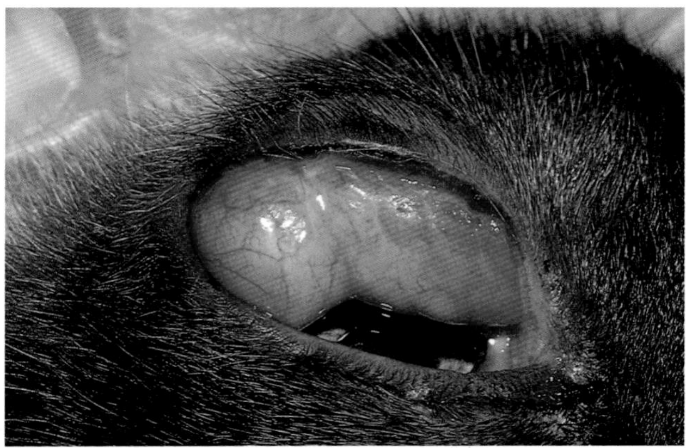

Fig. 5.22 *Systemic cryptococcosis in a 12-year-old Siamese cat imported to England after living in Venezuela and, later, New York. Cryptococcus neoformans was identified (culture and histopathology) from the upper eyelid of the right eye and chorioretinitis was present in the left eye (see Figures 12.49 and 12.50).*

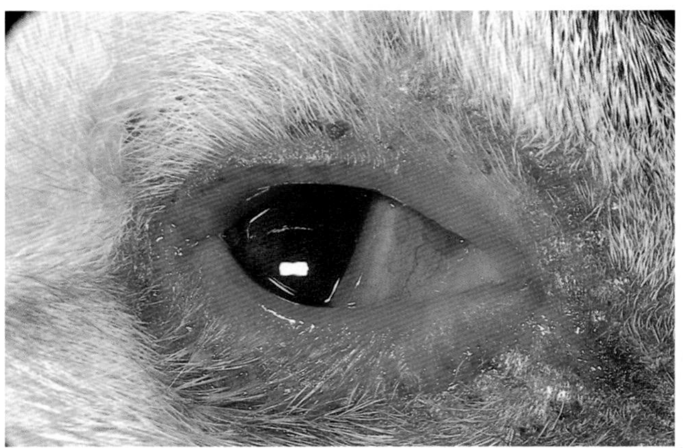

Fig. 5.23 *Bacterial blepharoconjunctivitis (bilateral) in a 9-month-old Siamese cat. The bacterial infection (Staphylococcus spp) may have been a complication of self mutilation.*

of the eyelid margins and ulceration may develop. Treatment includes warm water bathing to remove the exudate, followed by application of an emollient ophthalmic ointment. Systemic therapy with an appropriate broad-spectrum antibiotic (based on the results of culture and sensitivity testing) may need to be supplemented with oral corticosteroids when self-mutilation is a problem.

Mycobacterial diseases (classical tuberculosis, feline leprosy and atypical mycobacteriosis) are uncommon, but may present with cutaneous lesions such as swollen eyelids, together with regional lymphadenopathy (Gunn-Moore *et al.*, 1996).

Immune-mediated

Pemphigus foliaceus (periocular hyperkeratosis, crusting and alopecia) and pemphigus erythematosus (periocular erythematous macular dermatitis and excoriation) are very uncommon problems (Fig. 5.24). For both these conditions the nose, muzzle and pinnae are involved in addition to the periocular region. Biopsy is indicated to confirm the diagnosis and to rule out other possibilities. Systemic lupus erythematosus (periocular vesicles and papules) and drug eruptions to systemically administered drugs (pleiomorphic appearance) are rare immune-mediated problems in the cat.

Allergic

Allergies are rare in cats (Fig 5.25). Topical drugs (e.g. tetracycline, neomycin, antiviral agents and atropine) may be involved. Drug-related forms are usually relatively easy to diagnose, because the eyelid hyperaemia and erythema which typify the problem regress as soon as the drug is stopped; however, although rare, permanent depigmentation of the eyelid has been associated with topical tetracycline.

Food allergies are uncommon and may be associated with severe erythema and intense pruritis complicated by self-mutilation, but the cause of this type of blepharitis some-

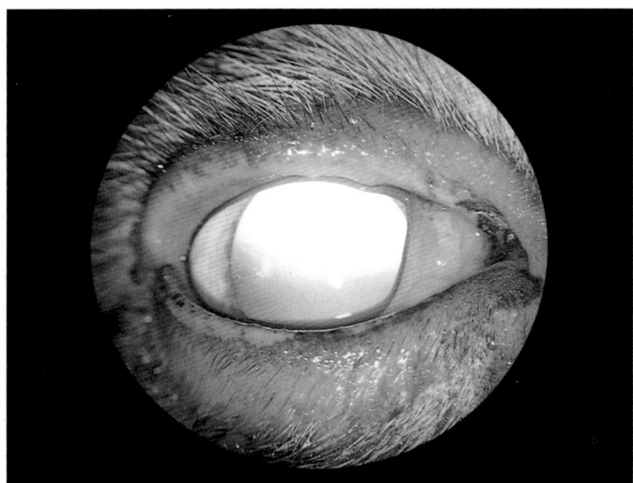

Fig. 5.24 *Pemphigus foliaceus (bilateral) in an 8-year-old Domestic shorthair.*

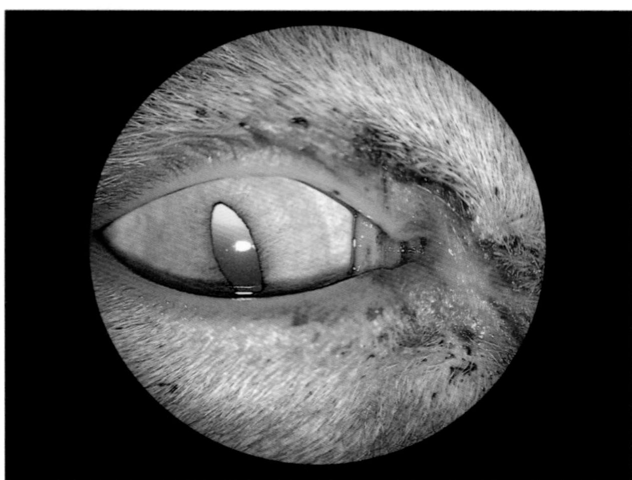

Fig. 5.25 *Allergic blepharitis (unilateral) apparently related to the use of topical tetracycline. The hyperaemia and discharge resolved within a few days of treatment being withdrawn.*

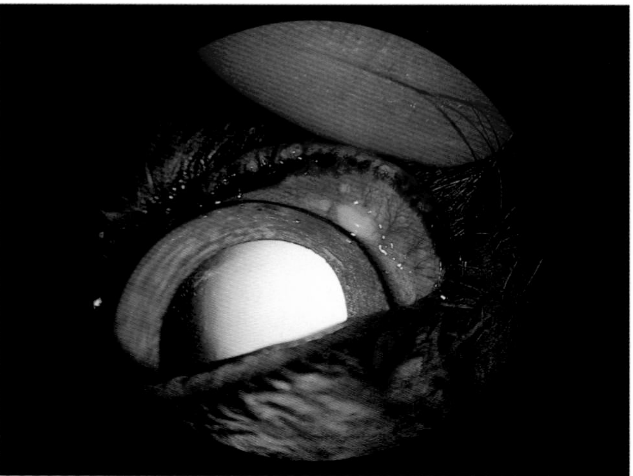

Fig. 5.26 *In this 5-year-old Persian crossbred, many of the meibomian gland openings are swollen and there are also focal swellings in the glands themselves. These changes are typical of meibomianitis. Both eyes were affected, the left eye is illustrated.*

times cannot be determined. Exclusion diets could be attempted in cats with suspected food allergies, but early referral to a dermatologist may be the best option.

Other dermatoses

Meibomianitis is occasionally encountered. Affected cats usually present with moderate ocular discomfort and an increased blink rate. Examination of the eyelid margin and the meibomian glands confirms the origin of the problem (Fig 5.26). In chronic cases lipid granulomas may develop in the meibomian glands and, as such, may be designated chalazia (Fig. 5.27). The underlying pathogenesis is obscure; however, the inspissated meibomian gland lipid of chalazia is

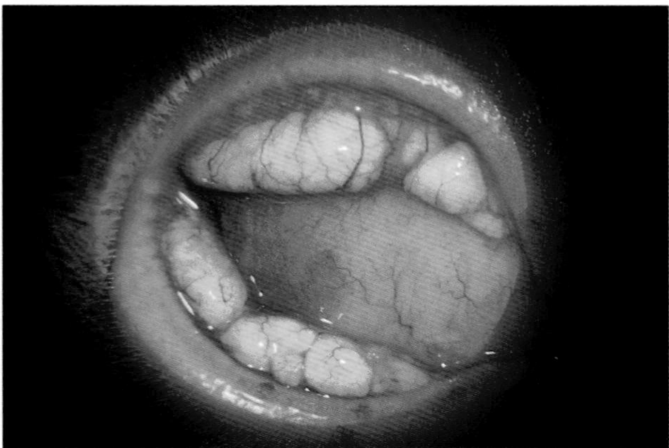

Fig. 5.27 *Chalazia affecting the upper and lower eyelids of both eyes in a 9-year-old Burmese. Note the secondary corneal pathology. The right eye is illustrated.*

of different origin from the lipid of xanthomas and the descriptions of xanthoma/xanthelasma are incorrect for such swellings at this site. Chalazia form firm, often caseous, swellings beneath the palpebral conjunctiva. When they become a source of chronic ocular discomfort the abnormal material should be removed by curettage via a conjunctival approach.

Creamy-white deposits and plaques can be associated with blepharitis in cats. These lesions are usually part of the presentation of proliferative (eosinophilic) keratoconjunctivitis (see Chapter 9). Eyelid cysts are encountered occasionally in Persian cats.

Xanthomatous plaques (see Chapter 9) are occasionally found in cats and are always associated with hyperlipoproteinaemia. They may be found anywhere on the body, including the periocular region.

Neoplasia

In cats, eyelid tumours are less common but more malignant than those of dogs. McLaughlin *et al.* (1993) have reviewed demograph data in relation to eyelid neoplasia. In most parts of the world squamous cell carcinoma is the most frequently encountered eyelid neoplasm, especially in white cats, those with white periocular fur, or those with nonpigmented eyelids (Figs 5.28–5.31). These tumours are of epidermal origin; they are invasive and potentially malignant (they initially spread to local lymph nodes and can metastasize to more distant sites), so careful examination of the whole animal is mandatory (see Fig. 4.26). Initially, there may be simply hyperaemia with a mild ocular discharge, but more characteristically they erode the eyelid margins producing nonhealing, red, eroded areas. The diagnosis should be confirmed by needle biopsy or excisional biopsy. Impression smears can be used to confirm the diagnosis, but the histological interpretation is more difficult.

A number of treatment regimes are available for the treatment of squamous cell carcinoma (SCC); for example

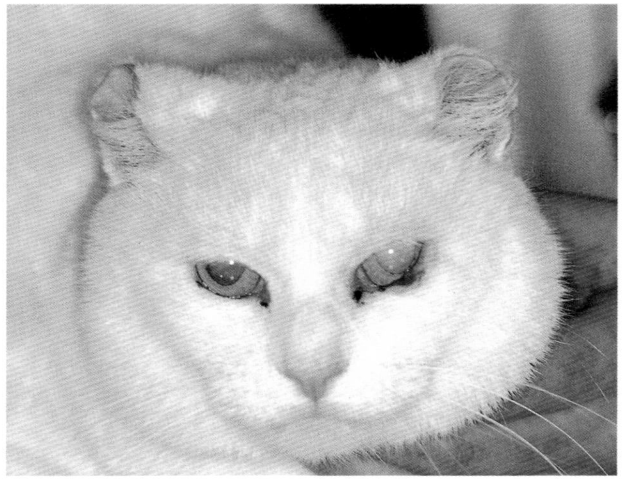

Fig. 5.28 *Squamous cell carcinoma affecting the lower eyelid of the left eye in a 7-year-old white Domestic shorthair. Note that there is also an early erosive lesion of the right lower eyelid and that both the ear tips have already been removed because of squamous cell carcinoma.*

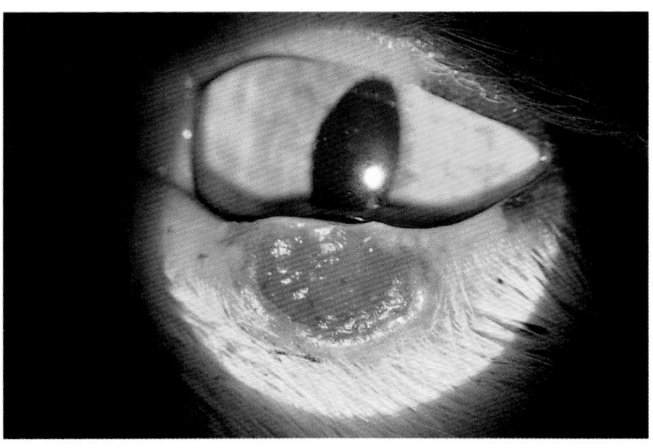

Fig. 5.29 *Squamous cell carcinoma of the lower eyelid in a 12-year-old black and white Domestic shorthair. The ulcer is eroding the eyelid, but is well circumscribed.*

cryotherapy may be used with and without wide-based surgical excision, although the excisional approach is best restricted to small lesions because of the complex nature of the blepharoplastic procedures which may be needed after surgery. SCC is also radiosensitive (e.g. β-irradiation from a strontium-90 applicator) and this method and laser therapy both give good results, often without the necessity for surgical excision. Hyperthermic techniques are also effective, but not generally available.

Blepharoplasty may be required when tumours are extensive; most can be simply performed by using a releasing incision technique at the lateral canthus, more complex techniques are needed when the tumour is extensive. The aims of surgery should always be to retain or restore the eyelid margins so that trichiasis with secondary keratitis do not produce long-term complications.

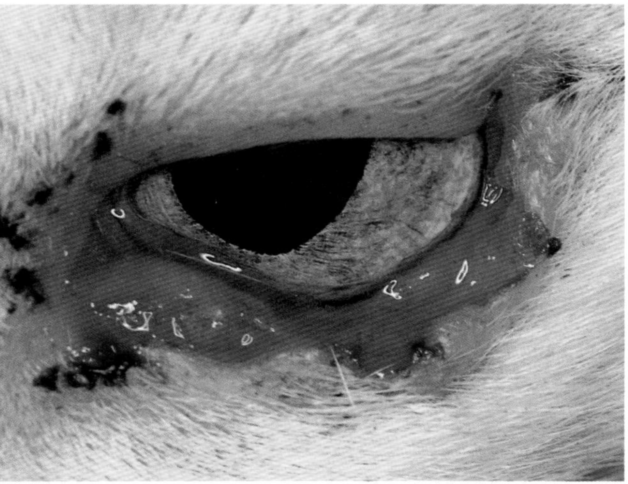

Fig. 5.30 *Domestic shorthair, 10 years old. More extensive squamous cell carcinoma affecting the whole of the lower eyelid in a white cat; there is no recognizable eyelid margin.*

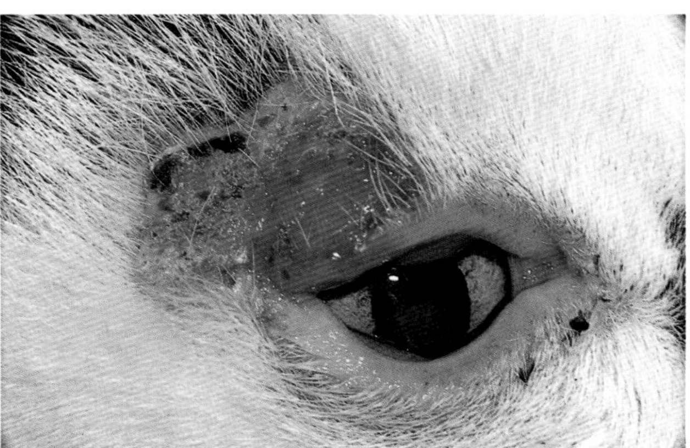

Fig. 5.31 *Squamous cell carcinoma affecting the upper eyelid in a 4-year-old white cat. Note the corneal oedema because of the thickened eyelid producing mechanical irritation. Both ear tips had also been removed because of squamous cell carcinoma.*

Other types of eyelid tumour are encountered; they include basal cell carcinoma, mast cell tumour (Fig. 5.32) and fibrosarcoma (Fig. 5.33) and, less commonly, papilloma, adenoma, adenocarcinoma, fibroma, neurofibroma, neurofibrosarcoma, melanoma, haemangioma, haemangiosarcoma and undifferentiated carcinoma (Williams *et al.*, 1981; Patnaik and Mooney, 1988). It is prudent to regard most feline eyelid tumours as potentially malignant, so histopathology is always indicated as a guide to management. Full-thickness wedge excision using an extended pentagon configuration or more complex blepharoplastic techniques (Peiffer *et al.*, 1987b: Collin, 1989; Mustardé, 1991; Gelatt and Gelatt, 1994) will be indicated, according to the extent of eyelid involvement.

Generalized neoplasia with eyelid involvement is rare; examples include lymphosarcoma and metastatic carcinoma (Fig 5.34) in cats of any age, whereas viral feline sarcoma is

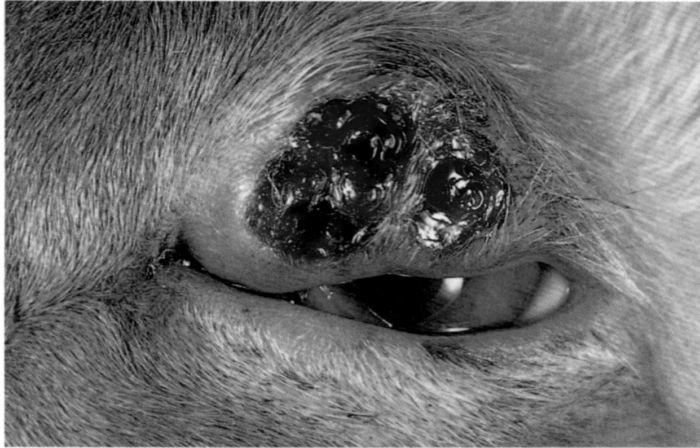

Fig. 5.32 *Mast cell tumour affecting the upper eyelid of a Domestic shorthair (courtesy of R. G. Jones).*

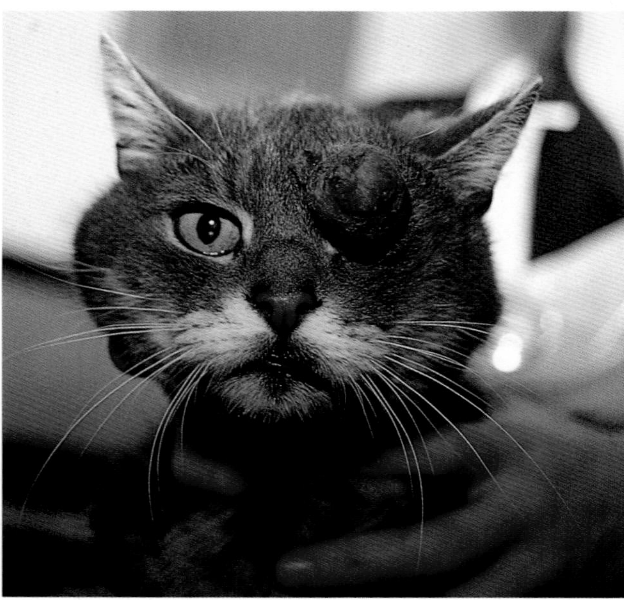

Fig. 5.33 *Fibrosarcoma of the upper eyelid in a Domestic shorthair (courtesy of R. Pontefract).*

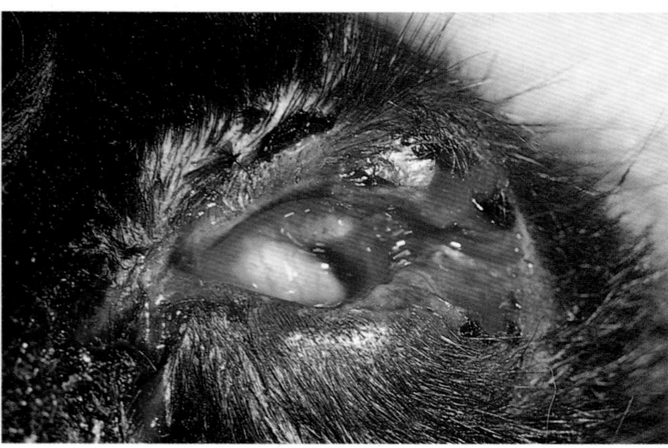

Fig. 5.34 *Metastatic mammary adenocarcinoma affecting the eyelids of a 14-year-old Domestic shorthair.*

a potential cause in young cats. In all such cases the prognosis is poor to grave.

REFERENCES

Barnett KC (1981) Ocular colobomata in the snow leopard *Panthera uncia*. *Journal of the Jersey Wildlife Preservation Trust* **18**: 83–85.

Bellhorn RW, Barnett KC, Henkind P (1971) Ocular colobomas in domestic cats. *Journal of the American Veterinary Medical Association* **159**: 1015–1021.

Bennett M, Gaskell CJ, Baxby D, Gaskell RM, Kelly DF, Naidoo J (1990) Feline cowpox virus infection. *Journal of Small Animal Practice* **31**: 167–173.

Collin JRO (1989) *A Manual of Systematic Eyelid Surgery*, 2nd edn. Churchill Livingstone, Edinburgh.

Dziezyc J, Millichamp NJ (1989) Surgical correction of eyelid agenesis in a cat. *Journal of the American Animal Hospital Association* **25**: 514–516.

Gelatt KN, Gelatt JP (1994) *Small Animal Ophthalmic Surgery, Vol. 1: Extraocular Procedures*. Pergamon, Oxford.

Gripenberg U, Blomqvist L, Pamillo P, *et al.* (1985) Multiple ocular coloboma in Snow Leopards *(Panthera uncia)*: clinical report, pedigree analysis, chromosome investigations and serum protein studies. *Hereditas* **103**: 221–229.

Gunn-Moore DA, Jenkins PA, Lucke VM (1996) Feline tuberculosis: A literature review and discussion of 19 cases caused by an unusual mycobacterial variant. *Veterinary Record* **138**: 53–58.

Hacker DV (1989) Ectopic cilia in a Siamese cat. *Companion Animal Practice* **19**: 29–31.

Hendy Ibbs PN (1985) Familial feline epibulbar dermoids. *Veterinary Record* **116**: 13–14.

Koch SA (1979) Congenital ophthalmic abnormalities in the Burmese cat. *Journal of the American Veterinary Medical Association* **174**: 90–91.

Martin CL, Stiles J, Willis M (1997) Feline colobomatous syndrome. *Veterinary and Comparative Ophthalmology* **7**: 39–43.

McLaughlin SA, Whitley RD, Gilger BC, Wright JC, Lindley DM (1993) Eyelid neoplasia in cats: A review of demographic data (1979–1989). *Journal of the American Animal Hospital Association* **29**: 63–67.

Mustardé JC (ed.) (1991) *Repair and Reconstruction in the Orbital Region*, 3rd edn. Churchill Livingstone, Edinburgh.

Patnaik AK, Mooney S (1988) Feline melanoma: A comparative study of ocular, oral and dermal neoplasms. *Veterinary Pathology* **25**: 105–112.

Peiffer RL, Nasisse MP, Cook CS, Harling DE (1987a) Surgery of the canine and feline orbit, adnexa and globe. Part 2: Congenital abnormalities of the eyelid and cilial abnormalities. *Companion Animal Practice* August: 27–37.

Peiffer RL, Nasisse MP, Cook CS, Harling DE (1987b) Surgery of the canine and feline orbit, adnexa and globe. Part 3: Other structural abnormalities and neoplasia of the eyelid. *Companion Animal Practice* September: 20–36.

Stades FC, Boeve MH, van der Woerdt A (1992) Palpebral fissure length in the dog and cat. *Progress in Veterinary and Comparative Ophthalmology* **2**: 155–161.

Wahlberg C (1978) A case of multiple ocular coloboma in the snow leopard. *International Pedigree Book of Snow Leopards* **1**: 108–112.

Williams LW, Gelatt KN, Gwinn RM (1981) Ophthalmic neoplasms in the cat. *Journal of the American Animal Hospital Association* **17**: 999–1008.

6 Third eyelid

Introduction

The third eyelid (synonyms are membrana nictitans, nictitating membrane; known colloquially as haw) is unobtrusive in the normal cat, particularly if the leading edge is unpigmented (Fig. 6.1). It consists of a semilunar fold of conjunctiva supported by a T-shaped piece of elastic cartilage curved to conform to the shape of the underlying globe. The nictitans gland which provides part of the aqueous portion of the pre-ocular tear film (ptf) surrounds the base of the cartilage (Fig. 6.2). Aggregates of lymphoid tissue are present on both the inner and outer aspects of the third eyelid.

In addition to supplying a portion of the ptf, the third eyelid functions to spread the tear film and protect the eye. The third eyelid sweeps across the cornea from ventromedial to dorsolateral to distribute the tear film. The cat is unique among the common domestic animals in possessing a mechanism for active protrusion of the third eyelid and the passive protective mechanism which comes into play when the globe is retracted by the retractor oculi muscles (innervated by the abducens nerve: CN VI). Active protrusion is effected by striated muscle fibres from the levator palpebrae superioris and lateral rectus muscle which attach to the third eyelid and these striated muscle fibres are also supplied by the abducens nerve. Sympathetic nerve fibres innervate the smooth muscle which is responsible for maintaining tonic retraction.

The third eyelid is a most important structure and should be preserved whenever possible. In practice this means that it is only removed when it is neoplastic and never when just traumatized or inflamed.

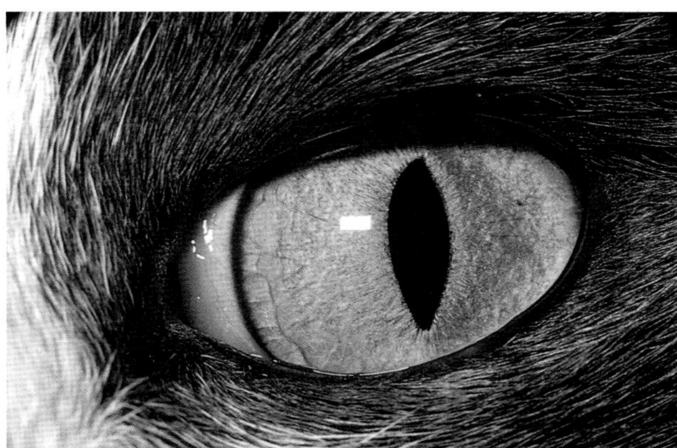

Fig. 6.1 *Left eye of a normal adult Domestic shorthair with a nonpigmented third eyelid.*

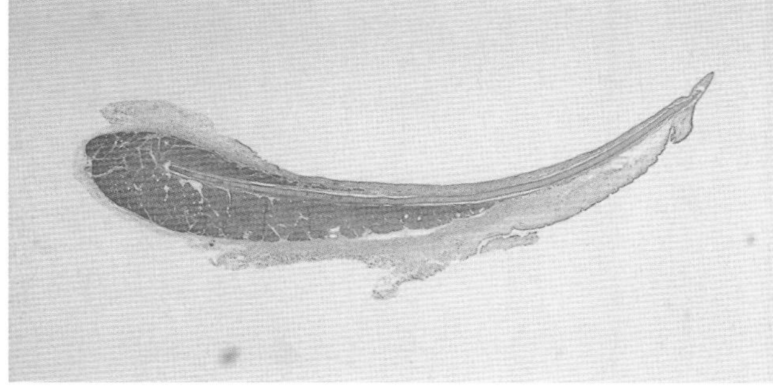

Fig. 6.2 *Histological section of the third eyelid (haematoxylin and eosin). The well-developed nictitans gland (dark staining) envelops the base of the supporting cartilage. Aggregates of lymphoid tissue are present in the conjunctiva which covers both the inner and outer surfaces.*

Disorders of the third eyelid

Protrusion of the third eyelid

Protrusion of the third eyelid is not unusual in this species (Nuyttens and Simoens, 1994) and is often associated with generalized problems, in which case the prominence is likely to be bilateral. The cause is not always apparent (Figs 6.3 and 6.4). There are a number of other conditions which may be associated with either unilateral or bilateral protrusion.

Interestingly, debility, weight loss and reduction in the amount of retrobulbar fat do not appear to be associated with third eyelid prominence in the cat as they are in the dog.

Generalized conditions associated with bilateral protrusion

Dysautonomia (see Chapter 15) may be associated with bilateral third eyelid protrusion, and may even be the presenting sign (Fig. 6.5), although absence of the pupillary light response with dilated pupils and normal vision is the most constant ocular feature (see Chapter 15).

Chronic diarrhoea is sometimes associated with a self-limiting, bilateral, third eyelid protrusion (Fig. 6.6), particularly affecting young cats (Muir *et al.*, 1990). Occasionally, it

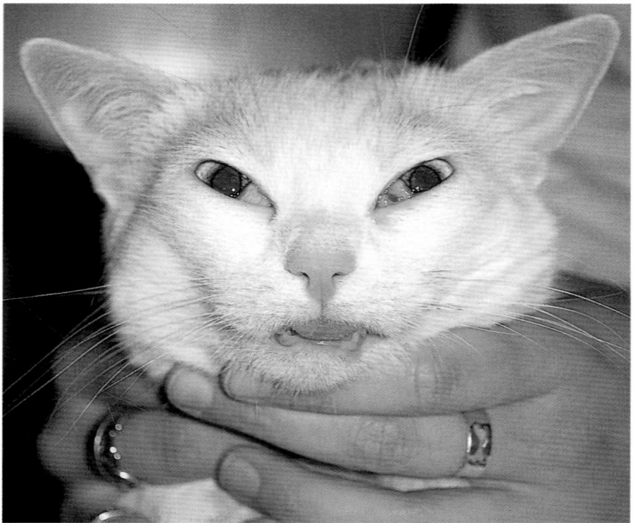

***Fig. 6.3** Domestic shorthair. Swelling of the head which developed within 6 h of endoscopy under general anaesthesia. Both eyes became progressively exophthalmic and the third eyelids more prominent, fundus examination indicated mild papilloedema and it was impossible to retropulse the globes into the orbit. There was also slight drooping of the jaw. Ultrasound examination of the eye and orbit supported the tentative diagnosis of orbital oedema. The cat was treated with systemic corticosteroids and diuretics.*

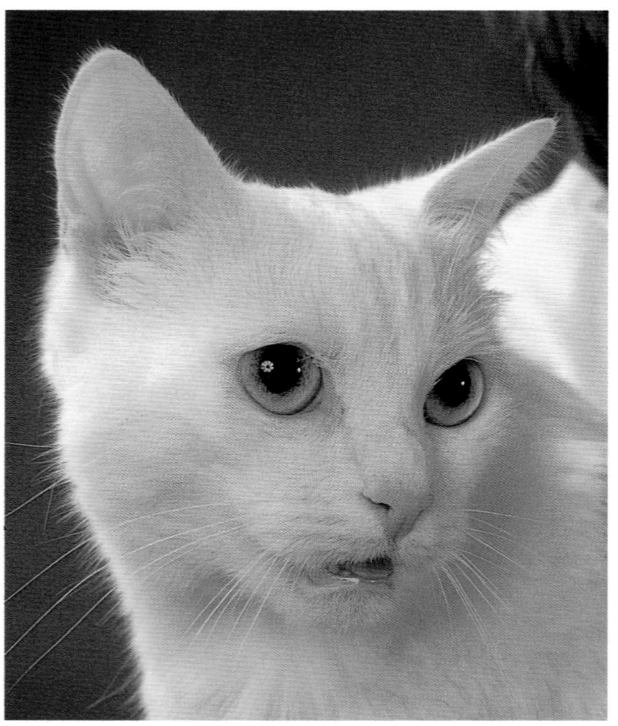

***Fig. 6.4** The same cat shown in Fig. 6.3 the following day. The ocular and orbital abnormalities have completely resolved and only the mild neuropraxia of the jaw remains, this resolved over the course of a few days.*

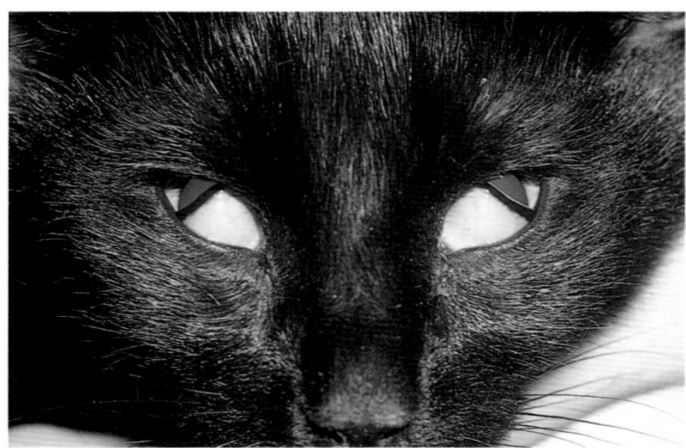

***Fig. 6.5** Bilateral third eyelid prominence and dilated pupils in a young adult cat with dysautonomia.*

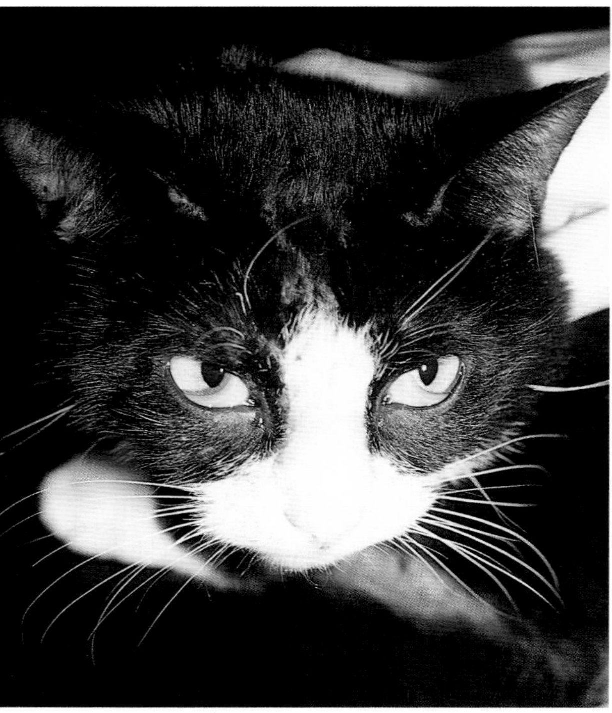

***Fig. 6.6** Bilateral third eyelid prominence associated with chronic diarrhoea.*

may have a protracted time course, but the cat is otherwise well and no treatment is required. The cause is unknown but an infectious agent (possibly a virus) is suspected. Topical administration of a sympathomimetic drug such as 10% phenylephrine produces retraction of the third eyelids within minutes, suggesting that postganglionic sympathetic denervation is part of the problem.

Tetanus may produce varying degrees of third eyelid protrusion (see Chapter 15). Drug-induced protrusion is a common, but temporary finding, after administration of, for example, phenothiazine tranquillizers.

Other causes of third eyelid protrusion

Microphthalmos (see Chapter 4), either bilateral or unilateral, is associated with protrusion of the third eyelid. *Phthisis bulbi* (see Chapter 4) is usually unilateral and is accompanied by protrusion of the third eyelid on the affected side.

Anterior segment pain produces globe retraction and consequent protrusion of the third eyelid, blepharospasm may obscure the underlying structures (Fig. 6.7). The condition may be unilateral or bilateral.

Symblepharon formation is a common reason for persistent protrusion of the third eyelid (Fig. 6.8) and may be unilateral or bilateral (see Chapter 8).

Third eyelid neoplasias (Fig. 6.9) whether primary tumours, which are rare (e.g. squamous cell carcinoma, fibrosarcoma, adenocarcinoma), or secondary tumours (e.g. squamous cell carcinoma, lymphosarcoma), which are uncommon, are causes of third eyelid protrusion (see below). They are usually unilateral when primary neoplasia is involved and may be unilateral or bilateral with secondary neoplasia.

Retrobulbar space-occupying lesions (Fig. 6.10 and see Chapter 4), because of inflammation or neoplasia are frequently associated with unilateral third eyelid protrusion and with exophthalmos. Strabismus may be present and the direction of the squint can provide helpful clues as to the site of the tumour (see Chapter 4).

Horner's syndrome has a variety of causes (see Chapter 15), although the fundamental abnormality is sympathetic denervation of the eye and adnexa (Kern *et al.*, 1989). The clinical presentation is of third eyelid protrusion, miosis, enophthalmos, ptosis and narrowing of the palpebral fissure. Most cases are unilateral.

Prolapse of the nictitans gland (Fig. 6.11) is a very uncommon condition in the cat which can give the spurious impression of a protruded third eyelid. It may occur in isolation, or in association with kinking of the third eyelid cartilage.

Conjunctival inflammation (Figs 6.12 and 6.13) may be associated with third eyelid prominence, usually in conjunction with generalized conjunctival involvement, but sometimes

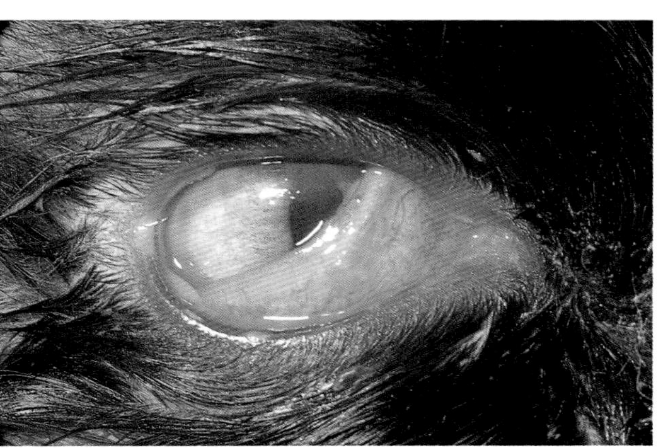

Fig. 6.7 *Unilateral third eyelid prominence associated with anterior segment pain (ulcerative keratitis).*

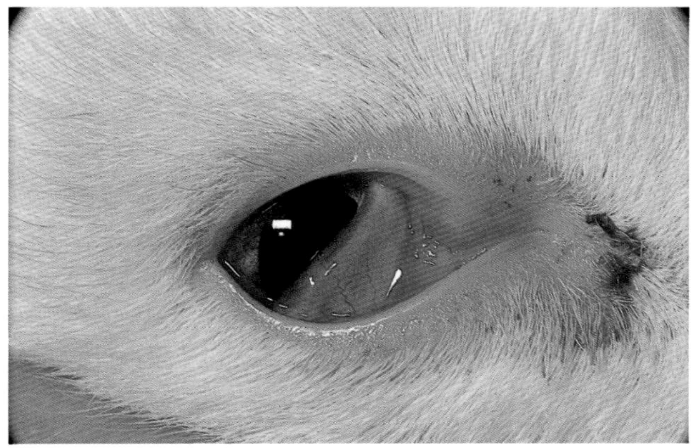

Fig. 6.9 *A neutered female, 7-year-old, Domestic shorthair. Unilateral third eyelid prominence associated with primary neoplasia at the base of the third eyelid.*

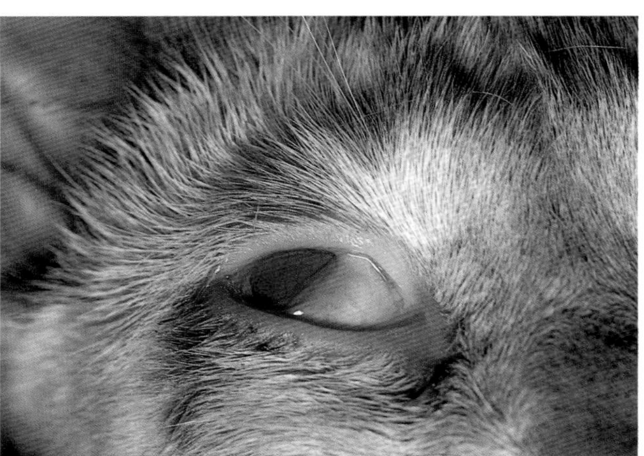

Fig. 6.8 *Unilateral third eyelid prominence associated with symblepharon. The third eyelid is adherent to the palpebral conjunctiva.*

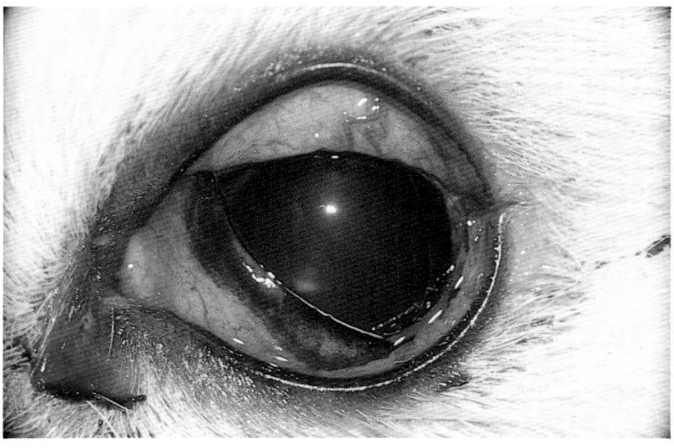

Fig. 6.10 *A neutered male, 7-year-old, Domestic shorthair. Third eyelid prominence associated with an intraorbital neoplasm. There is also conjunctival oedema (chemosis), congestion of visible vessels and a dilated, unresponsive pupil.*

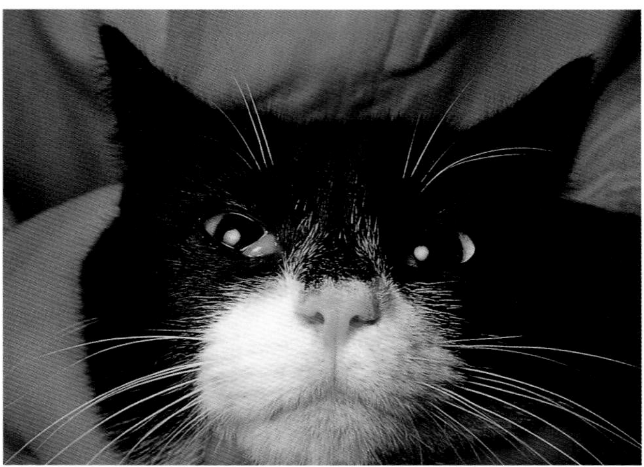

Fig. 6.11 Prolapse of the nictitans gland in a young cat, creating a spurious impression of third eyelid prominence on the right side.

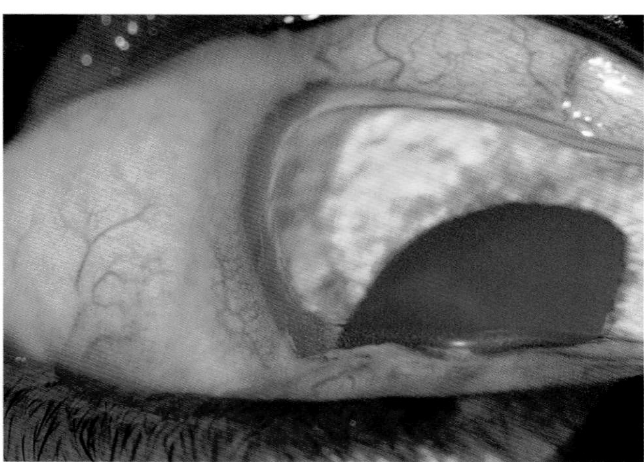

Fig. 6.12 An 11-year-old, Domestic shorthair. Prominence of the third eyelid (and also palpebral conjunctiva) as a consequence of oedema associated with conjunctivitis.

with involvement of the third eyelid alone and, very rarely, as a focal inflammation of the caruncle. Acute inflammation is typified by chemosis, chronic inflammation by gross thickening.

Trauma can damage the third eyelid (see Chapter 3), or the third eyelid may be prominent as a consequence of a head injury (see Chapter 15).

Symblepharon

See Chapter 8.

Eversion (kinking) of the third eyelid cartilage

This is a rare feline disorder, which may be a consequence of poor fascial attachments between the cartilage and deep orbital fascia. It is usually associated with concomitant pro-

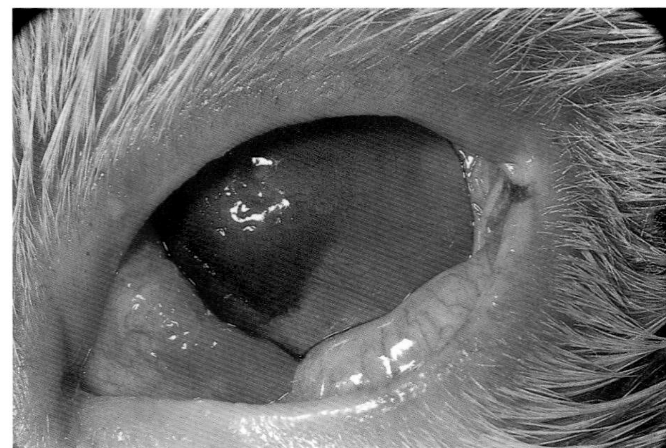

Fig. 6.13 Chronic conjunctival inflammation with gross thickening of the third eyelid in an adult Domestic short hair. The corneal erosion and chronic keratitis are a consequence both of the mechanical trauma from the thickened eyelids and the compromised eyelid function.

lapse of the nictitans gland. Of the two cases described in Burmese cats (Albert *et al.*, 1982), it was possible in one to relocate the gland by a surgical tie-down technique and this procedure straightened the everted cartilage; in the other it was necessary to incise the cartilage to straighten it. In both cases the nictitans gland was preserved but the third eyelid was immobilized.

Foreign bodies

See Chapter 3.

Neoplasia

Third eyelid neoplasia is rare (Fig. 6.9). Fibrosarcoma (Buyukmichi, 1975), squamous cell carcinoma, mast cell tumour and lymphosarcoma are the most likely tumours to be encountered (Williams *et al.*, 1981). Whereas fibrosarcoma is a primary tumour of the third eyelid, squamous cell carcinoma could have originated in the third eyelid, or extended there from neighbouring tissues. Mast cell tumours may extend from the upper or lower eyelids to involve the third eyelid.

Secondary tumours such as undifferentiated carcinomas and generalized lymphosarcoma may involve the third eyelid.

Chronic inflammation of the third eyelid (see below) should be differentiated from neoplasia by fine needle aspiration. Surgical excision is indicated for well circumscribed isolated tumours and, on occasion, the whole of the third eyelid may need to be removed. It is important to emphasize that this is the only indication for third eyelid removal. Absence of the third eyelid (Figs 6.14–6.16) may seriously compromise eyelid function in the cat.

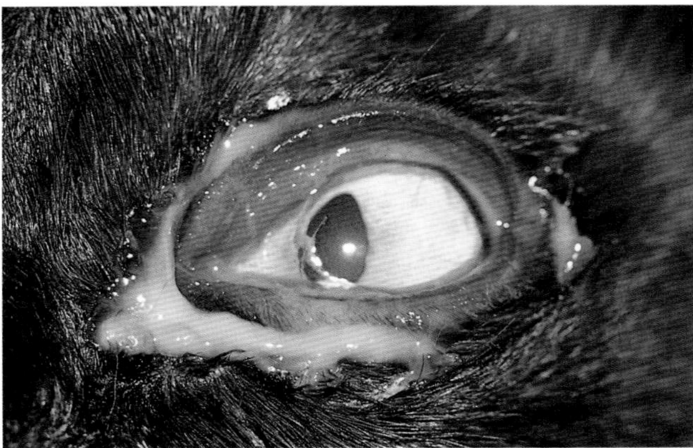

Fig. 6.14 *The third eyelid of this young cat had been removed for reasons unknown 1 year before. Note the intense conjunctival changes and prominent mucopurulent discharge.*

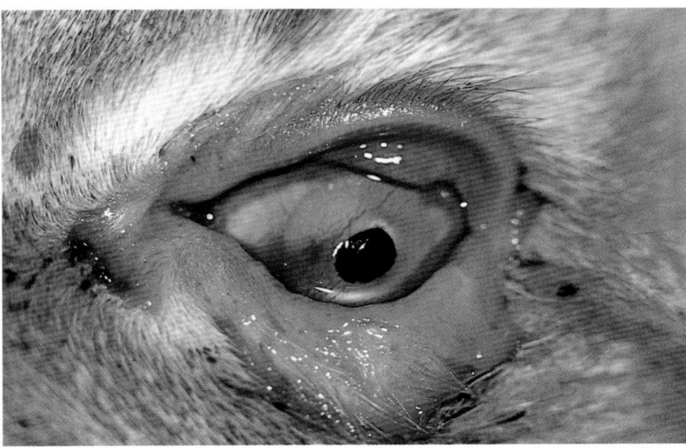

Fig. 6.15 *In this adult cat a sequestrum formed after third eyelid removal. The reasons for removal of the third eyelid were unknown.*

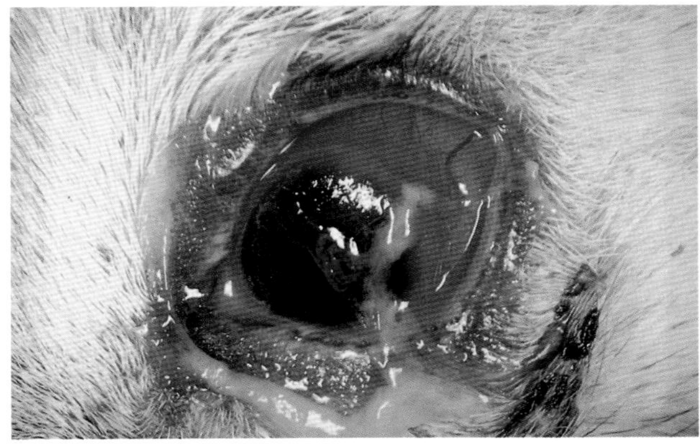

Fig. 6.16 *A 1-year-old, Persian crossbred, in which the third eyelid has been removed. The changes in this eye were so severe that the eye was subsequently removed. (Courtesy of J. R. B. Mould).*

THIRD EYELID FLAP

A third eyelid flap provides protection and support for corneal healing (Figs 6.17 and 6.18). Topical solutions can be administered with the flap in place and it is usual to leave the flap in place for a minimum of 10 days. Third eyelid

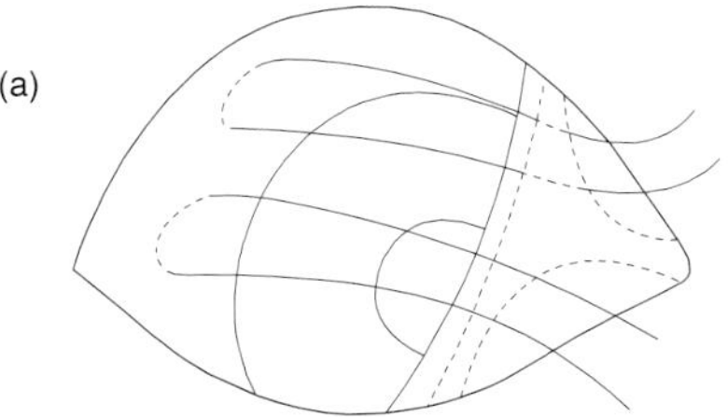

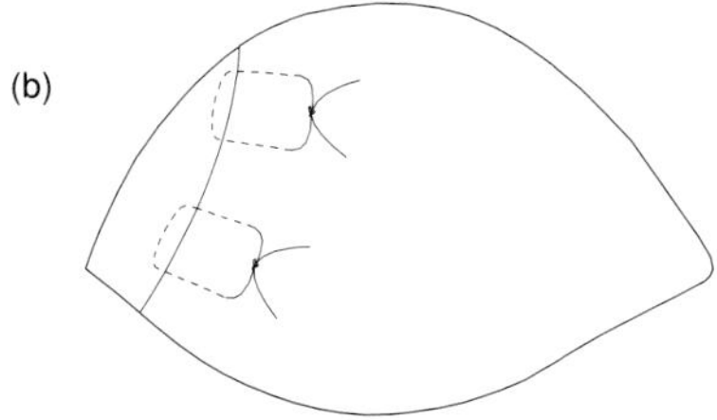

Fig. 6.17 *Third eyelid flap.*
(a) Two horizontal mattress sutures are laid as illustrated, avoiding the free border of the third eyelid. The inner surface of the third eyelid should be checked to ensure that the sutures have not penetrated the entire thickness of the third eyelid before the sutures are tied.
(b) the third eyelid has been sutured to the bulbar conjunctiva and underlying Tenon's capsule close to the limbus. The flap should be left in place for a minimum of ten days and the sutures can be removed after topical application of local anaesthetic.

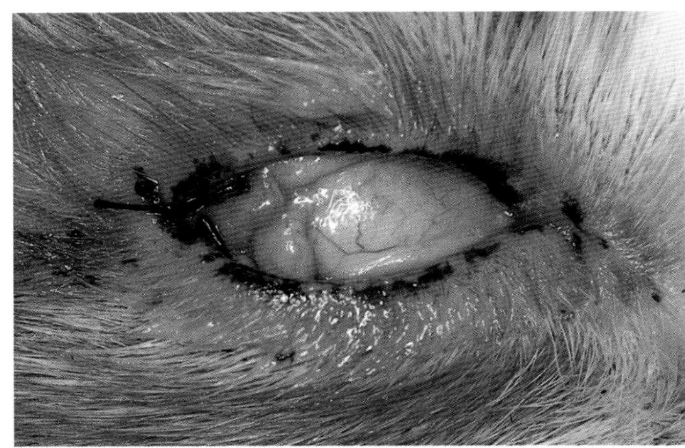

Fig. 6.18 *Right eye, third eyelid flap which has been secured to the bulbar conjunctiva and Tenon's capsule.*

flaps have, to some extent, been replaced by therapeutic soft contact lenses and pedicle grafts, which both offer the advantage of easier monitoring of the healing process by direct visualization. Healing will also be more rapid with a pedicle graft rather than a third eyelid flap.

References

Albert RA, Garrett PD, Whitley RD (1982) Surgical correction of everted third eyelid in two cats. *Journal of the American Veterinary Medical Association* **180**: 763–766.

Buyukmichi N (1975) Fibrosarcoma of the nictitating membrane in a cat. *Journal of the American Veterinary Medical Association* **167**: 934–935.

Kern TJ, Aramondo MC, Erb HN (1989) Horner's syndrome in cats and dogs: 100 cases (1975–1985). *Journal of the American Veterinary Medical Association* **195**: 369–373.

Muir P, Harbour DA, Gruffydd-Jones TJ, Howard PE, Hopper CD, Gruffydd-Jones EAD, Broadhead HM, Clarke CM, Jones ME (1990) A clinical and microbiological study of cats with protruding nictitating membrane and diarrhoea: isolation of a novel virus. *Veterinary Record* **127**: 324–330.

Nuyttens J, Simoens P (1994) Protrusion of the third eyelid in cats. *Vlaams Diergeneeskundig Tijdschrift* **63**: 80–86.

Williams LW, Gelatt KN, Gwinn RM (1981) Ophthalmic neoplasms in the cat. *Journal of the American Animal Hospital Association* **17**: 999–1008.

7 Lacrimal system

Introduction

The lacrimal system or lacrimal apparatus (Poels and Simoens, 1994) consists of two components, a secretory component and an excretory component. The secretory component produces the pre-ocular tear film (ptf), a trilaminar structure 7 μm thick (Carrington *et al.*, 1987) which consists of lipid produced by the meibomian (tarsal) glands; aqueous, produced by the lacrimal and nictitans glands; and mucin, which is produced by the conjunctival goblet cells. The lipid tear film prevents undue evaporation of the middle aqueous portion and contributes to the stability of the tear film as does the adsorptive capacity of the thick mucin component.

The tear film covers the ocular surface and is distributed partly by blinking of the upper and lower eyelids and mainly by third eyelid movement combined with globe retraction. Some loss of tears occurs because of evaporation and some from drainage into the excretory component of the lacrimal system. The excretory portion of the lacrimal system consists of upper and lower puncta and their respective canaliculi which conjoin at the rudimentary lacrimal sac and continue as the nasolacrimal duct. The nasolacrimal duct passes into the lacrimal bone via the lacrimal foramen, passes along the medial surface of the maxilla and exits in the vestibule of the nasal cavity beneath the ventral concha.

The openings of the upper and lower puncta are located just inside the eyelids close to the medial canthus and can be examined by slightly everting the eyelid margins in this region; the tissue in their immediate vicinity is usually unpigmented. Tears pass into the drainage system by a process of gravity feed, capillary attraction and the pumping effect of orbicularis oculi muscle contraction during blinking.

Investigation

Investigations of the lacrimal apparatus consist of the assessment of production, distribution and drainage of the pre-ocular tear film and careful inspection of the ocular surface. Some of the techniques used are described in Chapter 1.

Production

In all cases in which abnormal production is suspected it is important to observe the eye carefully (Fig. 7.1), to assess the blink rate, to note the appearance of the ocular surface and associated pre-ocular tear film, to check that the eyelid margins and meibomian gland openings are normal and to try and make some assessment of tear film quality and quantity. Pre-ocular tear film dysfunction of any one component (lipid, aqueous, mucin) may adversely affect the other components (Johnson *et al.*, 1990).

There are no accurate means of assessing the quality and quantity of the lipid contribution from the meibomian glands in cats. In cats with congenitally defective eyelid development (see Chapter 5) meibomian gland openings may be poorly defined, even absent, in the abnormal region. Meibomianitis (see Chapter 5) is not uncommon and inspection of the meibomian gland openings should be routine because it is likely that both acute and chronic inflammatory problems will have some effect on the meibomian gland lipids and thus on the tear film itself.

In clinical practice it is the aqueous component of the ptf which is assessed most frequently by means of a Schirmer I (STT I) or Schirmer II (STT II) tear test. Mean readings obtained in the normal cat are not as high as those recorded for normal dogs (see Chapter 1) but, with the exception of cats less than 12 months old, a reading of at least 8 mm/min should be obtained.

Abnormal production of mucin is recognized less frequently in cats than dogs and there has been no critical evaluation of tests which attempt to establish tear film

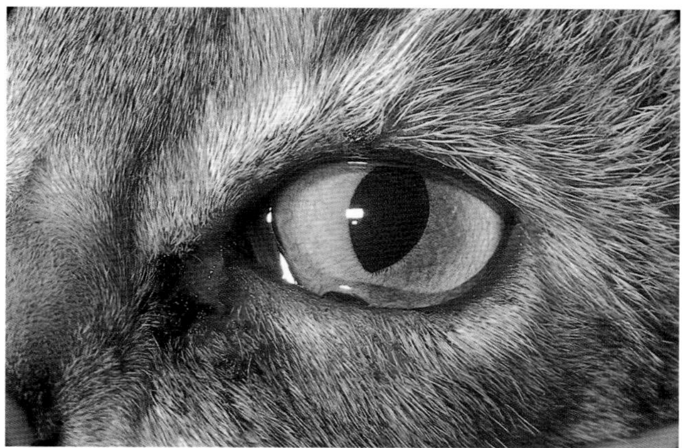

Fig. 7.1 *An 11-month-old Abyssinian cat with acquired obstruction of the nasolacrimal duct to show the prominent meniscus of the lacrimal lake.*

stability or aim to assess the nature and quantity of the mucin component.

Distribution

Because anatomical eyelid abnormalities are less frequent in cats than dogs, there are fewer ptf distribution problems in most breeds of cat. The exception is any type of flat-faced cat, especially some Persians (Fig. 7.2), in which the eyelids are closely apposed to the eye so that the lacrimal lake is shallow. If there is also a tendency to entropion and a wick effect from hairs at the medial canthus, poor distribution and drainage of the tear film results and epiphora is the obvious presenting sign. No specific investigative procedures other than careful observation are required to make the diagnosis.

Drainage

Drainage problems are investigated as described in Chapter 1. The protocol adopted is to start with visual inspection, then measurement of tear production, followed by collection of samples, if they are indicated. The patency of the system can be assessed somewhat imperfectly with fluorescein dye, allowing adequate time between application to each side to avoid confusing results.

If there is doubt about patency of the system it is logical to proceed next to cannulation of the upper punctum and canaliculus as a means of investigating the entire drainage system. When it is impossible to irrigate the system via the upper or lower punctum then dacryocystorhinography can be performed, or the examiner may decide to try and pass a very fine catheter through the entire system; either technique will indicate the site of obstruction and both techniques are usually attempted via the upper punctum and canaliculus.

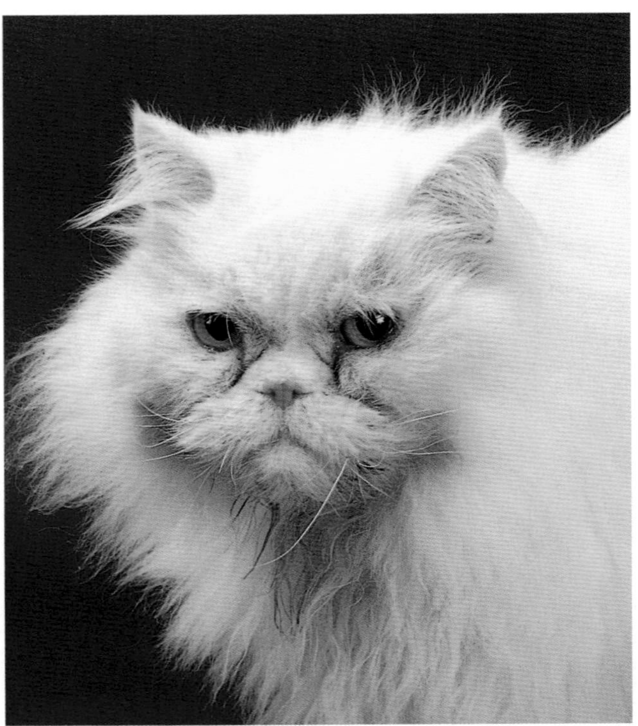

Fig. 7.2 *A young adult Persian cat showing typical facial appearance and mild epiphora.*

Diseases of the Lacrimal System

Diseases of the lacrimal system may be a consequence of abnormal production (secretory component) or inadequate drainage (excretory component), inflammation and neoplasia (may affect both components).

Tear production

Paradoxical Lacrimation

There is a single case report of this phenomenon in the cat (Hacker, 1990). Excessive lacrimation from one eye ('crocodile tears') was associated with eating; no cause was established.

Keratoconjunctivitis Sicca

Dry-eye syndromes (Figs. 7.3–7.8) are far less common in cats than dogs and the aetiology is not always easy to determine. Keratoconjunctivitis sicca (kcs) may be a consequence of feline herpesvirus infection, particularly following severe conjunctivitis when conjunctival cicatrization can affect the function of the lacrimal ductules. Orbital trauma, direct trauma to the lacrimal gland and damage to the parasympathetic division of the facial nerve will affect tear production, as will removal of the nictitans gland or third eyelid. The effects of lacrimotoxic drugs (both systemically and topically) are not as well documented in cats as dogs, but certain drugs known to be lacrimotoxic in the dog do not affect tear secretion in the cat. A proportion of old cats may have reduced tear production without obvious precipitating cause.

Feline dysautonomia, an autonomic polygangliopathy (see Chapter 15), produces widespread effects on organs innervated by parasympathetic nerves and keratoconjunctivitis sicca may be one of the presenting signs, although other

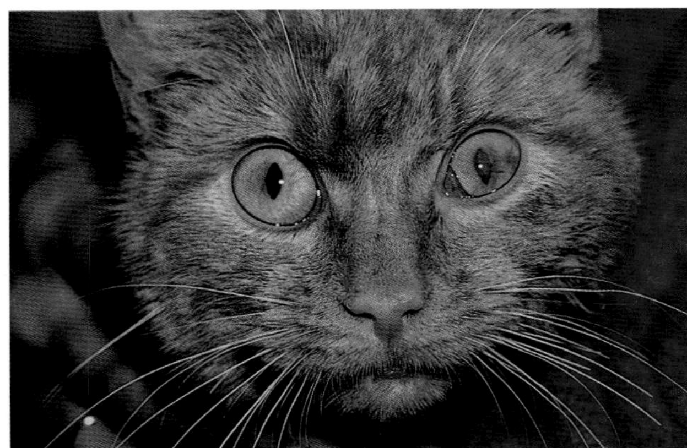

Fig. 7.3 *Adult Domestic shorthair. Keratoconjunctivitis sicca affecting the left eye.*

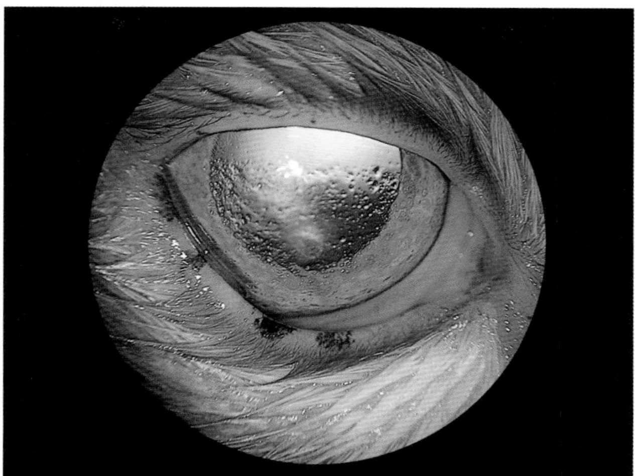

Fig. 7.4 *An 8-year-old Domestic shorthair. Multiple tear film abnormalities in a cat with suspected immune-mediated polyarthritis and glossitis. There was reduced tear production and meibomian gland dysfunction; the latter was associated with excessive particulate matter in the tear film and inadequate barrier function on the eyelid margins.*

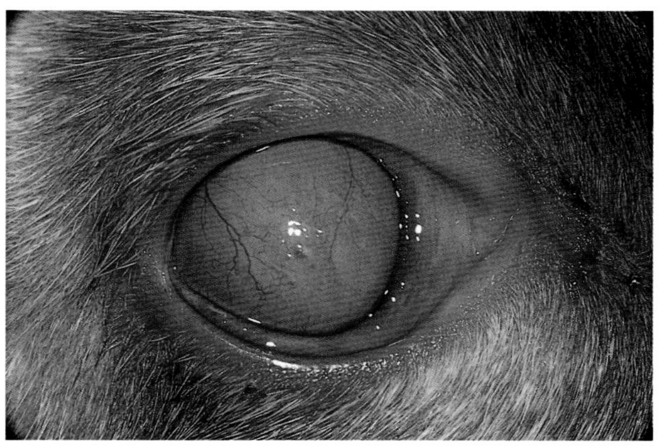

Fig. 7.5 *A ten-month-old Siamese cat with severe conjunctivitis, presumed to be a consequence of feline herpesvirus infection as a kitten. Symblepharon, keratoconjunctivitis sicca and ocular surface failure were present (see also Fig. 8.14).*

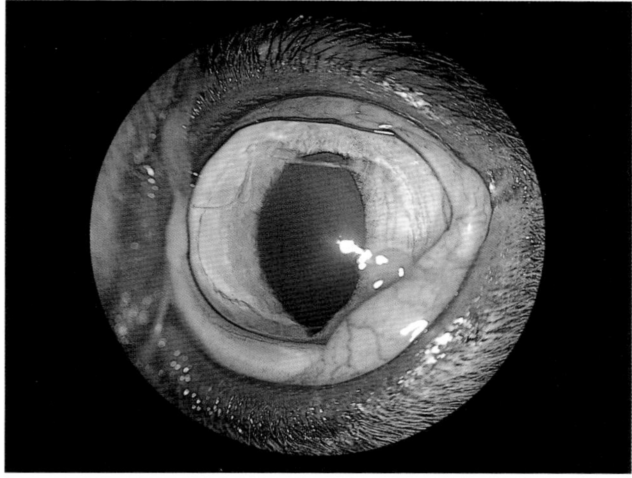

Fig. 7.6 *Chronic unilateral keratoconjunctivitis sicca of unknown cause in a 4-year-old Domestic shorthair. There is chemosis, a rather dull cornea, with disruption of the corneal reflex and a scanty ocular discharge.*

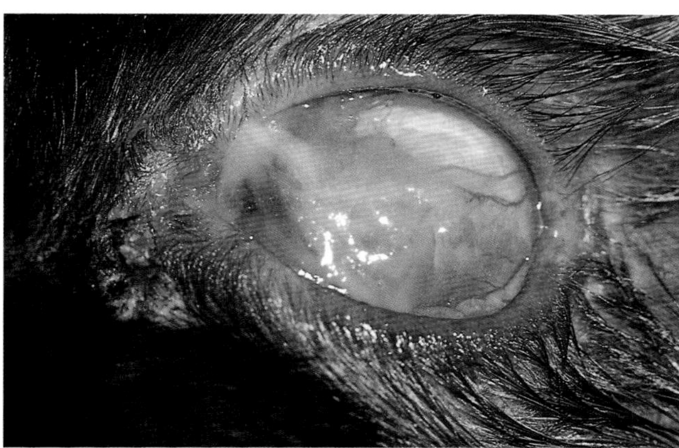

Fig. 7.7 *An 11-year-old Persian cat with bilateral keratoconjunctivitis sicca of unknown cause. Note the tacky ocular discharge and vascular keratitis.*

ocular features such as prominent third eyelids, dilated, unresponsive pupils (with normal vision) may be more obvious in the acute phase. Tear replacement therapy (e.g. 0.2% polyacrylic acid; Viscotears CIBA Vision; 0.2% w/w Carbomer 940; GelTears Chauvin) will be needed to mitigate the effects of reduced tear production.

Clinical signs of keratoconjunctivitis sicca, whatever the initiating cause, include some or all of the following: an increased blink rate, conjunctival hyperaemia, or frank conjunctivitis and a dull, lack-lustre cornea. There is often only a scant ocular discharge. Early in the course of the disease the eye may look remarkably normal on brief examination and the diagnosis is easily missed if a Schirmer tear test is not performed. Affected animals have Schirmer I (STT I) tear test values of less than 8 mm/min, usually less than 5 mm, and values of 0 are not uncommon in eyes which look almost normal. In more chronic cases corneal vascularization, opacification and ulceration may occur and in those cases associated with chronic feline herpesvirus (FHV) infection ocular surface disease will be obvious (see Chapter 9).

Treatment aims to identify and eliminate the cause when this is possible, but in many cases treatment tends to be palliative rather than curative. For cases of neurogenic origin treatment consists of one drop of 0.5% or 1% pilocarpine solution given well mixed in food, usually twice daily. Unfortunately, many cats will not eat adulterated food and pilocarpine on its own is not well tolerated orally. Topical pilocarpine may have some beneficial effect, but has not been clinically evaluated.

For keratoconjunctivitis sicca of non-neurogenic origin, tear replacement therapy applied to the eye three to four

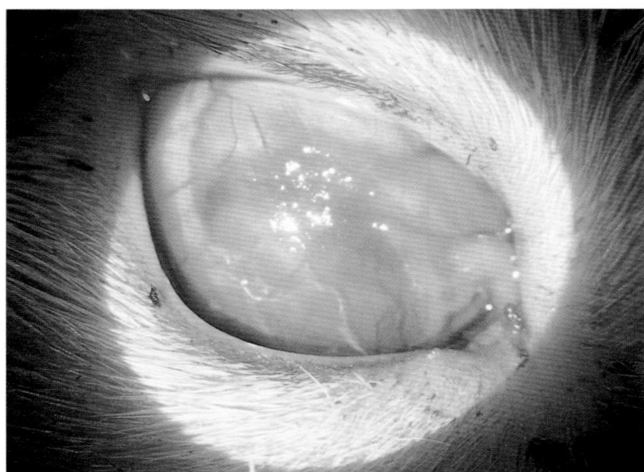

Fig. 7.8 *A 6-year-old Domestic shorthair with early sequestrum formation and keratoconjunctivitis sicca.*

times daily, is usually the treatment of choice, although ocular inserts have also been used. Cyclosporin does not appear to be an effective treatment for cats with keratoconjunctivitis sicca. Occasionally, parotid duct transposition should be considered for irreversible cases, the surgery is more difficult in cats than dogs, but nevertheless is possible and successful (Gwin *et al.*, 1977).

Topical corticosteroids (usually dexamethasone, betamethasone or prednisolone) are useful in the initial stages of treatment if corneal vascularization is present. However, the usual precautions apply and it is important to ensure that no corneal ulceration is present.

Tear drainage

Atresia and Hypoplasia

Partial or complete absence of parts of the nasolacrimal drainage system is an unusual congenital problem in cats (Figs 7.9–7.14). The upper or lower punctum is usually absent, and the associated canaliculus may occasionally be missing; the punctum is sometimes misplaced. In cats, the upper punctum and canaliculus is most frequently involved, whereas in the dog it is usually the lower punctum which is imperforate or hypoplastic (micropunctum) and there are no associated defects of the canaliculus.

The presenting clinical sign is epiphora, although in chronic cases there may be a mucoid, or even mucopurulent, ocular discharge. The breed most commonly affected is the Persian and since this breed may also suffer epiphora as a consequence of its head conformation (poorly defined orbit, prominent globe, shallow lacrimal lake, misalignment of the puncta, kinking of the canaliculus, tight apposition between the eyelid and eye) it is important to check that the puncta are present at the initial clinical examination. When there is poor head conformation the nasolacrimal drainage system may become blocked secondarily; consequently, irrigation of the drainage system will produce only

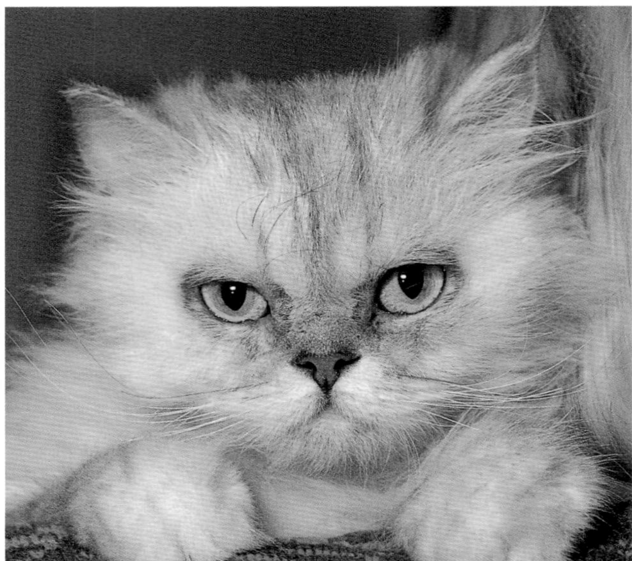

Fig. 7.9 *A 1-year-old Persian cat with mild epiphora, the epiphora of the right eye was slightly more marked than that of the left. In addition to the usual features of Persian anatomy, this cat had upper punctal aplasia on the right side.*

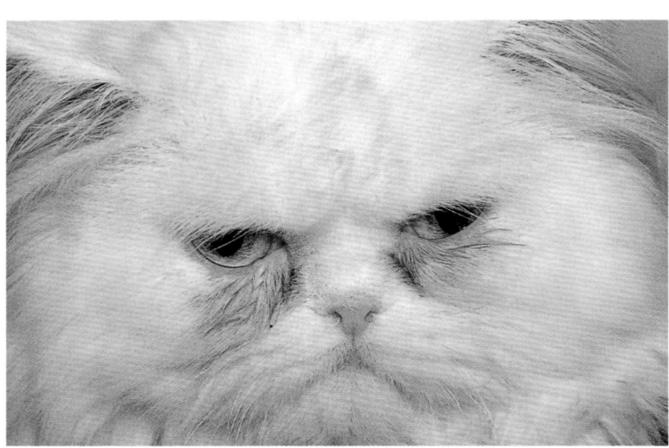

Fig. 7.10 *A 7-month-old Persian cat with bilateral epiphora photographed after fluorescein administration. There was absence of the upper punctum, but a lower punctum of normal size and position was present.*

temporary improvement unless the primary problem is also addressed.

If examination reveals that the upper or lower punctum is absent, the other punctum should be cannulated and the system irrigated as described in Chapter 1. If the only defect is caused by a sheet of mucous membrane covering the punctum then a transient bleb may form in this area and simple excision of the overlying mucous membrane will be all that is required to establish patency. Patency is maintained by applying a topical antibiotic–corticosteroid ophthalmic solution to the punctum for 5–7 days after surgery to minimize scar formation.

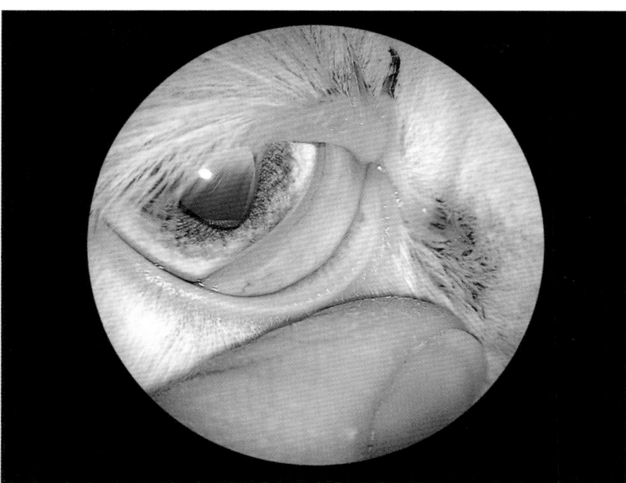

Fig. 7.11 *The same cat as illustrated in Fig 7.10, demonstrating the lower punctum.*

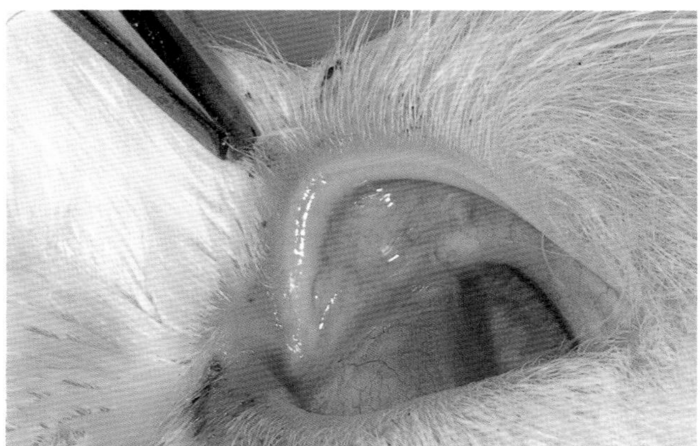

Fig. 7.12 *A 1-year-old Persian cat with bilateral epiphora and upper punctal aplasia of both eyes; the left eye is illustrated and no upper punctum can be seen.*

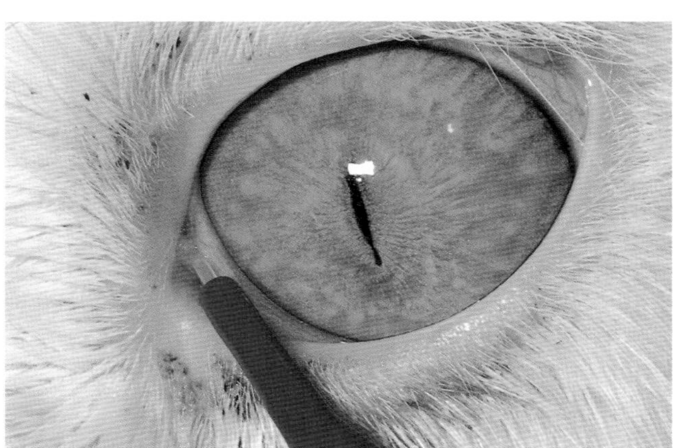

Fig. 7.13 *The same cat as illustrated in Fig. 7.12. A nasolacrimal cannula has been placed in the lower punctum to demonstrate that it is abnormally located.*

When simple punctal occlusion is not the only defect then dacryocystorhinography may help to establish the extent of the problem; treatment to produce an alternative drainage route may be required. It is sometimes possible to create an absent canaliculus and punctum by feeding a fine, malleable, lacrimal cannula via the normal punctum, canaliculus and lacrimal sac to the affected area. The conjunctiva over the tip of the cannula is excised to create a punctum and fine nylon is then passed through the lumen of the cannula. The cannula is withdrawn, the nylon is retained in place with butterfly sutures and should remain *in situ* for some 3–4 weeks until canalization is assured (Figs 7.15 and 7.16).

Other techniques create an alternative outflow channel, but the provision of alternative drainage routes using bypass techniques such as conjunctivo-rhinostomy and conjunctivo-oralostomy are not always easy procedures in the cat and the

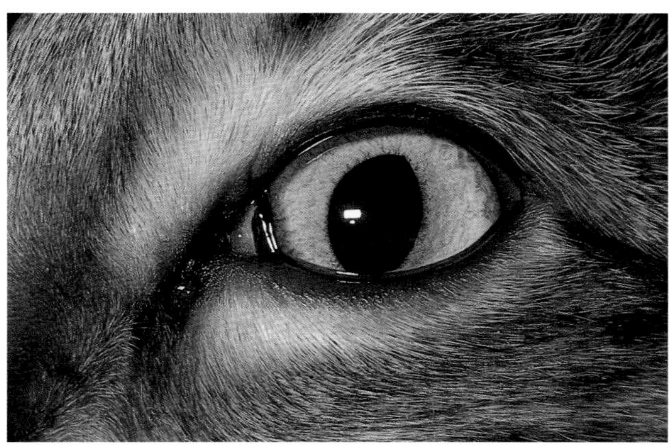

Fig. 7.14 *A 7-month-old Bengal cat with bilateral epiphora. The upper punctum was present, but the lower punctum and part of the canaliculus was missing on the left side.*

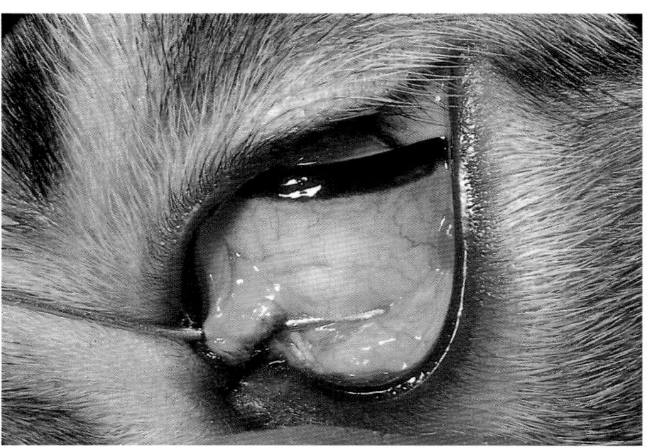

Fig. 7.15 *The same cat as illustrated in Fig. 7.14 after a fine silver probe has been passed via the upper punctum, canaliculus and lacrimal sac to the region of the lower canaliculus. The lower punctum and canaliculus has been recreated by blunt dissection to the probe.*

long-term results can be disappointing (Gelatt and Gelatt, 1994). Surgery should therefore be reserved for those cases in which epiphora, from whatever cause, is producing serious problems for the patient (Fig. 7.17) as, for example, marked staining of the hair, skin excoriation, periocular infection and chronic dacryocystitis (dacryocystitis is, strictly speaking, inflammation of the lacrimal sac, but in domestic animals it usually implies inflammation of the nasolacrimal drainage system).

Acquired Obstructions of the Lacrimal Drainage System

Acquired partial or complete obstruction (Figs 7.18–7.22) may be a consequence of inflammation, trauma, abnormalities external to the drainage system (e.g. medial canthus, nose, sinuses and teeth roots) or within it (e.g. foreign bodies, infection). Comprehensive investigation is required to establish the cause and may include visual inspection, nasolacrimal and nasal flushes for cytology and culture, dacryocystorhinography and imaging techniques. Epiphora is the commonest presenting sign, but occasionally a more florid ocular discharge is present, usually when dacryocystitis complicates the presentation.

The commonest cause of acquired stenosis or occlusion is previous ophthalmia neonatorum where symblepharon formation obliterates one or both the punctal openings (Fig. 7.18). The diagnosis of this problem is easy on close examination of the medial canthus, but treatment is difficult as adhesions reform rapidly whatever surgical technique is adopted.

Other causes of obstruction or partial obstruction may be less obvious (Figs 7.19–7.22) and include nasal problems

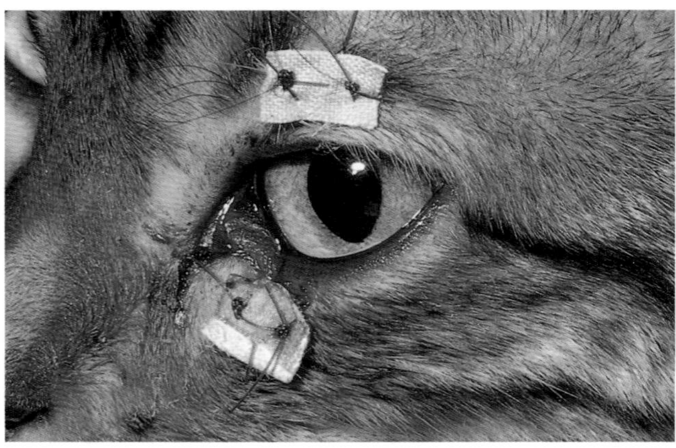

Fig. 7.16 *The same cat as illustrated in Figs 7.14 and 7.15 with monofilament nylon in situ to maintain patency during healing.*

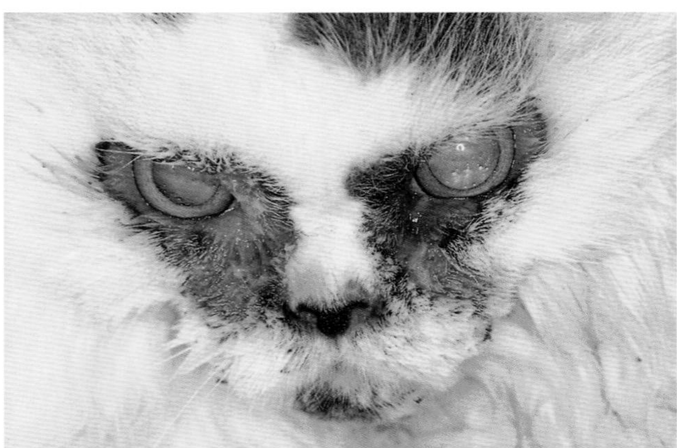

Fig. 7.17 *Periorbital dermatitis in a 2-year-old Persian with bilateral absence of the upper puncta.*

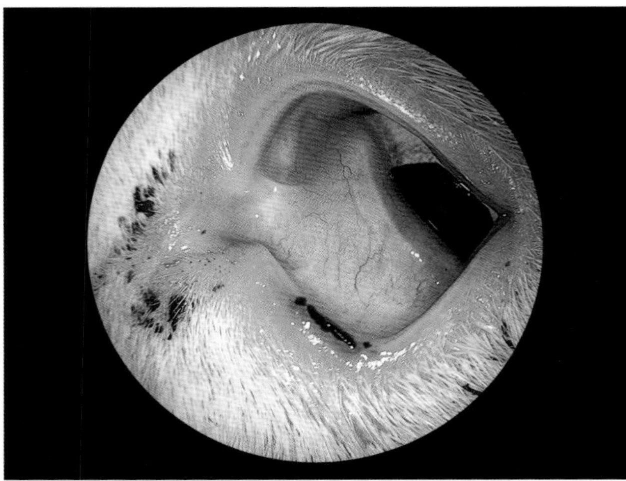

Fig. 7.18 *A 15-month-old Domestic shorthair with acquired blockage of the upper and lower puncta as a result of extensive symblepharon formation (FHV infection).*

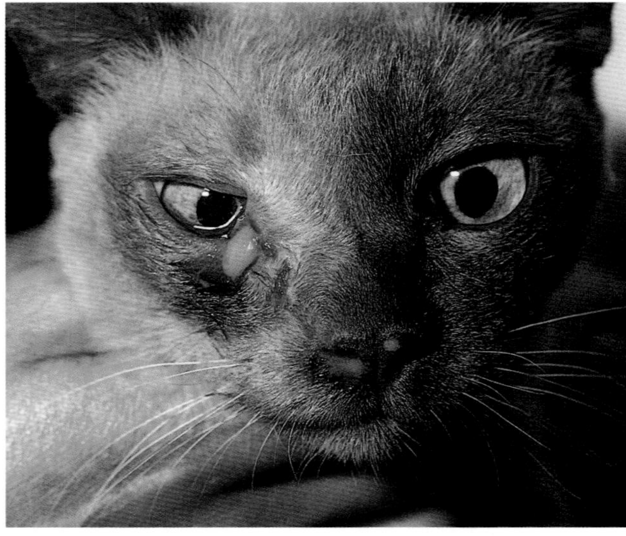

Fig. 7.19 *A 17-year-old Burmese cat which presented with severe epistaxis and pus issuing from the lower punctum and nostril on the right side. Investigations revealed a nasal polyp on the right side which was surgically extirpated after preoperative preparations which included blood transfusion because the laboratory findings included a haematocrit of 8. The cat made an uneventful recovery.*

such as previous upper repiratory tract infections, chronic rhinitis, nasal polyps and neoplasia, dental disease (especially tooth root problems), and, rarely, inflammatory and neoplastic diseases of the sinuses. Local neoplasia (e.g. squamous cell carcinoma) may involve the nasolacrimal system and produce partial or complete obstruction (Peiffer *et al.*, 1978). It is not always possible to establish a specific cause.

Traumatic injury, especially cat claw injuries which involve the medial canthus, can also interfere with tear drainage. Primary repair of canalicular injuries requires facilities for microsurgery. Chronic complications of unrecognized damage in this region include dacrocystitis, abscessation, bone sequestration and formation of a draining sinus below the medial canthus.

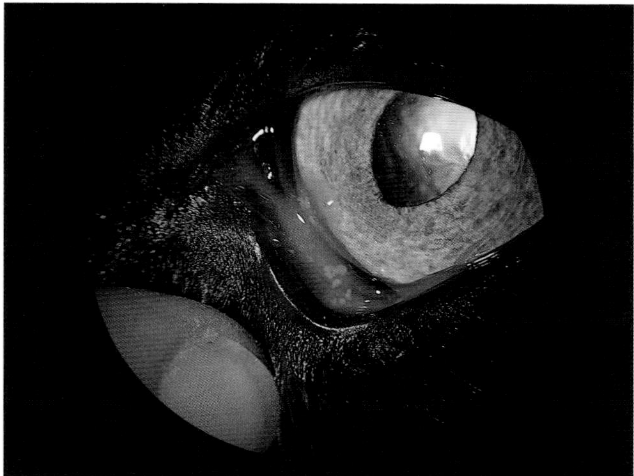

Fig. 7.20 *A 6-year-old Domestic shorthair with left sided dacryocystitis as a complication of chronic rhinitis. At initial presentation a flocculent discharge emanating from the lower lacrimal punctum was present.*

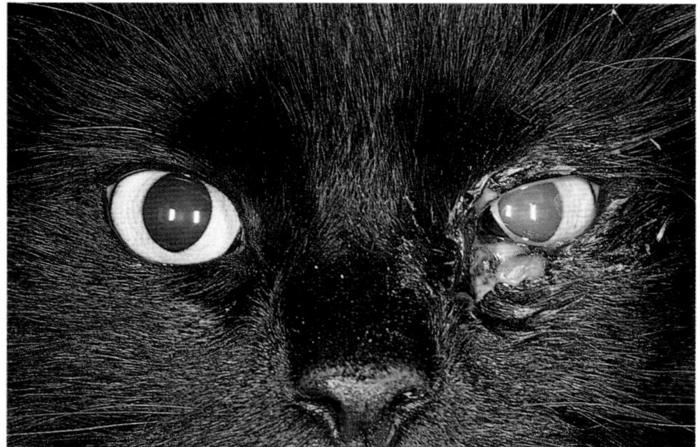

Fig. 7.21 *Same cat as shown in Fig. 7.20, with a more florid ocular discharge at the time of referral. Investigation demonstrated that there was communication between the left nasolacrimal duct and nasal cavity and also between the right and left nasal cavities because of chronic destructive changes associated with rhinitis. Initial culture had revealed Bacteroides spp., later culture demonstrated anaerobic Gram-negative cocci. On the basis of culture and sensitivity results, she was given a 3-week course of topical and oral tetracycline, to which she responded well. (Courtesy of J. R. B. Mould.)*

Dacryocystitis is a likely sequel to established obstructive disease, whatever the initiating cause, and clinical signs are typical. There is usually an ocular or periocular discharge which may be profuse and purulent, especially in chronic cases (Figs 7.20–7.22). It is often possible to see that the discharge emanates from the puncta and gentle digital pressure at the medial canthus in the region of the lacrimal sac usually expresses purulent material. There may be slight reddening in the medial canthus area.

The primary reason for dacryocystitis should be identified and eliminated whenever possible. Irrigation of the drainage system allows the discharge to be cultured both aerobically and anaerobically and antibiotic sensitivity to be established. Appropriate systemic antibiotic and topical antibiotic solution should be given for 7–10 days in uncomplicated cases. More complex situations may require antibiotic treatment for at least 1 month, with or without cannulation of the entire system.

In the event of abscessation or sinus formation, surgery (for drainage of the abscess and removal of necrotic tissue and fistulous tract) may be required. Surgical bypass of the affected area may also be necessary.

Other diseases of the lacrimal system

Dacryoadenitis

Dacryoadenitis (inflammation of the lacrimal gland) is uncommon in the cat. Eosinophilic granuloma of the orbit and tuberculosis of the lacrimal gland have been recorded as causes of dacryoadenitis (Roberts and Lipton, 1975).

Neoplasia

Neoplasia of the lacrimal and nictitans gland is rare; squamous cell carcinoma and adenocarcinoma are the most likely

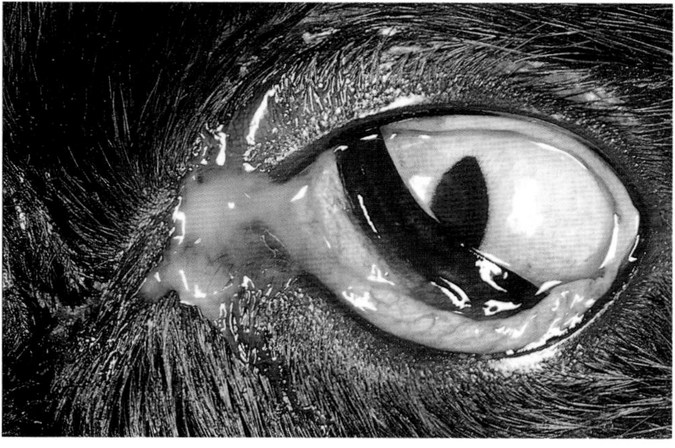

Fig. 7.22 *Close-up of same cat as shown in Figs 7.20 and 7.21. (Courtesy of J. R. B. Mould.)*

tumours to be encountered. Involvement of the drainage system is often secondary to neoplasia in neighbouring structures (e.g. squamous cell carcinoma, lymphosarcoma and adenocarcinoma involving, for example, the medial canthus, nasopharynx and sinuses).

References

Carrington SD, Bedford PGC, Guillon JP, Woodward EG (1987) Polarised light biomicroscopic observations on the pre-corneal tear film III. The normal tear film of the cat. *Journal of Small Animal Practice* **28**: 821–826.

Gelatt KN, Gelatt JP (1994) Small Animal Ophthalmic Surgery, Volume 1: Extraocular Procedures, pp. 132–134. Pergamon: Oxford.

Gwin RM, Gelatt KN, Peiffer RL (1977) Parotid duct transposition in a cat with keratoconjunctivitis sicca. *Journal of the American Animal Hospital Association* **13**: 42–45.

Hacker DV (1990) 'Crocodile tears' syndrome in a domestic cat: Case report. *Journal of the American Animal Hospital Association* **26**: 245–246.

Johnson BW, Whiteley HE, McLaughlin SA (1990) Effects of inflammation and aqueous tear film deficiency on conjunctival morphology and ocular mucus composition in cats. *American Journal of Veterinary Research* **51**: 820–824.

Peiffer RL, Spencer C, Popp JA (1978) Nasal squamous cell carcinoma with periocular extension and metastasis in a cat. *Feline Practice* **8**: 43–46.

Poels P, Simoens P (1994) The lacrimal apparatus of cats. *Vlaams Diergeneeskundig Tijdschrift* **63**: 87–89.

Roberts ST, Lipton DE (1975) The eye. In Catcott EJ (ed.) Feline Medicine and Surgery, 2nd Edn. American Veterinary Publications, Santa Barbara.

8 Conjunctiva, limbus, episclera and sclera

Introduction

Commencing at the limbus, conjunctiva covers a portion of the anterior globe (bulbar conjunctiva), reflects at the fornices to line the inner surface of the upper and lower eyelids (palpebral conjunctiva) and both surfaces of the third eyelid (nictitating conjunctiva). In the normal cat there is very little exposed conjunctiva, except for that of the third eyelid medially and a small area of bulbar conjunctiva which may be visible at the lateral canthus (see Figs 1.1–1.3). *Staphylococcus* spp. can often be isolated from the conjunctival sac of normal cats (Espinola and Lilenbaum, 1996).

The conjunctiva is a typical mucous membrane of semitransparent nature. It consists of an outer nonkeratinized epithelial layer which contains mucin-producing goblet cells and an underlying substantia propria which contains blood vessels, nerves, lymphatics and accessory lacrimal glands (Fig. 8.1). Conjunctival-associated lymphoid tissue (CALT) is implicated in immune-mediated conjunctival responses. Dendritic Langerhans cells, important in antigen presentation to the immune system, may be present at the limbus and between the peripheral corneal epithelial cells (Carrington, 1985).

The episclera and sclera are located beneath the bulbar conjunctiva and may be considered together. Tenon's capsule is comparatively well developed and all four rectus muscles have fascial extensions from their insertion on the globe to the limbal region, the dorsal and ventral oblique muscles pass beneath these fascial extensions. The sclera is thinner posteriorly than anteriorly and appears darker as the choroidal pigment shows through. The lamina cribrosa is almost as thick as the adjacent sclera. Anteriorly, the sclera is thicker and white, except where it approaches the limbal region where heavy pigmentation imparts a blue colour to the perilimbal zone in many cats. At the limbus there is usually a very clearly defined narrow rim of pigment which delineates the junction of the 'white' of the eye with the clear cornea (Figs 1.1–1.3).

Disorders of the conjunctiva

Epibulbar dermoid

Epibulbar dermoids (see also Chapter 5) or choristomas are described in Chapter 5. Those which arise on conjunctiva are usually found in the region of the lateral canthus (Figs 8.2–8.5), where they sometimes involve the skin of the lateral canthus and some encroach onto the cornea. Epibulbar dermoids may also be found at other conjunctival sites. They are removed by surgical excision as previously described and a lateral canthotomy may help to provide adequate surgical exposure for those situated in the region of the lateral canthus.

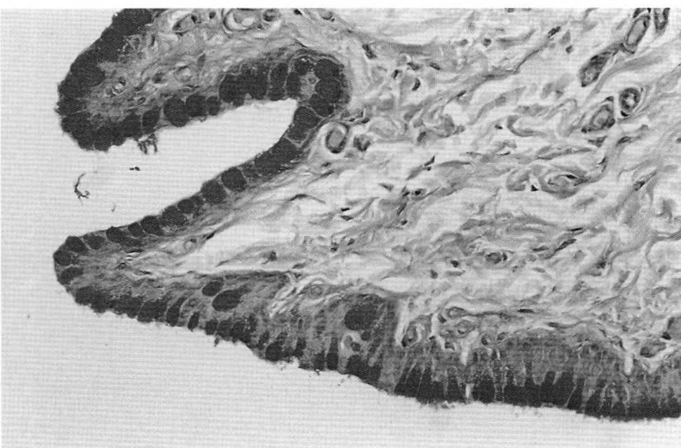

Fig. 8.1 *Histological section of the conjunctiva stained with Periodic acid–Schiff reagent to demonstrate the profuse goblet cells in the conjunctival epithelium.*

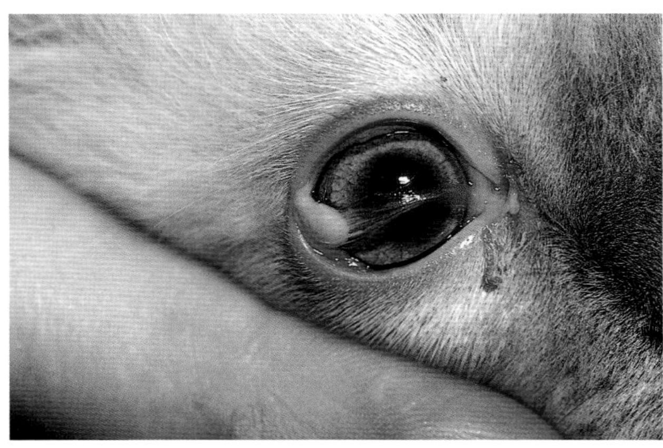

Fig. 8.2 *An 8-week-old female Birman kitten with epibulbar dermoid involving the lateral canthus.*

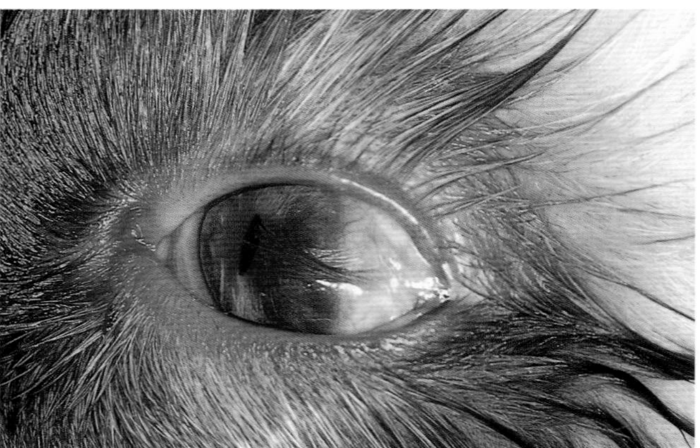

Fig. 8.3 *A 4-month-old male Birman cat with epibulbar dermoid involving the conjunctiva of the lateral limbus. The cat had been operated upon as a kitten for removal of the dermoid, but removal was incomplete. A lateral canthotomy improved exposure for the second attempt and the dermoid was excised by starting in the limbal region and dissecting laterally.*

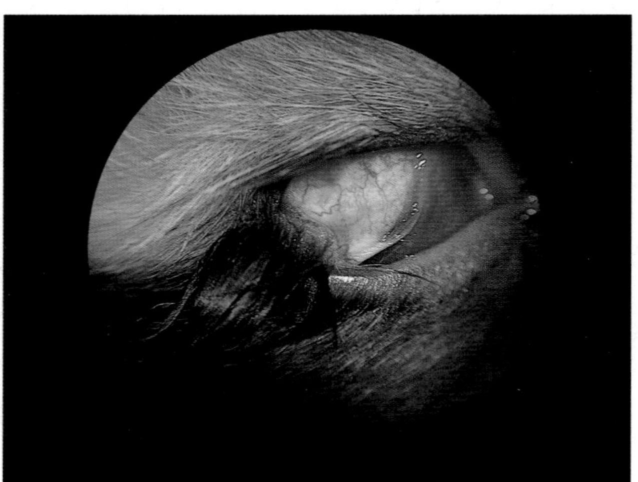

Fig. 8.4 *Young colourpoint with an extensive dermoid of the lateral canthus, involving the eyelids and bulbar conjunctiva. The canthus required repair following surgical removal.*

SYMBLEPHARON

Conjunctival adhesion of palpebral, bulbar, or nictitating conjunctiva, to each other, or to the cornea is termed symblepharon and, while very rare in dogs, it is extremely common in cats. Symblepharon is occasionally of congenital origin, but most frequently follows neonatal infection, most commonly that due to feline herpesvirus and, less frequently, can be a complication of other types of severe conjunctival inflammation, chemical and thermal injuries (Figs 8.6–8.20).

Symblepharon may be seen as a distinct entity or in conjunction with other ocular defects such as microphthalmos.

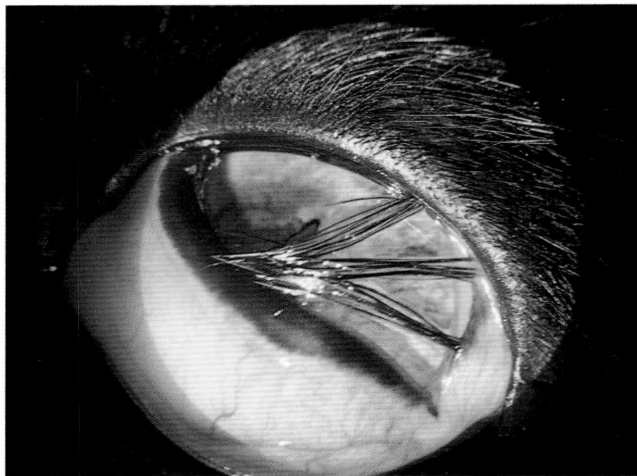

Fig. 8.5 *Unusual epibulbar dermoid in a young adult Domestic shorthair. There are three separate dermoids producing hairs in the perilimbal conjunctiva.*

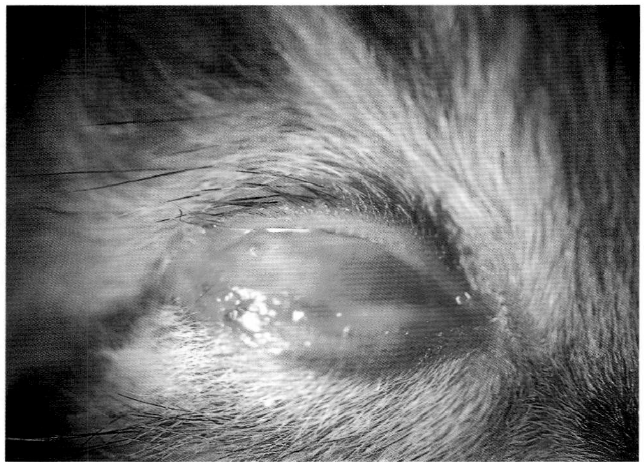

Fig. 8.6 *A 14-day-old Domestic shorthair kitten with severe conjunctival inflammation and symblepharon formation with feline herpesvirus infection. The other eye was unaffected.*

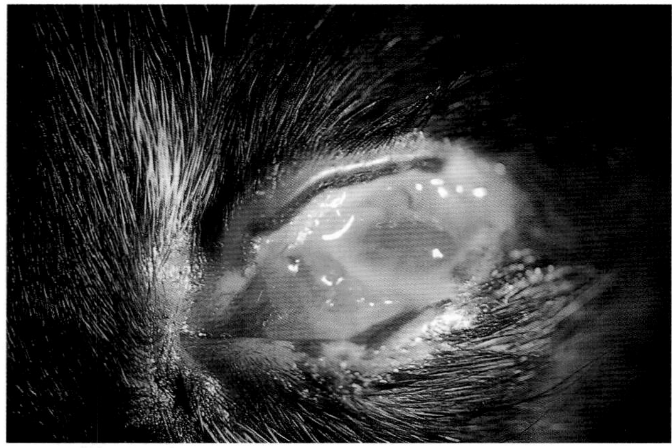

Fig. 8.7 *A 5-week-old Domestic shorthair kitten with severe keratoconjunctivitis and symblepharon formation with feline herpesvirus infection. The other eye was less severely affected.*

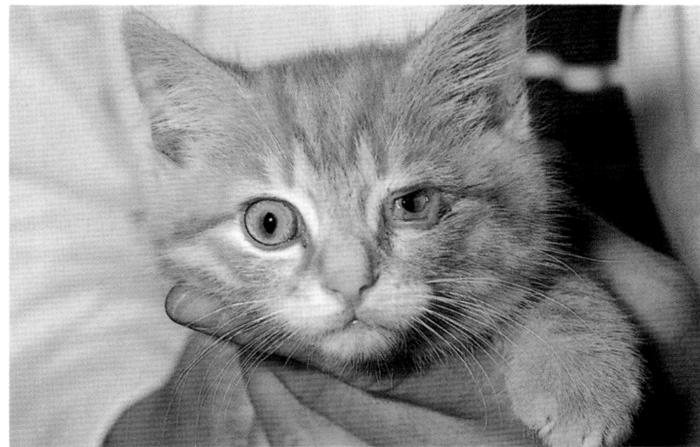

Fig. 8.8 *A 3 month-old Domestic shorthair kitten with unilateral symblepharon following ophthalmia neonatorum. The right eye is unaffected. The left eye has normal vision despite the adhesions between the conjunctival surfaces (mainly third eyelid and bulbar conjunctiva). Note the mild cicatricial ectropion and the rather poor eyelid apposition in the left eye.*

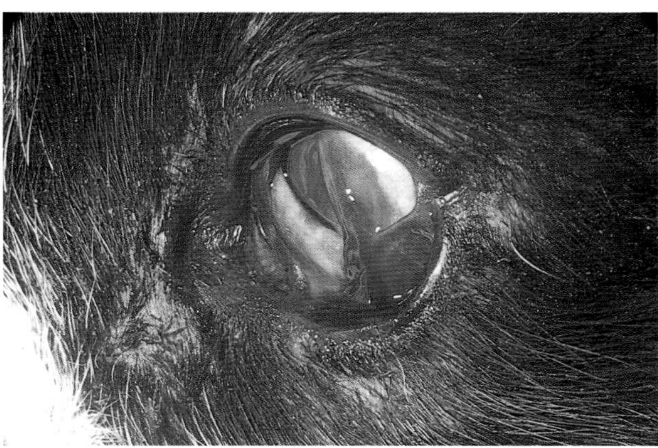

Fig. 8.10 *Close up of the left eye of the cat shown in Fig. 8.9. There is extensive symblepharon between the lateral palpebral and bulbar conjunctiva, the third eyelid and palpebral conjunctiva and there is also opacification of the dorsal cornea. Despite the fact that the ventral fornix is obliterated, the cat had no serious clinical problems as a result of these adhesions and there was no necessity to operate.*

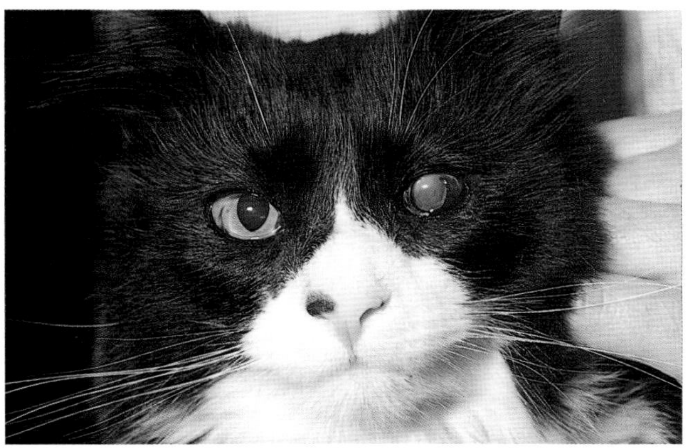

Fig. 8.9 *A 1-year-old Domestic shorthair neutered male with bilateral symblepharon; the left eye was more severely affected than the right, but there were no obvious effects on vision.*

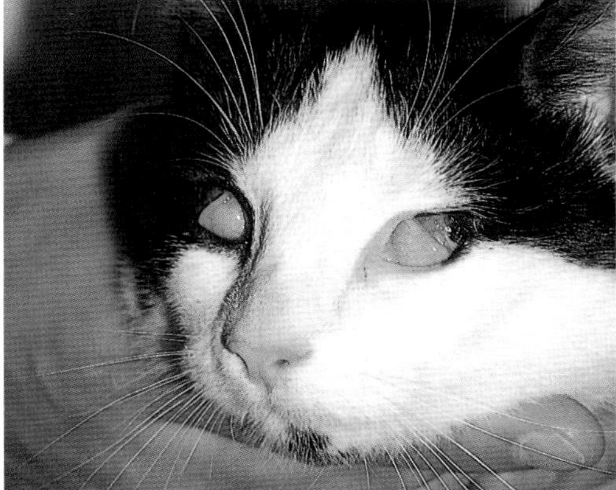

Fig. 8.11 *A 6-month-old Domestic shorthair. Severe symblepharon affecting both eyes and affecting vision. This cat had originally been less severely affected, but the symblepharon had been exacerbated by a number of unsuccessful surgical procedures.*

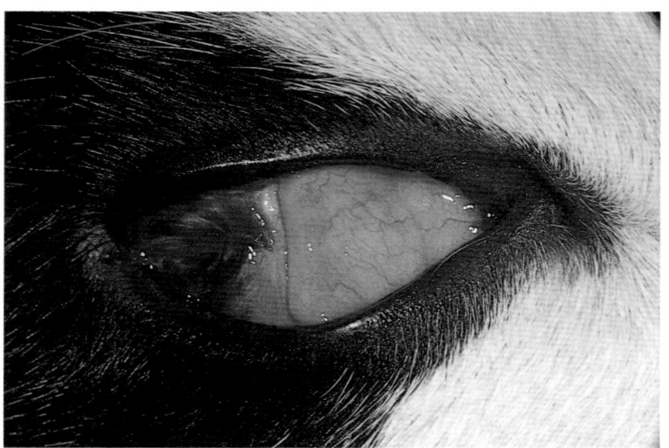

Fig. 8.12 *Close-up of the right eye of the cat shown in Figure Fig. 8.11. A small area of pigmented cornea laterally is the only area where light perception and 'vision' is possible. Elsewhere, there are extensive attachments between conjunctival surfaces (including the third eyelid) to each other and to the cornea.*

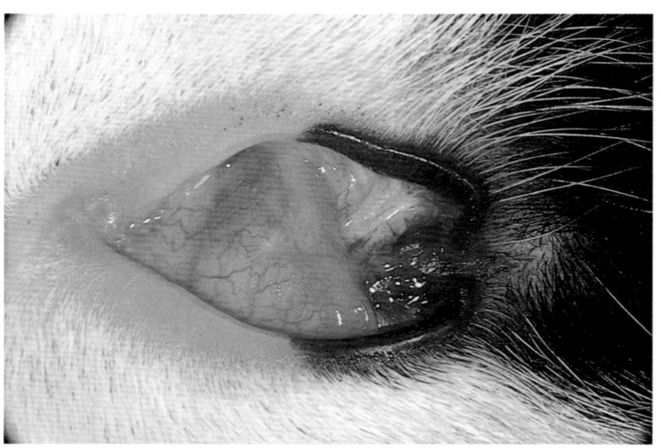

Fig. 8.13 *Close-up of the left eye of the cat shown in Fig. 8.11. Symblepharon formation has completely obliterated any view of the underlying cornea and this eye is blind. Rather than further compromise the very imperfect vision of the right eye the left eye was operated upon.*

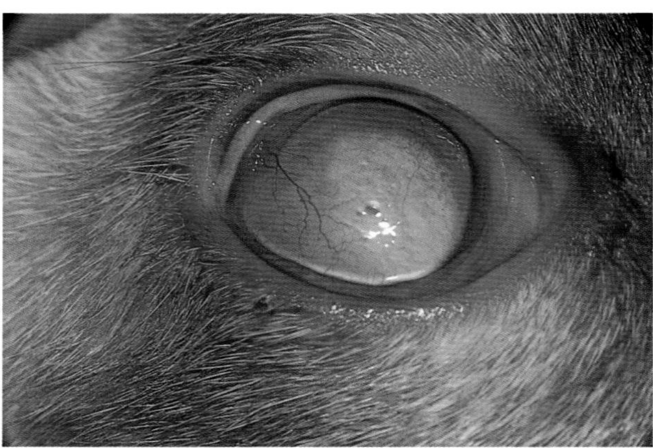

Fig. 8.14 *A 10-month-old Siamese female. This cat had severe bilateral conjunctivitis as a kitten, presumed to be a consequence of feline herpesvirus infection. In addition to symblepharon formation, the right eye demonstrates classical ocular surface failure with corneal epithelial defects and vascularization. Tear production was abnormally low (see Fig. 7.5)*

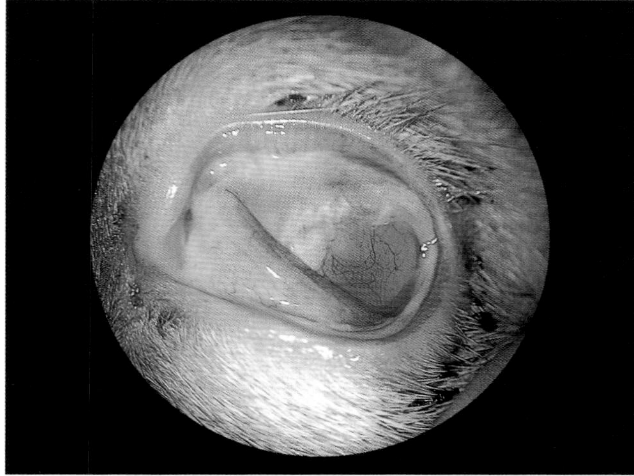

Fig. 8.15 *The left eye of the cat shown in Fig. 8.14. Ocular surface failure, including corneal epithelial defects, vascularization and conjunctival overgrowth is apparent. Symblepharon formation has resulted in obliteration of the fornices. The abnormalities present emphasize the complications which arise when the normal limbal stem cell population has been destroyed.*

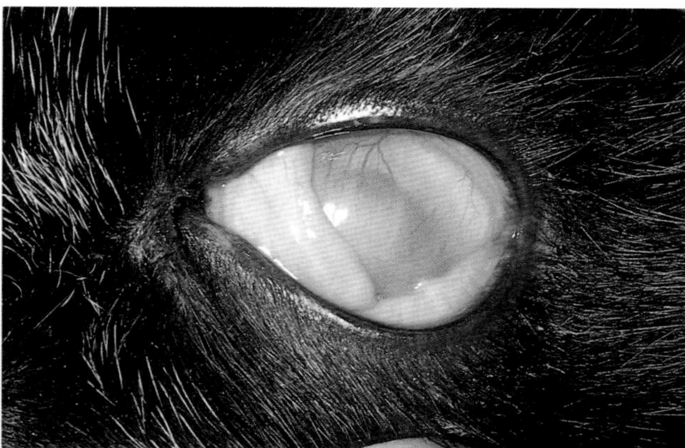

Fig. 8.16 *Adult Domestic shorthair. Symblepharon formation as a consequence of an alkali burn. This eye is also illustrated at the time of the acute injury (Fig. 3.42)*

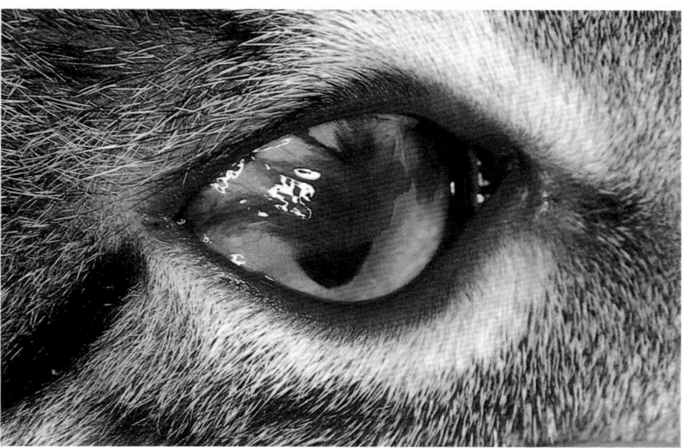

Fig. 8.18 *Young adult Domestic shorthair. Pigmented conjunctiva covering some two-thirds of the cornea with, in addition, obliteration of the dorsal fornix.*

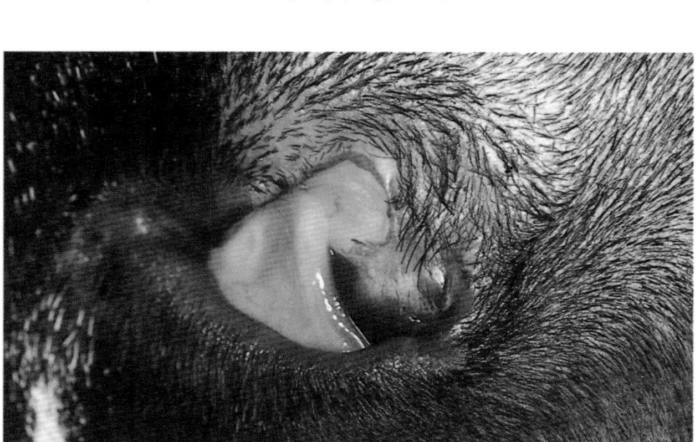

Fig. 8.17 *Young adult Domestic shorthair. This cat had been one of a large cat population on a farm and the cause of the symblepharon was unknown. On the right side there was a phthitic sightless eye and normal eyelids. On the left side, the eye was visual but symblepharon was extensive and the problem had been exacerbated by excision of the upper eyelid margin in a failed attempt to mobilize the eyelid. The case was treated successfully by removing the damaged right eye and then switching the undamaged lower eyelid of the right eye to replace the abnormal eyelid region of the left eye.*

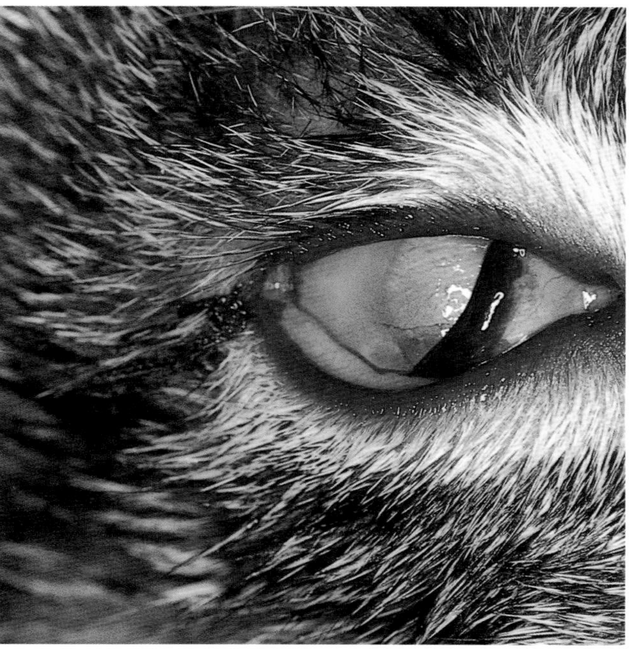

Fig. 8.19 *The same cat as shown in Fig. 8.19 immediately after performing the Arlt technique (Mustardé, 1991) to treat the symblepharon. The postoperative appearance was good immediately after surgery, but further corneal opacification developed some months later.*

The problems caused by symblepharon in relation to eyelid motility and the production and drainage of the pre-ocular tear film are described in Chapters 5–7.

No treatment is required unless the effects of symblepharon are severe (e.g. some or all of poor or absent vision, impaired eyelid and globe mobility). Surgical section of the adhesions is a simple procedure, but the adhesions reform rapidly, are often more severe than those of the original symblepharon and the corneal clarity achieved at surgery is soon lost. To minimize reattachment it is necessary to use complex surgical procedures (Mustardé, 1991) and therapeutic soft contact lenses (Figs 8.17–8.21), but even with these techniques the long-term prognosis is poor. These disappointing results reflect the pathogenesis, notably the destruction of limbal stem cells at the time of acute inflammation. Consequently, corneal epithelium cannot be generated for repair and conjunctival epithelium resurfaces the cornea; thus 'conjunctivalization' of the cornea results. The clinical picture is of ocular surface failure characterized by conjunctival overgrowth, corneal epithelial defects, vascularization and scarring. Recent advances in autotransplantation of limbal stem cells from a normal limbus, usually of the fellow eye, offers an exciting and more rational approach for problems of this type.

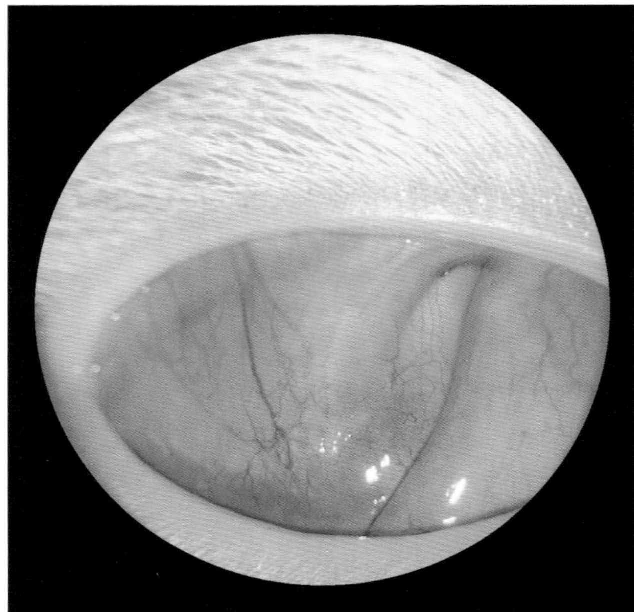

Fig. 8.20 An 11-month-old Domestic shorthair. Symblepharon formation similar to that shown in Fig. 8.18, but the conjunctiva is nonpigmented.

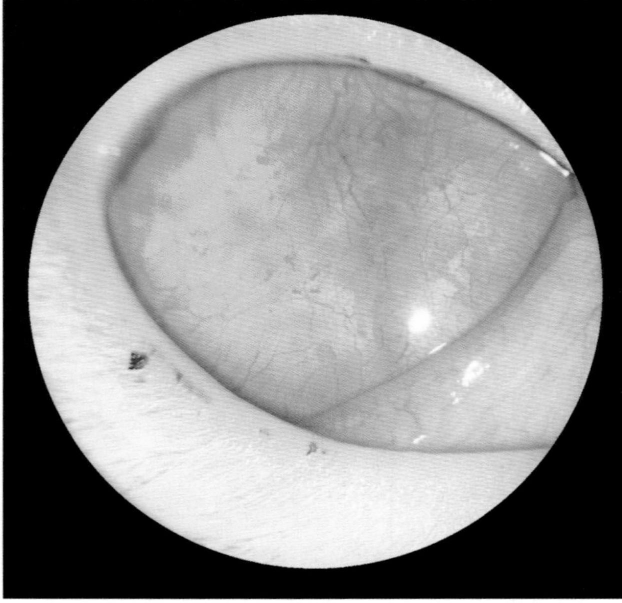

Fig. 8.21 The same cat as shown in Fig. 8.20 2 weeks after superficial keratectomy and fitting a therapeutic soft contact lens. The corneal clarity was retained with the contact lens in place, corneal opacification developed once the lens was removed.

Conjunctival cysts

Conjuctival cysts (Fig 8.22) may be associated with symblepharon, or may arise independently of symblepharon as epithelial inclusion cysts; both types are treated by surgical excision.

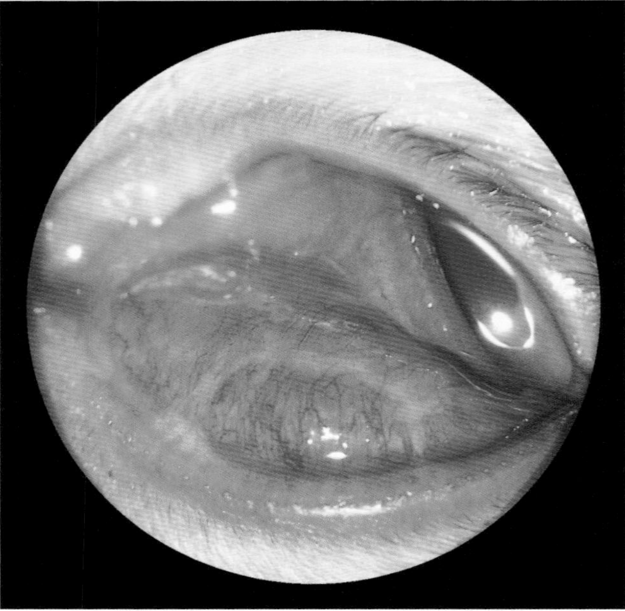

Fig. 8.22 A 10-month-old Siamese. Large conjunctival cyst associated with symblepharon. The cyst was surgically excised.

Subconjunctival haemorrhage

Subconjunctival haemorrhage is bright red when fresh and is usually a consequence of trauma to the head (Fig. 4.29). In such cases the eye should be examined carefully in case there has been internal damage to the globe. The possibility of globe rupture should always be considered when there has been severe blunt injury to the globe and orbit (see Chapter 3).

In uncomplicated cases the haemorrhage is resorbed over several days and no treatment is necessary. When haemorrhage is extensive the swollen conjunctiva can quickly become dessicated and lagophthalmos predisposes to secondary corneal pathology (e.g. exposure keratopathy and corneal ulceration). Ocular lubrication using a commercial tear replacement solution, with or without a temporary tarsorrhaphy, will be required in these cases.

Chemosis

Because the cat has an extensive and loosely arranged conjunctiva, conjunctival oedema (chemosis) may be of spectacular appearance and chemosis is a ubiquitous accompaniment to many types of conjunctival disease (Fig. 8.23). In addition to addressing the underlying problem it is important to prevent conjunctival dessication, as described above.

Conjunctivitis

Conjunctivitis is a common condition in the cat and may be unilateral or bilateral. The classical signs of acute conjunctivitis are active hyperaemia (redness) of the conjunctival vessels, chemosis and an ocular discharge which may be serous, mucoid, purulent, haemorrhagic or combinations of these

(Figs 8.23–8.31). Redness of the eye is not synonymous with conjunctivitis and may occur in a number of other situations; for example, as a consequence of the local effect of impeded venous return because of an orbital mass (Fig. 4.22), as part of a systemic vascular response (Fig. 8.32), or associated with cardiovascular disease (Fig. 8.33).

Chronic conjunctivitis is associated with follicle formation, conjunctival thickening and a persistent ocular discharge (Fig 8.34).

The aetiology of conjunctivitis in cats is most commonly infection, particularly of the respiratory tract viruses (e.g. feline herpesvirus and calicivirus), bacteria such as *Chlamydia psittaci* (which is the commonest isolate from feline conjunctivitis cases in the UK) and *Mycoplasma* spp. Viral and bacterial conjunctivitis are discussed in greater detail below.

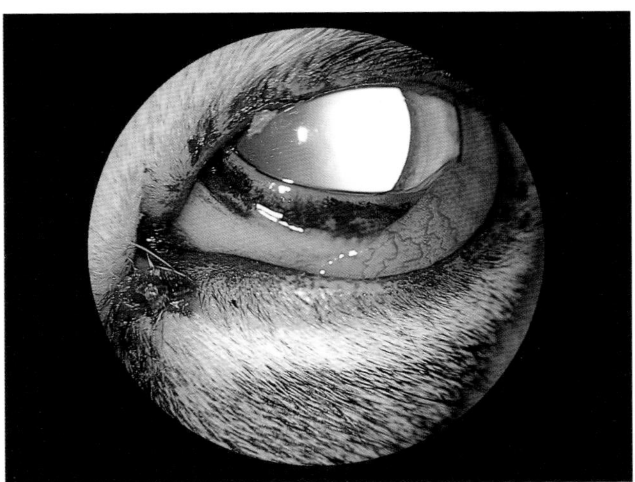

Fig. 8.23 *A Domestic shorthair, approximately 3 months old, with acute conjunctivitis. Note the conjunctival hyperaemia, chemosis and ocular discharge.*

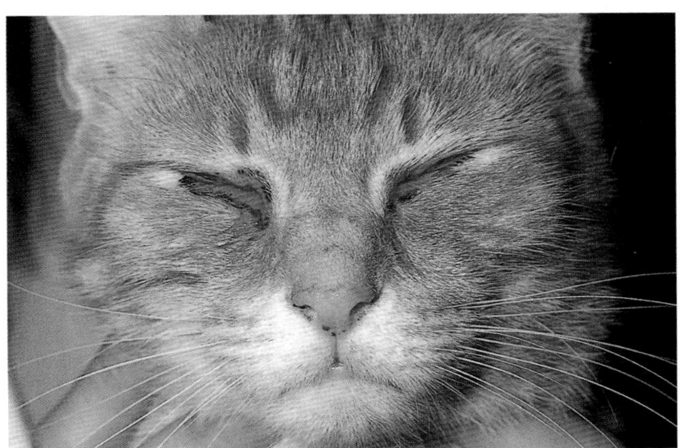

Fig. 8.24 *A 5-month-old Domestic shorthair with FHV-1 conjunctivitis. Note that there is some lacrimation and obvious ocular discomfort.*

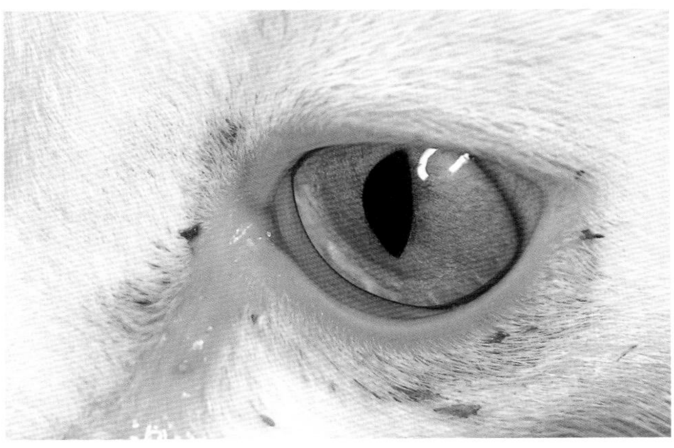

Fig. 8.25 *A 4-month-old Domestic shorthair with FHV-1 conjunctivitis. Both eyes were affected, the left eye is shown. Note that there is much less discomfort than in the previous figure and that the discharge is becoming more mucoid.*

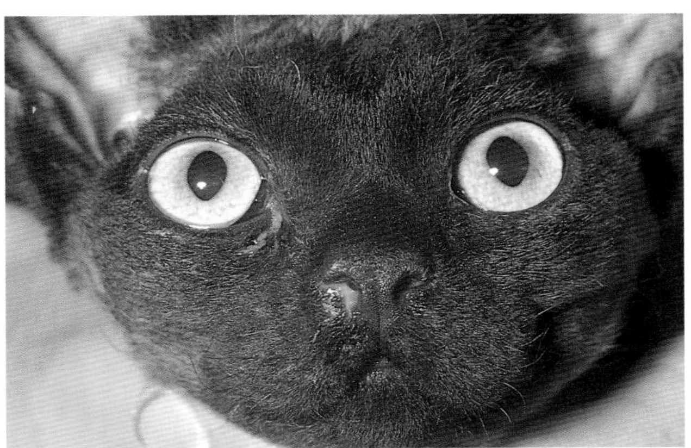

Fig. 8.26 *An 8-month-old Devon Rex with calicivirus conjunctivitis. Mild ocular discharge from the right eye, however, the most prominent feature is the nasal discharge.*

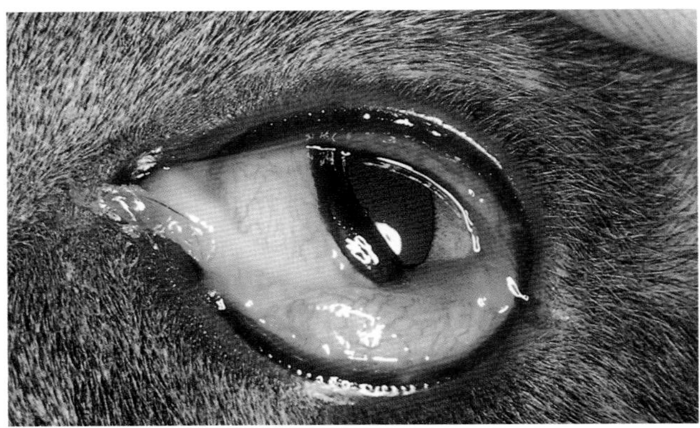

Fig. 8.27 *A 6-month-old Foreign Blue with conjunctivitis associated with calicivirus and Chlamydia psittaci infection.*

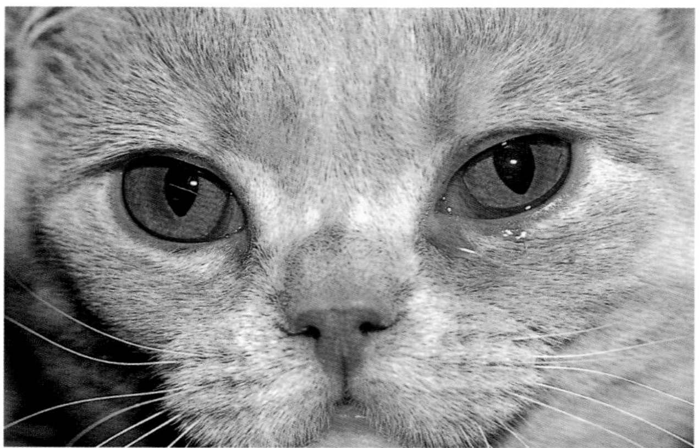

Fig. 8.28 *A 4-month-old British Silver Tabby with Chlamydia psittaci infection as a cause of conjunctivitis. The left eye is affected at this early stage, if left untreated, the right eye will also become affected within a matter of days.*

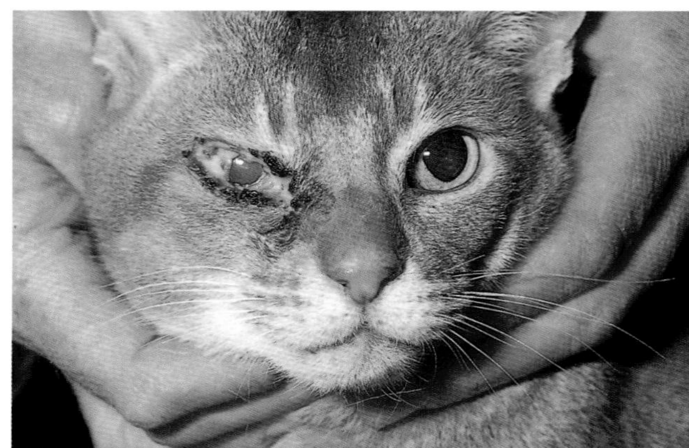

Fig. 8.31 *A 9-year-old Abyssinian. Mycoplasma felis was isolated from the right eye. The most notable feature of this case is the white pseudodiphtheritic membrane and the lack of obvious ocular discomfort.*

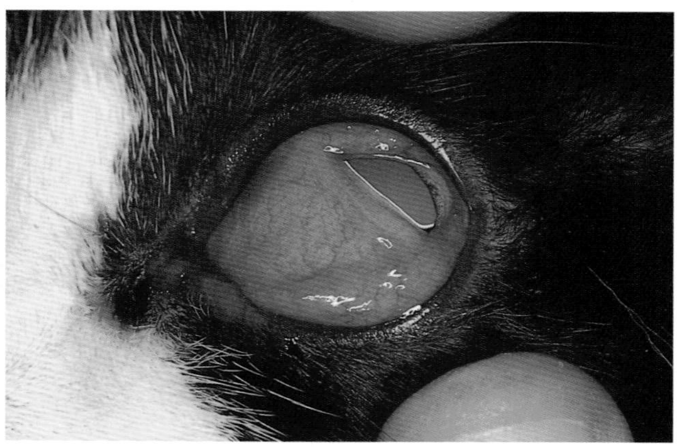

Fig. 8.29 *A 2-month-old Domestic shorthair with a more severe chlamydial conjunctivitis.*

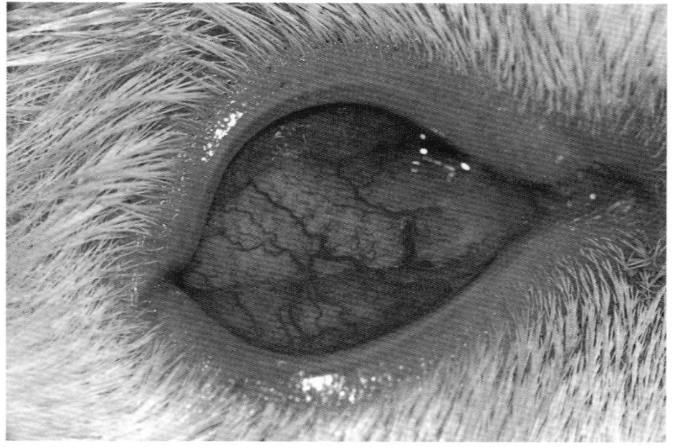

Fig. 8.32 *A 5-year-old Siamese with conjunctival reddening. The cat had a liver tumour and the appearance of the conjunctival vessels may be a result of the release of vasoactive substances by the tumour.*

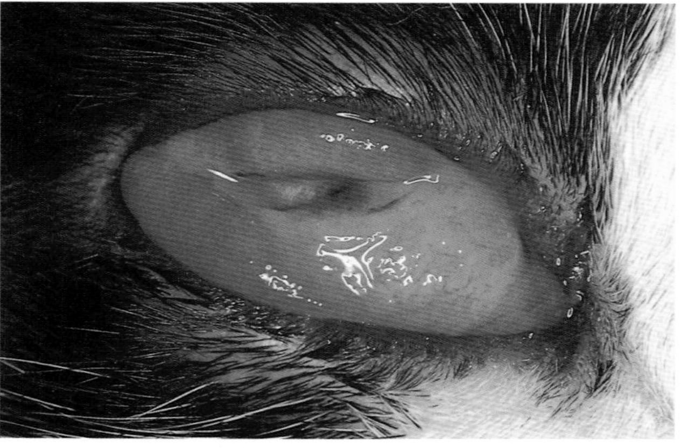

Fig. 8.30 *An 8-month-old Domestic shorthair. Acute unilateral conjunctivitis associated with Mycoplasma felis. Note the marked chemosis, conjunctival hyperaemia and conjunctival thickening.*

Mycotic conjunctivitis is occasionally seen in climates which support fungal growth and disseminated infections may also involve the eyelids and conjunctiva. Biopsy and culture are the easiest means of confirming the diagnosis and systemic treatment should be given with appropriate antifungal drugs. Predisposing factors include prolonged corticosteroid and antibiotic usage and treatment with these drugs should be withdrawn.

Thelaziasis caused by the nematode *Thelazia californiensis* has been identified in the western USA and can cause conjunctival irritation and hyperaemia (Knapp *et al.*, 1961). The thread-like worms can be removed with fine forceps after topical local anaesthesia.

Allergic conjunctivitis (Fig. 8.35) is most frequently encountered as a response to topically applied drugs, as previously described for allergic blepharitis and, less commonly, as a reaction to insect venom. Long-term treatment with

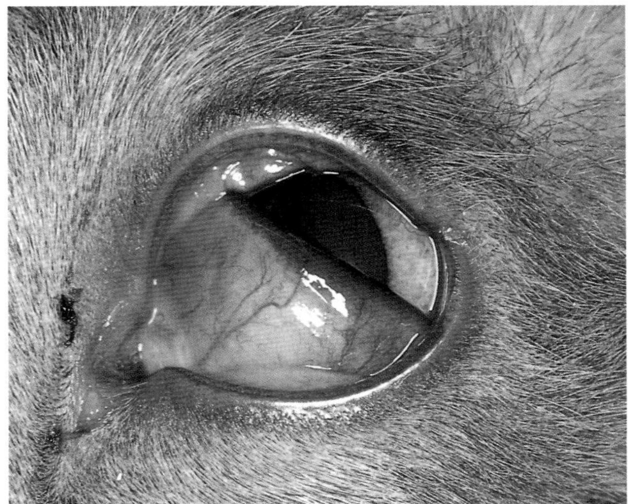

Fig. 8.33 A 10-month-old Domestic shorthair. Cyanosis in a cat with tetralogy of Fallot. Polycythaemia (packed cell volume 62) was present. The fundus of this cat is illustrated in Fig. 14.38.

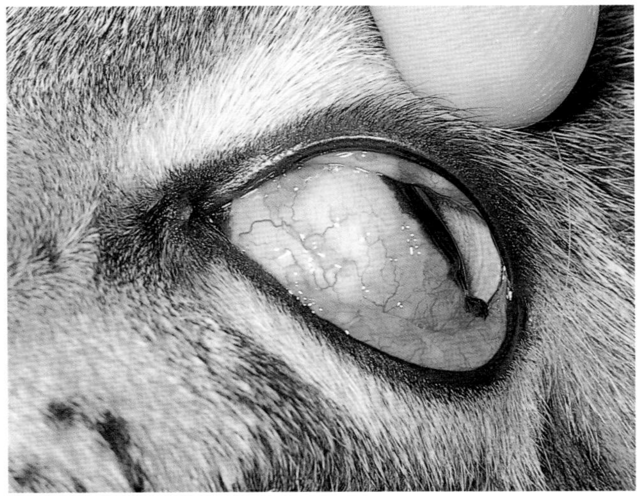

Fig. 8.34 An 8-month-old Domestic shorthair with chronic conjunctivitis. Note the numerous lymphoid follicles which are obvious on the palpebral and nictitating conjunctiva. This appearance is not pathognomonic for any specific type of conjunctivitis, it simply indicates chronicity.

topical preparations (e.g. tetracycline) is sometimes associated with periocular poliosis (see Chapter 5). Treatment consists of avoiding the allergen; topical antihistamines or corticosteroids can be given, but most cases have resolved completely by 12–48 h after removal from the allergen.

Foreign bodies, thermal and chemical insults constitute other causes of conjunctivitis (see Chapter 3). Thermal injuries are usually associated with the crippling effects of smoke inhalation and palliative therapy with a bland ophthalmic ointment is all that is required to prevent dessication of the conjunctiva and cornea while the more serious lung

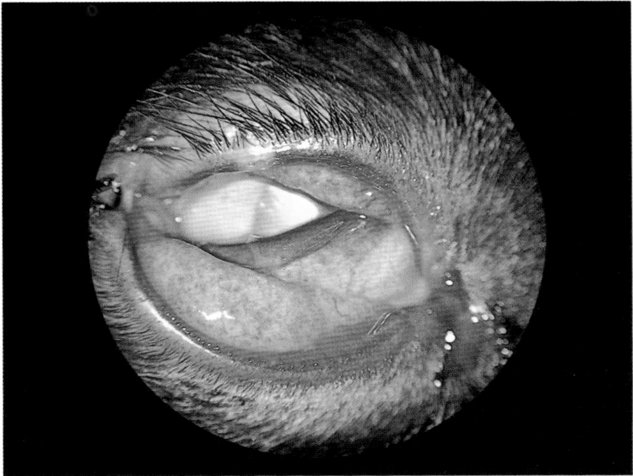

Fig. 8.35 A 2-year-old Burmese. Allergic conjunctivitis, an apparently acute hypersensitivity response to topical idoxuridine.

problems are treated. Chemical injuries are uncommon in cats and alkali burns usually damage the conjunctiva and cause symblepharon formation (Fig. 8.16).

Other primary causes of conjunctivitis are rare in cats, but the conjunctiva may become secondarily involved because of disease in neighbouring structures – for example, secondary to endophthalmitis, panophthalmitis, pre-ocular tear film abnormalities of production such as keratoconjunctivitis sicca and of drainage such as dacryocystitis, eyelid abnormalities, including iatrogenic absence of the third eyelid, sinusitis, orbital fractures and inflammatory diseases of the orbit.

The diagnosis of conjunctivitis is not difficult, but effective management depends upon establishing the precise aetiology and it is important to emphasize that respiratory tract viruses are widespread in the cat population and the presence of the virus must correlate with the clinical presentation and history. The history should include an assessment of the cat's age, vaccination status and lifestyle and whether there are other cats at risk or affected. Clinical appearance may be helpful, but is likely to be remarkably similar with a range of different causes.

Viral Conjunctivitis

Feline herpesvirus type 1 (FHV-1) is a common cause of ocular disease in the cat (Nasisse, 1982, 1990) and primary infection is associated with respiratory signs such as rhinitis, tracheitis and bronchopneumonia (feline viral rhinotracheitis) and also a range of ocular signs, which may be very mild or so severe that affected eyes are lost. Herpetic keratitis is described in Chapter 9.

In neonates (up to 4 weeks old) FHV-1 infection presents most commonly as bilateral conjunctivitis *(ophthalmia neonatorum)* and sometimes keratitis, and usually affects the entire litter (see Chapters 4 and 5). Microdendritic lesions are the only pathognomonic feature of primary infection but they are not always present and are difficult to visualize without magnification and staining with Rose Bengal, which should be applied after other diagnostic tests have been performed.

Complications of neonatal infection may be severe and include symblepharon formation as a result of conjunctival epithelial necrosis (Figs 8.6 and 8.7), corneal ulceration, corneal perforation, keratoconjunctivitis sicca, occluded lacrimal puncta and obliteration of the fornices (because of symblepharon), endophthalmitis and panophthalmitis.

Acute, usually bilateral, conjunctivitis is the most frequent ocular manifestation in older kittens and cats (Figs 8.24 and 8.25). Initially, the ocular discharge is serous but becomes purulent within a week of the onset of the clinical signs. Most cases also show signs of upper respiratory tract infection. Uncomplicated infections usually take about 2 weeks to resolve.

About 80% of affected cats become latently infected (Gaskell and Povey, 1977). Chronic asymptomatic carriers are relatively common and FHV-1 may be isolated from a small proportion of healthy cats (Coutts *et al.*, 1994); for numerous reasons it may be difficult to confirm feline herpesvirus in chronic cases.

Recrudescence of infection is a particular problem in chronically infected cats and any form of stress (e.g. rehoming, cat shows, introduction of new cats, lactation, general anaesthesia and surgery), endogenous immunosuppression (e.g. FeLV and FIV) and exogenous immunosuppression (e.g. corticosteroids, cyclosporin and chemotherapy) may produce a relapse. The clinical signs in chronically affected cats are diverse; they include epiphora, low-grade conjunctivitis and ulcerative and nonulcerative keratitis (see Chapter 9).

Commonly used diagnostic laboratory tests have limitations (e.g. immunofluorescence and serology), usually because of their lack of sensitivity, especially in relation to chronic infections. Viral isolation can provide definitive diagnosis of acute infections, but is not sufficiently sensitive for chronic infections. The polymerase chain reaction (PCR) is a sensitive and specific technique for identifying FHV-1 DNA (Nasisse and Weigler, 1997) and a positive PCR result for FHV-1 probably equates with naturally occurring herpetic conjunctivitis (Stiles *et al.*, 1996). PCR is used to identify FHV-1 DNA in the USA, but not, at present, in the UK.

The treatment of conjunctivitis associated with primary infection is largely supportive (rehydration and careful nutrition) and symptomatic. Topical antiviral treatment is not indicated for acute conjunctivitis. Nasal and ocular discharges should be removed by regular, gentle cleaning and topical antibiotic applied to control secondary bacterial infection. White petroleum jelly can be smeared below the eyes to prevent skin excoriation. A systemic broad-spectrum antibiotic (e.g. amoxicillin by mouth) will also be needed when secondary bacterial infection is present. The treatment regimes for chronic infections are described in Chapter 9.

If keratoconjunctivitis sicca is present, tear replacement therapy (e.g. 0.2% polyacrylic acid; 0.2% w/w Carbomer 940) will be required until tear production is adequate. Occasionally, parotid duct transposition is needed in the long term.

Feline calicivirus (FCV) can affect cats of all ages, but infection is more common and most severe in young kittens. It typically presents as a serous conjunctivitis and rhinitis, secondary bacterial infection often complicates the situation (Figs 8.26 and 8.27). Mouth and nasal ulcers are common but ulcers may be present in other sites, such as the feet, on rare occasions.

Definitive diagnosis is obtained by isolation of the virus from conjunctival and oropharyngeal swabs. Infected animals continue to excrete virus for protracted periods and chronic carrier states can occur, such that FCV can be isolated from a proportion of healthy cats (Coutts *et al.*, 1994). Because the virus is excreted constantly it is relatively easy to confirm infection in animals which have the clinical signs outlined above.

The treatment of conjunctivitis associated with feline calicivirus is similar to the symptomatic treatment described for acute FHV-1.

Feline pox virus is an unusual cause of conjunctivitis (see Chapter 5).

Bacterial Conjunctivitis

Chlamydia psittaci (an obligate intracellular bacterium) is the most important of the feline conjunctival pathogens and the clinical signs may be observed in cats from 4 weeks old onwards (Wills, 1988). Clinical signs are of a unilateral conjunctivitis initially, which becomes bilateral several days later (Figs 8.28 and 8.29). Initially, there is a serous discharge with obvious chemosis and conjunctival hyperaemia, later the discharge can become mucopurulent and other organisms may be isolated. There is no corneal involvement and no primary respiratory disease, although mild rhinitis may be present. In a proportion of cases both respiratory tract viruses and *Chlamydia psittaci* will be isolated. Lymphoid follicle formation is common in chronic cases.

Diagnosis is confirmed by chlamydial isolation from swabs taken into VCTM and from conjunctival scrapings to demonstrate intracytoplasmic inclusion bodies in Giemsa and Gram-stained material. Intracytoplasmic inclusion bodies can be difficult to differentiate from intracytoplasmic pigment granules. Serology is of limited value in unvaccinated cats and of no value in vaccinated animals.

Treatment consists of topical tetracycline or systemic doxycycline for some 3–4 weeks. Oral treatment with doxycycline (25 mg/kg in divided doses) is well tolerated and effective.

A proportion of previously infected cats become chronic carriers and may be a possible source of infection for other cats (the organism can be isolated from the urogenital and gastrointestinal tract). This may pose problems in catteries, especially for breeding colonies. In this type of environment all the cats will require systemic tetracyline, erythromycin or doxycycline for at least 4 weeks. Systemic doxycycline is probably the drug of choice and is also suitable for younger cats.

Mycoplasma felis is recorded as an occasional cause of conjunctivitis, although the pathogenicity of the organism is equivocal, particularly as the condition is self-limiting and usually resolves within 30 days, although the cat may remain infectious for up to 60 days. *Mycoplasma felis* can be isolated from the conjunctiva of both normal cats and those with conjunctivitis, so it is important to ensure that no other potential pathogens are present in suspect cases. The clinical appearance is often spectacular as chemosis, hyperaemia and conjunctival thickening are marked (Fig. 8.30). Slit lamp examination may reveal papillary hypertrophy in the initial stages. In an untreated case the hyperaemia becomes less obvious after 14 days and the conjunctiva becomes pale with a friable white diphtheritic membrane (pseudomembrane) as an obvious feature (Fig. 8.31).

Confirmation of the diagnosis is usually obtained by culturing the organism from conjunctival swabs, but it is important to inform the diagnostic laboratory that *Mycoplasma* spp. is suspected so that the correct culture medium is selected. The samples should also be checked for respiratory viruses and *C. psittaci*. Mycoplasma is sensitive to topical tetracylines or systemic doxycline which shorten the clinical course to less than 1 week.

Other bacteria identified such as *Pasteurella* spp., *Staphylococcal* spp., *Streptococcus* spp., *Salmonella* spp., *Moraxella* spp.) are of uncertain pathogenicity. Any underlying primary problem should be identified and eliminated and appropriate antibiotic therapy initiated for the bacterial conjunctivitis.

MEIBOMIANITIS

See Chapter 5.

KERATOCONJUNCTIVITIS SICCA

See Chapter 7.

PROLIFERATIVE KERATOCONJUNCTIVITIS

See Chapter 9.

CONJUNCTIVAL TRAUMA AND FOREIGN BODIES

See Chapter 3.

CONJUNCTIVAL NEOPLASIA

A number of tumours may involve the conjunctiva (they can also involve the eyelids); they include squamous cell carcinoma (see Chapter 5), papilloma, adenoma, adenocarcinoma, fibrosarcoma (Fig. 8.36), haemangioma, haemangiosarcoma and primary melanoma (Williams *et al.*, 1981; Cook *et al.*, 1985).

Lymphosarcoma is the commonest secondary neoplasm to infiltrate the conjunctiva and involvement may be bilateral (Figs 8.37–8.39).

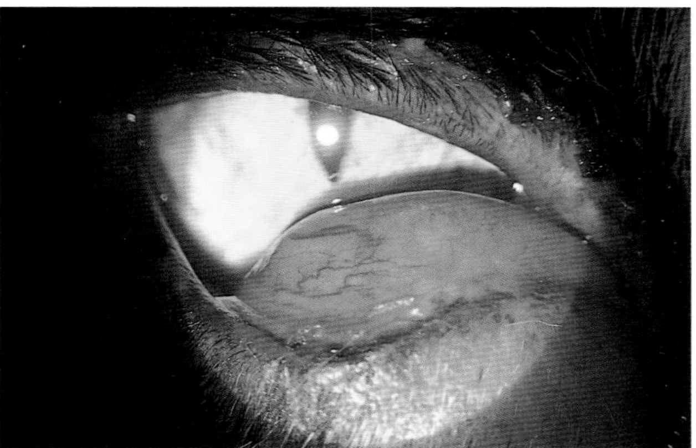

Fig. 8.36 *A 10-year-old Domestic shorthair with a fibrosarcoma of the conjunctiva of the lower eyelid.*

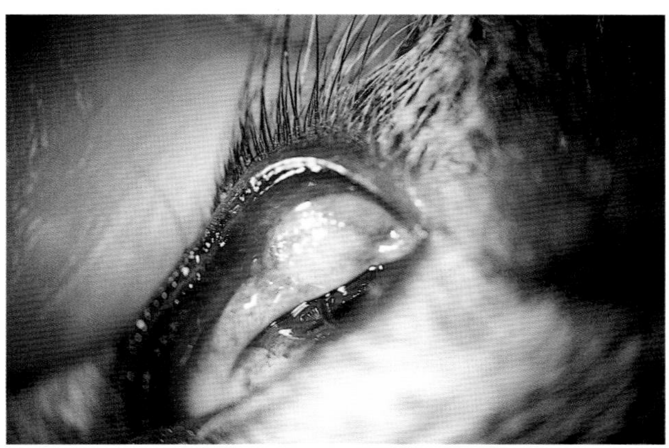

Fig. 8.37 *A 3-year-old Domestic shorthair with generalized lymphosarcoma, with infiltration of the conjunctiva of the outer aspect of the upper eyelid (see also Fig. 14.79 of the same cat).*

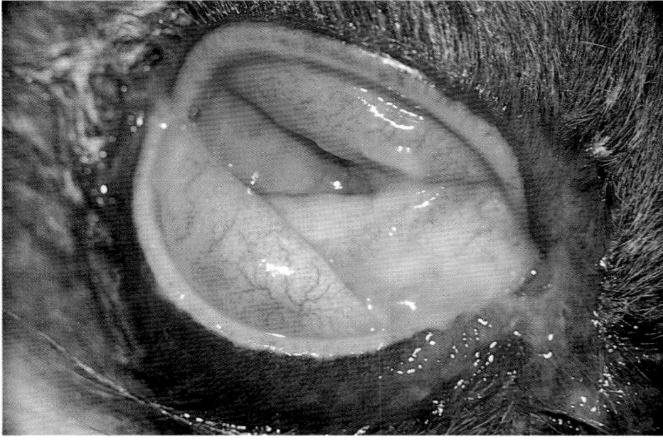

Fig. 8.38 *An 8-year-old Persian neutered male. Generalized lymphosarcoma with infiltration of the conjunctiva, sclera and cornea. In addition, Chlamydia psittaci was isolated from the conjunctival sac and the cat was also FeLV positive.*

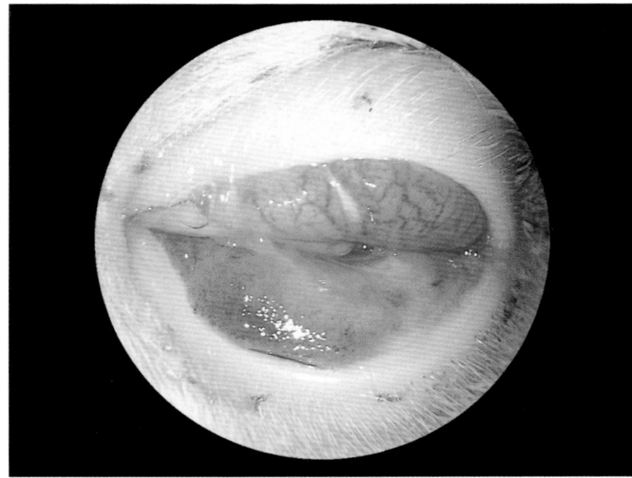

Fig. 8.39 A 13-year-old British white. Generalized lymphosarcoma with infiltration of the conjunctiva.

Assessment depends upon careful examination of the eye, adnexa and the rest of the animal.

For primary neoplasia the treatment is usually surgical excision, debulking, or biopsy combined with other therapy (e.g. radiotherapy, cryotherapy, laser therapy). For secondary neoplasia, treatment other than palliative treatment may not be a realistic option.

Disorders of the limbus, episclera and sclera

The limbus is an important transition zone between the ordered austerity of the transparent cornea and the 'white' of the eye (Fig. 1.3) which is composed of semitransparent bulbar conjunctiva overlying the predominantly collagenous episclera and sclera (Fig. 8.40). It is the site of the pluripotential limbal stem cells which play such a critical role in the healing processes of the ocular surface.

Abnormal limbal appearance

The poor differentiation of the limbus associated with symblepharon has been discussed above and there are other problems of differentiation, most notably inherited connective tissue disorders and anterior segment dysgenesis which affect this area (Fig. 8.41).

Excessive limbal pigmentation is sometimes an incidental finding in cats which have suffered nonspecific perinatal insult and chronic keratitis (Fig. 8.42).

Inflammatory problems

Limbal-based inflammations are rare in cats (Fig. 8.43) and unlike humans and dogs, episcleritis and scleritis do not appear as specific disease entities in cats. Eosinophilic infiltrates occur at a variety of sites, including the conjunctiva; they are discussed in Chapter 9.

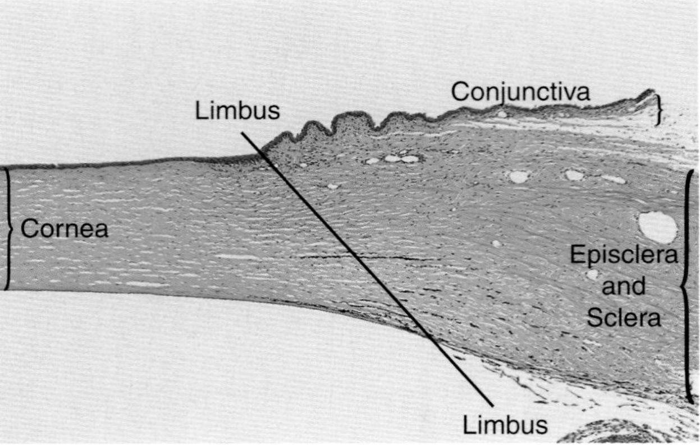

Fig. 8.40 Histological section of the normal feline limbus stained with haematoxylin and eosin. The cornea is to the left and the conjunctiva with underlying episclera and sclera to the right. There is a fairly abrupt transition between the smooth corneal epithelium and the corrugated conjunctival epithelium at the limbus. Blood vessels and sparse pigmentation are obvious on the right, they are absent on the left. Portions of pectinate ligament are apparent in the bottom right hand corner of the figure.

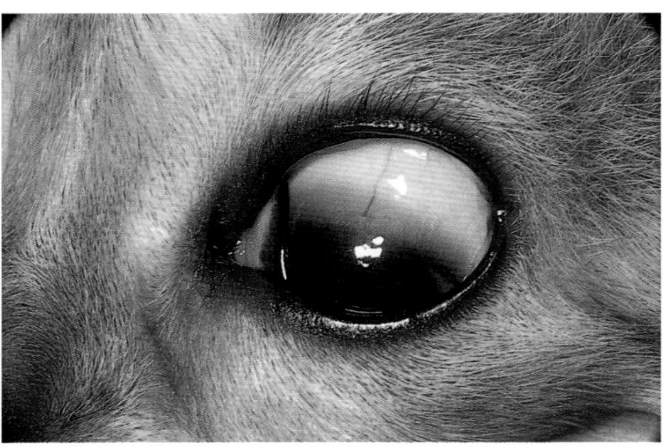

Fig. 8.41 A 4-month-old Bengal female with anterior segment dysgenesis. Note the poor limbal differentiation and the single conjunctival vessel traversing this area. Histopathology indicated that goblet cells were present in the peripheral cornea.

Trauma

see Chapter 3.

Neoplasia

The limbus is a rare site for primary neoplasia. Limbal epibulbar melanoma (scleral shelf melanoma) is the most frequently encountered neoplasm and is a benign, well-circumscribed and slow-growing tumour (Figs 8.44 and 8.45). Other tumours in this region are very rare and include fibrosarcoma (Fig. 8.46).

Regular observation, with intervention if size increases, using radiotherapy (β irradiation), laser therapy or cryotherapy after excisional biopsy, or complete excision, are the

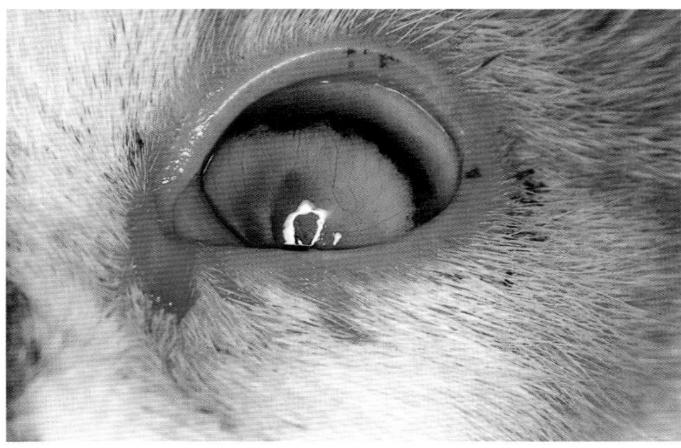

Fig. 8.42 *A 3-year-old Domestic shorthair, with pigmentation at the limbus associated with chronic keratitis (previous penetrating injury) and ocular surface changes. The pigmentation is at the level of the sparse pigment described in Figure 8.40.*

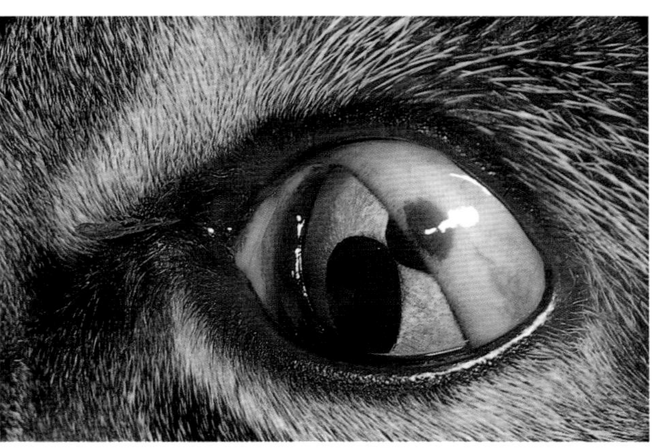

Fig. 8.44 *A 3-year-old Domestic shorthair with limbal epibulbar melanoma. Treated by surgical bebulking and cryotherapy with liquid nitrogen.*

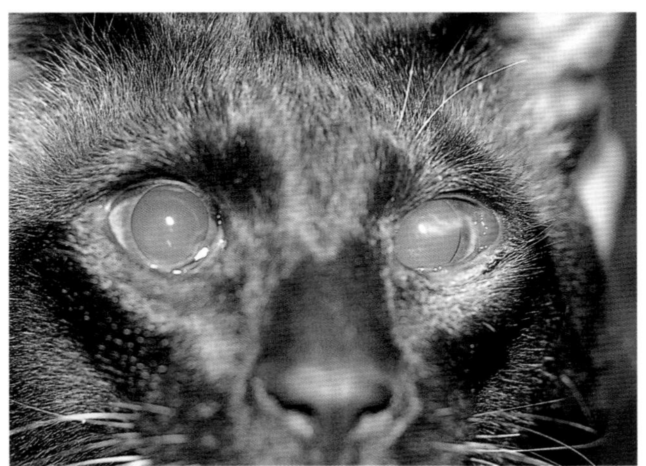

Fig. 8.43 *A 13-year-old Siamese neutered male with nodular inflammation at the lateral limbus of the left eye. The cause was unknown. Excisional biopsy indicated a granulomatous inflammation. Complete resolution followed a short course of topical corticosteroid.*

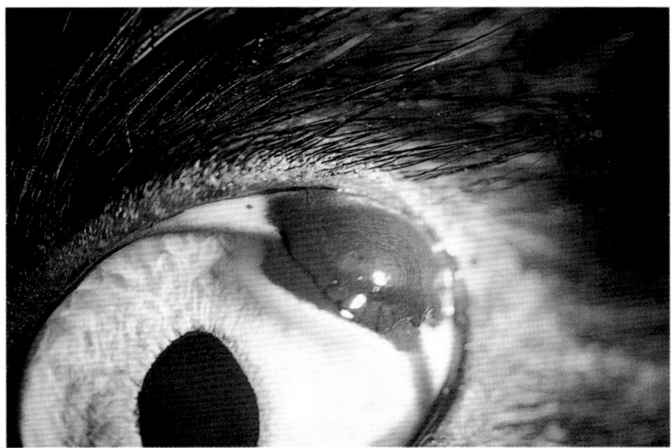

Fig. 8.45 *An 11-year-old Domestic longhair with limbal epibulbar melanoma. Treated with β-irradiation.*

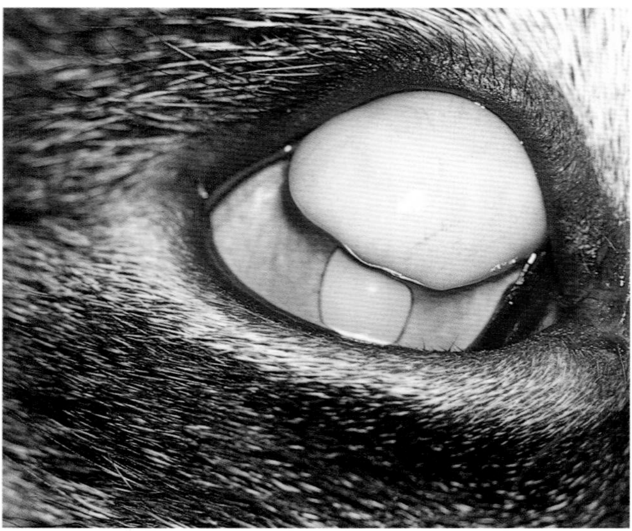

Fig. 8.46 *A 4-year-old Domestic shorthair. Fibrosarcoma arising in the dorsal perilimbal region and invading the cornea; the mass had been removed previously without histology being performed and it had returned within 1 month. The tumour was removed surgically (keratectomy and conjunctivectomy) and no recurrence was reported.*

possible ways of managing scleral shelf melanoma. Other tumours in this region should be assessed and treated according to their size and growth pattern.

Lymphosarcoma is the commonest secondary tumour encountered in this region. For example, scleral deposits of lymphosarcoma can occur, but are often obscured by similar deposits in the conjunctiva (Fig. 8.38). Affected eyes are red and painful and biopsy is diagnostic.

References

Carrington SD (1985) Observations on the structure and function of the feline cornea. Ph.D. thesis, University of Liverpool, UK.

Cook CS, Rosenkrantz W, Peiffer RL, MacMillan A (1985) Malignant melanoma of the conjunctiva in a cat. *Journal of the American Veterinary Medical Association* **186**: 505–506.

Coutts AJ, Dawson S, Willoughby K, Gaskell RM (1994) Isolation of feline respiratory viruses from clinically healthy cats at UK cat shows. *Veterinary Record* **135**: 555–556.

Espinola MB, Lilenbaum W (1996) Prevalence of bacteria in the conjunctival sac and on the eyelid margin of clinically normal cats. *Journal of Small Animal Practice* **37**: 364–366.

Gaskell RM, Povey RC (1977) Experimental induction of feline viral rhinotracheitis virus re-excretion in FVR-recovered cats. *Veterinary Record* **100**: 128–133.

Knapp SE, Bailey RB, Bailey DE (1961) Thelaziasis in cats and dogs – a case report. *Journal of the American Veterinary Medical Association* **138**: 537–538.

Mustardé JC (ed.) (1991) *Repair and Reconstruction in the Orbital Region, 3rd edn.* Churchill Livingstone, Edinburgh.

Nasisse MP (1982) Manifestations, diagnosis and treatment of ocular herpesvirus infection in the cat. *Compendium on Continuing Education for the Practicing Veterinarian* **4**: 962–970.

Nasisse MP, Weigler BJ (1997) The diagnosis of ocular feline herpesvirus infection. *Veterinary and Comparative Ophthalmology* **7**: 44–51.

Nasisse MP (1990) Feline herpesvirus ocular disease. *Veterinary Clinics of North America: Small Animal Practice* **29**: 667–680.

Stiles J, McDermott M, Willis M, Martin C, Roberts W, Greene C (1996) Use of nested polymerase chain reaction to identify feline herpesvirus in ocular tissue from clinically normal cats and cats with corneal sequestra or conjunctivitis. *Proceedings of the American College of Veterinary Ophthalmologists* **27**: 82.

Weigler BJ, Babinaeu CA, Sherry B, Nasisse M. (1997) A polymerase chain reaction for studies involving the epidemiology and pathogenesis of feline herpesvirus type 1. *Veterinary Record* **140**: 335–338.

Williams LW, Gelatt KN, Gwinn RM (1981) Ophthalmic neoplasms in the cat. *Journal of the American Animal Hospital Association* **17**: 999–1008.

Wills JM (1988) Feline chlamydial infection (feline pneumonitis). *Advances in Small Animal Practice* **1**: 182–190.

9 Cornea

Introduction

The cornea and sclera consist predominantly of collagen and it is this fibrous 'tunic' which maintains the shape of the globe (Fig. 1.1). Whereas the sclera is white, the cornea is transparent (Figs 1.2–1.3) and this remarkable appearance is largely achieved by very precise spacing between the uniform diameter collagen fibrils that make up the lamellae of the corneal stroma.

The adult cat's cornea is almost circular with a mean horizontal diameter of 16.5 mm (SD ± 0.60 mm), which is slightly greater than the vertical diameter of 16.2 mm (SD ± 0.61 mm) (Carrington, 1985). There is some variation with age, breed and sex. The cornea fills most of the palpebral aperture and has a marked convexity (radius of curvature approximately 9 mm). Corneal thickness, as measured with ultrasonic pachymetry, is not uniform, being thicker temporally and subperiaxially and thinnest in the dorsonasal quadrant (Schoster *et al.*, 1995). Corneal thickness is approximately 0.75 mm in the normal deturgescent state (Carrington and Woodward, 1986).

The cornea is derived embryologically from surface ectoderm and mesenchyme. There is experimental evidence in other species that some at least of the mesenchyme is derived from pluripotent neural crest cells. Structurally, the cornea comprises an outer epithelium of approximately six layers thick, composed of a basal layer of epithelial cells which become relatively more flattened (stratified squamous) as they move anteriorly. A basement membrane separates the epithelial cell layer from the underlying stroma (substantia propria). Stroma accounts for some 90% of the corneal thickness and is composed of orthogonally arranged bundles or lamellae of collagen fibrils which cross the entire diameter of the cornea from limbus to limbus. A proteoglycan ground substance separates the collagen fibrils and both the ground substance and collagen are produced by stromal fibroblasts (keratocytes). The posterior surface of the cornea is formed by a single layer of endothelial cells and these cells produce a collagenous basement membrane known as Descemet's membrane located between the substantia propria and the endothelial cell layer (Fig. 9.1). The entire epithelium turns over in about 7 days whereas the endothelial cells have a very limited regenerative capacity.

The normal cornea is free of obvious opacity and is of lustrous appearance; there should be no disruption of a reflected image (the corneal reflex) anywhere on its surface (Fig. 1.3); an abnormal corneal reflex indicates a pre-ocular tear film and/or corneal abnormality. While the normal cornea is devoid of blood vessels and lymphatics, there is a rich supply of fine unmyelinated nerves derived from the ophthalmic division of the trigeminal nerve. Pain is often a prominent feature of corneal disease.

Normal epithelium is impermeable to water, electrolytes, nutrients, metabolites and most micro-organisms, but is

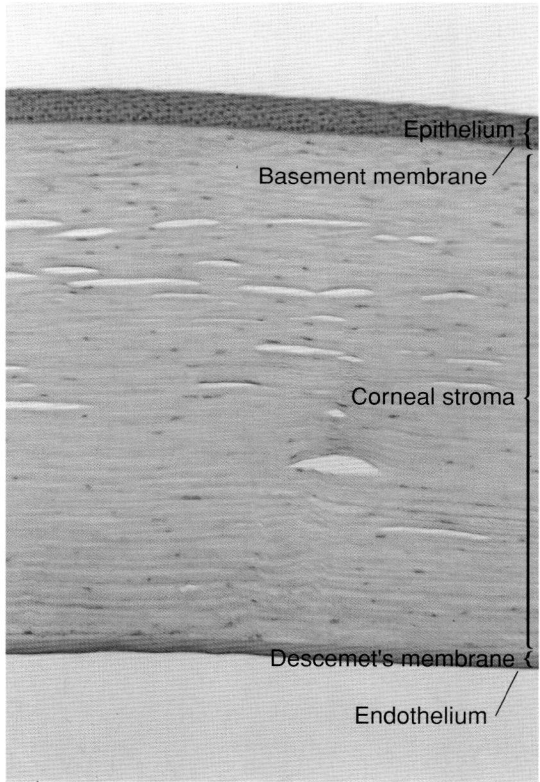

Fig. 9.1 *Histological section of the normal feline cornea. The anterior epithelium is 5–6 cell layers thick and rests on an inconspicuous basement membrane. The majority of the cornea consists of the stroma which consists of collagen, ground substance and keratocytes. A single layer of closely packed endothelial cells comprise the posterior limiting layer. Descemet's membrane, the basement membrane of the endothelium, is obvious but thin in this young cat; it will become thicker with age.*

permeable to oxygen and carbon dioxide. The endothelium is semipermeable, allowing nutrients to enter and metabolites to leave. Corneal nutrition is therefore derived from the aqueous and perilimbal vessels and not from the tear film, whereas gaseous diffusion can take place via the tear film, aqueous and perilimbal vessels.

The epithelium and endothelium are the most actively metabolizing layers of the cornea. The endothelium is more active than the epithelium because it has large energy requirements to sustain the pump mechanism which transports water out of the stroma and so maintains corneal transparency. An active pumping mechanism in the corneal endothelial cells is critical in maintaining the cornea in a slightly dehydrated state and the epithelium may also possess a similar, but less important, water-pumping activity. If the endothelial pump fails to work properly then stromal oedema develops; the affected cornea becomes thicker and less transparent as water enters, and the oedema is resolved only if normal endothelial function is restored to pump the water out through the posterior surface of the cornea. Minor trauma to the epithelium produces mild stromal oedema beneath the lesion which resolves once epithelial integrity returns. Oedema is a feature of many corneal abnormalities but is not a specific disease entity.

Corneal wound healing

Epithelial damage is repaired by sliding of the outer stratified squamous cells; these migrate across the stroma as a flattened sheet of single cells within hours of the injury. Hemidesmosomes and intercellular contacts also reform during the early stages of re-epithelialization, but the anchoring fibrils which ensure firm adhesion between epithelium, basement membrane and anterior stroma do not appear for days and this may explain, in part, the phenomenon of recurrent erosion. Epithelial mitosis largely takes place at the limbus where the mitotic activity of limbal stem cells is crucial.

Stromal damage is repaired with help from the epithelial cells (which fill the defect) and by generation from the stromal elements (fibroblasts derived from resting keratocytes produce collagen and ground substance). The type of collagen which is laid down in damaged stroma differs from the original collagen in type and orientation so the transparency of the cornea is lost in the affected area. Neovascularization is usual when the stroma is damaged by, for example, infection, trauma or chemicals. Clean wounds of the cornea heal by avascular scarring. More fibrous tissue is laid down when neovascularization accompanies wound healing.

Descemet's membrane is highly elastic in cats and a descemetocoele represents the anterior bulging of the intact membrane, whereas rupture is followed by retraction due also to the membrane's elastic nature. Reduplication can occur from endothelial cells which slide in over the injured area.

Endothelial damage is repaired by hypertrophy and migration of the single layer of cells; there is no capacity for mitotic regeneration in the adult cat. It is, however, important to emphasize that the functional reserve of the endothelium is considerable and it has been suggested that up to 80% of the cells may be lost in the human cornea before corneal decompensation becomes inevitable.

Diseases of the cornea

Epibulbar dermoid

While the commonest site for dermoids is skin and conjunctiva in the region of the lateral canthus (see Chapters 5 and 8), corneal involvement is not unusual (Fig. 9.2) and can be extensive in area, but not in depth, allowing these masses to be removed by superficial keratectomy. The surgery is simplified if a bridle suture is passed through the dermoid to allow easy manipulation. Suturing is not required unless a lateral canthotomy has been performed to improve exposure.

Microcornea and megalocornea

Problems of this type are unusual as distinct entities because, by definition, no other ocular abnormalities can be present. Microcornea is a cornea which is smaller than normal and megalocornea is a cornea which is larger than normal. In both conditions the abnormalities are congenital, bilateral and nonprogressive.

Other ocular diseases such as microphthalmos (see Chapter 4), or buphthalmos (see Chapter 10) associated with congenital glaucoma, commonly result in corneas which are smaller or larger than normal, respectively. The effects of infectious agents (e.g. FHV-1) should be considered when litters are born with multiple ocular anomalies which include corneal abnormality.

The cornea may also look abnormally small when there are limbal and perilimbal anomalies; for example, some

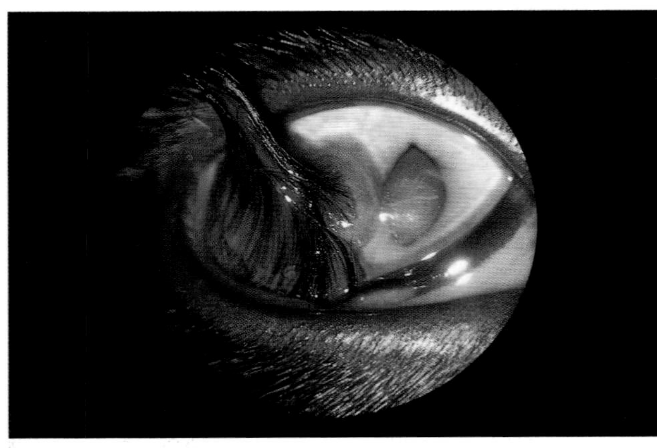

Fig. 9.2 *A 16-week-old Domestic shorthair with a large epibulbar dermoid involving the lower lateral conjunctival limbus and lateral cornea. The dermoid was surgically removed.*

forms of anterior segment dysgenesis (see Chapter 8) and inherited connective tissue disorders (Fig. 9.3).

Persistent pupillary membrane

Persistent pupillary membrane remnants (see Chapters 2 and 12) may sometimes attach to the posterior cornea, producing localized, or more generalized, opacity at the point of contact. They are usually of no significance and should be left alone.

Keratoconus and keratoglobus

Keratoconus, a consequence of bilateral central thinning of the cornea, has been reported sporadically as a possible primary corneal dystrophy, or in association with other ocular defects such as lenticonus.

Keratoglobus is usually a consequence of limbal to limbal corneal thinning such that the cornea protrudes (Fig. 9.4). Both keratoconus and keratoglobus may develop in cases of endothelial dystrophy (see below).

Lysosomal storage disorders

Diffuse corneal clouding is a feature of a number of neurometabolic storage diseases (Figs 9.5 and 9.6); including mucopolysaccharidosis I, mucopolysaccharidosis VI, mucopolysaccharidosis VII, GM_1 gangliosidosis, GM_2 gangliosidosis and mannosidosis. Specific enzyme deficiencies lead to the accumulation of abnormal products within the cell lysosomes and the disorders are classified according to the substrate that accumulates (Haskins and Patterson, 1987).

Diagnosis is made on clinical grounds (mainly neurological and ocular signs, although facial dysmorphia may also be part of the clinical picture in mucopolysaccharidosis I, VI, VII and mannosidosis), from examination of peripheral blood smears for lymphocyte vacuolation and microscopic examination of biopsy material. Enzyme activity analysis of peripheral leukocytes and cultured fibroblasts can provide definitive diagnosis.

The prognosis is poor as these disorders are progressive and debilitating. Gene therapy offers the only means of attempting to correct the underlying enzyme defect in affected animals; however, the use of oral evening primrose oil, if started early, may ameliorate the severity of the clinical signs in some cases.

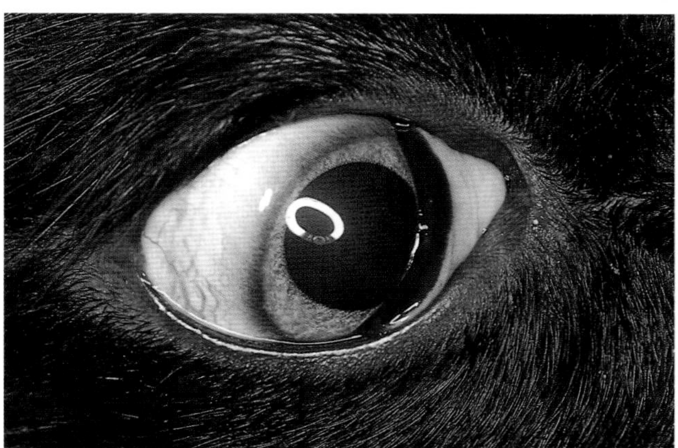

Fig. 9.3 *A 6-month-old Domestic shorthair with cutaneous asthenia, in this case caused by deficient procollagen peptidase activity. Both eyes are affected, the cornea is smaller than normal (microcornea) and the sclera in the perilimbal region blue.*

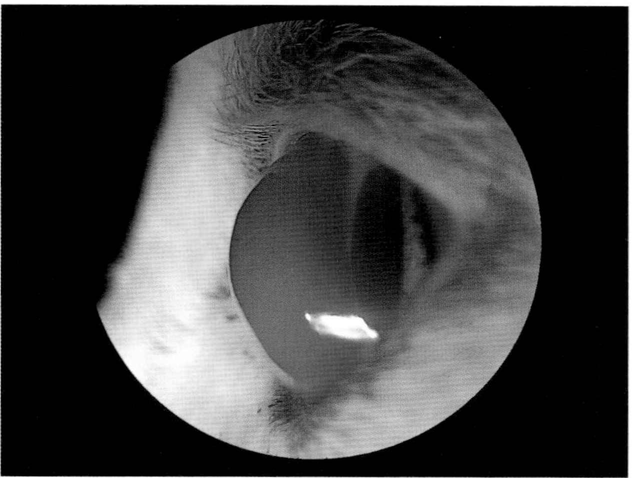

Fig. 9.4 *An 11-month-old Domestic shorthair with keratoglobus associated with endothelial dystrophy. In this case the peripheral cornea is still clear, whereas the central cornea is oedematous. (Courtesy of D.D. Lawson)*

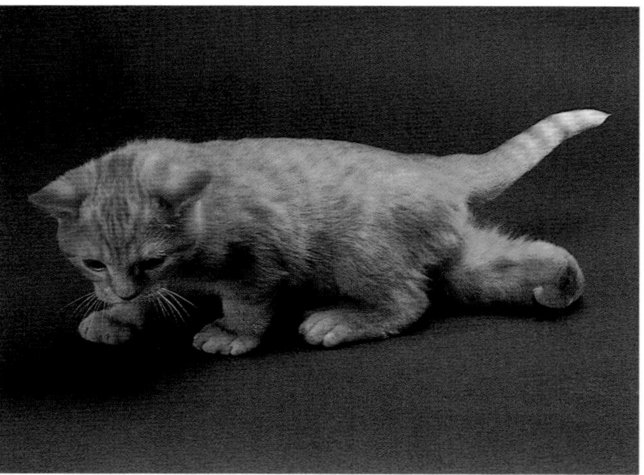

Fig. 9.5 *A male 3-month-old Domestic shorthair with lysosomal storage disease. In this kitten with mucopolysaccharidosis there is corneal clouding, facial dysmorphia (a broad, flattened face) and the paws appear disproportionately large. The kitten was small relative to normal litter mates, there was an abnormal hindlimb gait at the time of presentation and proprioceptive reflexes were slow (see also Chapter 15).*

Stromal corneal dystrophy in the Manx cat

A progressive form of corneal dystrophy which is apparently inherited as a simple autosomal recessive has been described in a group of closely inbred Stump-tailed Manx cats (Bistner *et al.*, 1976).

The dystrophy is first apparent at about 4 months old, when bilateral corneal clouding becomes evident. Over a period of months the whole of the cornea may become oedematous and, in some cases, bullous keratopathy with subsequent erosion of the epithelium can occur.

The most obvious histopathological feature is oedema of the anterior corneal stroma with swelling and disintegration of the collagen fibrils. Changes also occur in the corneal epithelium and basement membrane but these are thought to be secondary to the stromal oedema. Extensive vesicle formation may be observed in the epithelium with coalescence of the small vesicles to form large vacuoles, so that epithelial oedema is particularly marked in the central, axial, region of the cornea. The endothelium is of normal appearance.

There is no specific treatment, although penetrating keratoplasty may be of benefit.

Endothelial corneal dystrophy in the Domestic shorthair

A progressive, bilateral and severe endothelial dystrophy is occasionally encountered in short-haired Domestic cats. While cases have only been seen in inbred animals the mode of inheritance is unknown. Only the cornea is affected and the cats are normal in other respects (Crispin, 1982).

Stromal oedema may be detected as early as 3–4 weeks, beginning centrally and spreading towards the limbus, but with perilimbal sparing. Keratoconus (central stromal thinning) and keratoglobus (limbus-to-limbus stromal thinning) are frequent complications (Figs 9.4 and 9.7).

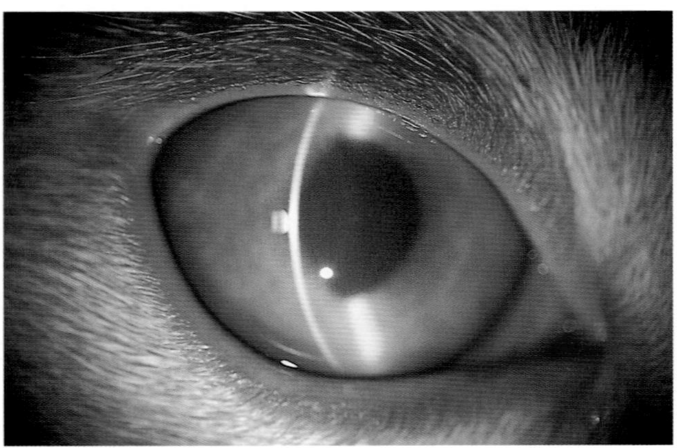

Fig. 9.6 *The same kitten as shown in Fig. 9.5. Corneal clouding (because of the abnormal accumulation of mucopolysaccharides in corneal cells) is an important clinical feature of the condition and the slit lamp appearance is illustrated here.*

The earliest pathological change is probably in the central corneal endothelium. The cytoplasm of the endothelial cells becomes vacuolated (a change which is especially marked in the endothelial cytoplasm closest to Descemet's membrane). Towards the limbus the endothelial cells are of normal appearance.

Endothelial dysfunction results in stromal oedema and an increase in stromal thickness. The corneal epithelium shows no abnormality early in the disease but later becomes thinner than normal with a reduced number of layers; a change of corneal profile is clinically evident at this stage. Bullous keratopathy is a late complication and corneal decompensation may follow.

There is no specific treatment but penetrating keratoplasty may be of benefit.

Acute bullous keratopathy

In this syndrome there is acute, severe, bullous keratopathy of unknown aetiopathogenesis (Fig. 9.8). Young cats are most commonly affected and the problem is usually

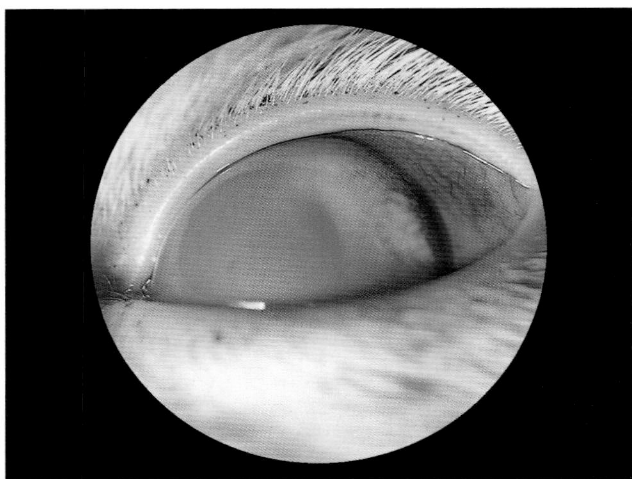

Fig. 9.7 *Endothelial dystrophy (the same cat as shown in Fig. 9.4). (Courtesy of D.D. Lawson)*

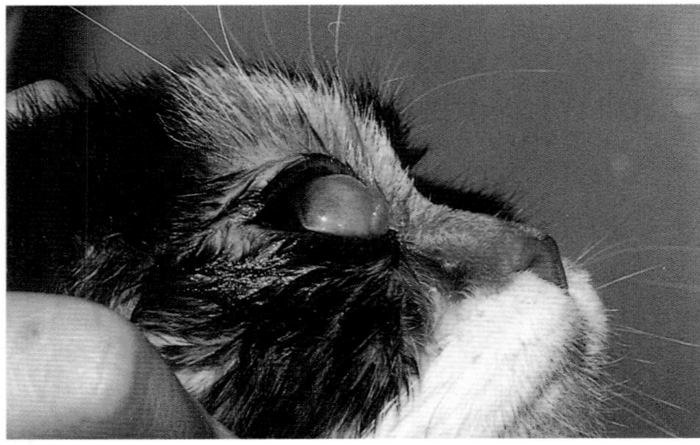

Fig. 9.8 *Domestic shorthair. Bullous keratopathy (courtesy of M. C. A. King).*

bilateral. The lesions either resolve with little or no scarring or progress rapidly to corneal perforation. A conjunctival pedicle graft is usually an effective means of preventing corneal perforation if applied sufficiently early (Glover *et al.*, 1994). Thermokeratoplasty may also be of benefit.

Feline keratitis

Keratitis (inflammation of the cornea) may be ulcerative and nonulcerative in type. Both types are relatively common in cats. There are a number of important differences between keratitis in the cat and dog. The level of corneal vascularization is easy to appreciate in dogs, as superficial vessels arising from conjunctival vessels may be followed to the cornea where they cross the limbus, but deep vessels arising from the ciliary plexus are only visible once they are within the cornea. In the cat both superficial and deep vessels may only be apparent as they enter the cornea (Fig. 9.9) and careful observation is necessary to determine the level of vascularization. Chemosis is often dramatic in cats because of the loose nature of the feline conjuctiva (see Chapter 8). Corneal pigmentation as a response to insult is rare in cats, except for the changes in limbal pigment which are sometimes a feature of perinatal problems and chronic keratitis (see Chapter 8). Scarring of the cornea tends to be less severe in cats than dogs. Lipid deposition is much less common in cats than dogs and, when it does occur, it is almost always in the form of lipid keratopathy.

Feline herpesvirus-1 (FHV-1) is a primary corneal pathogen in the cat, there is no primary pathogen in the dog. Proliferative (eosinophilic) keratoconjunctivitis and sequestrum formation are both relatively common feline problems without a canine equivalent.

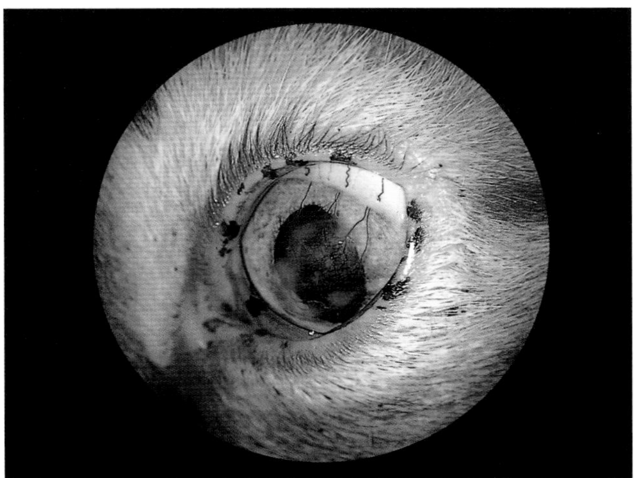

Fig. 9.9 *A 5-year-old Domestic shorthair. Superficial vascularization associated with multiple ulcers and stained with fluorescein. Note that the blood vessels are only apparent when they have entered the cornea, they branch dichotomously within it.*

Indolent ulceration (epithelial erosion)

An indolent or refractory type of superficial ulceration (epithelial erosion) of unknown cause is seen occasionally in cats (Figs 9.10–9.13). It has been observed in association with keratoconjunctivitis sicca, herpetic keratitis, proliferative keratoconjunctivitis, sequestrum formation, uveitis, glaucoma, FIV and FeLV infections. These associations may be genuine or accidental.

Affected animals exhibit mild blepharospasm and lacrimation. The ulcer is superficial, surrounded by a rim of nonadherent corneal epithelium and shows little initial evidence of active healing processes. Fluorescein stains the whole area of corneal ulceration and underruns the

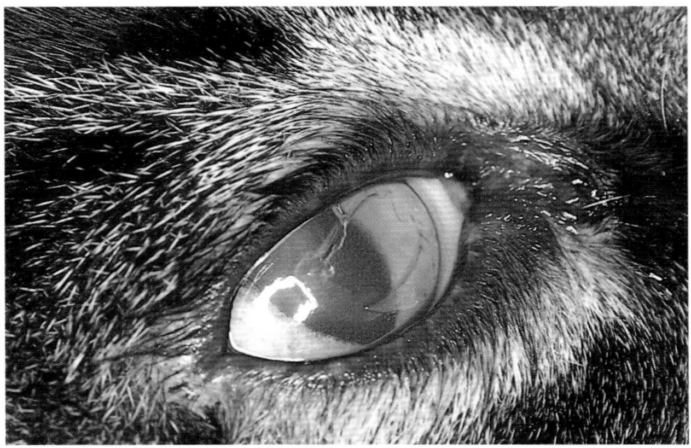

Fig. 9.10 *A 7-year-old Domestic shorthair with epithelial erosion, possibly a consequence of recrudescent FHV infection. The cat had been treated with topical corticosteroids for unilateral anterior uveitis and was also positive for FIV. Note the unattached epithelium at the periphery of the erosion.*

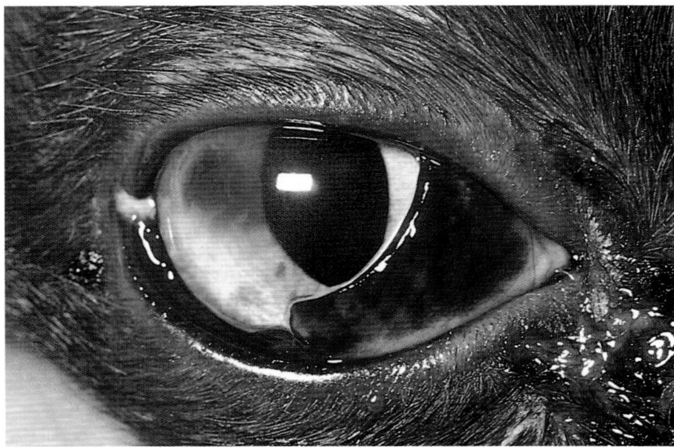

Fig. 9.11 *A 6-year-old Burmese cat. Sequestrum formation in the region of epithelial erosion. Note the defect in the third eyelid and the scar at the lateral canthus as a result of a cat fight injury. There was inadequate cover of the cornea in the region of the epithelial erosion because of the third eyelid defect, suggesting that this had contributed to the corneal pathology. The tears were stained brown.*

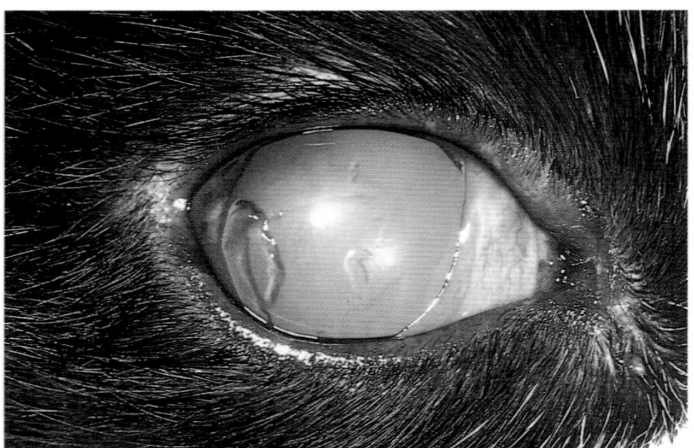

Fig. 9.12 A 12-year-old Domestic shorthair with multiple epithelial erosions, the cat had glaucoma secondary to idiopathic anterior uveitis.

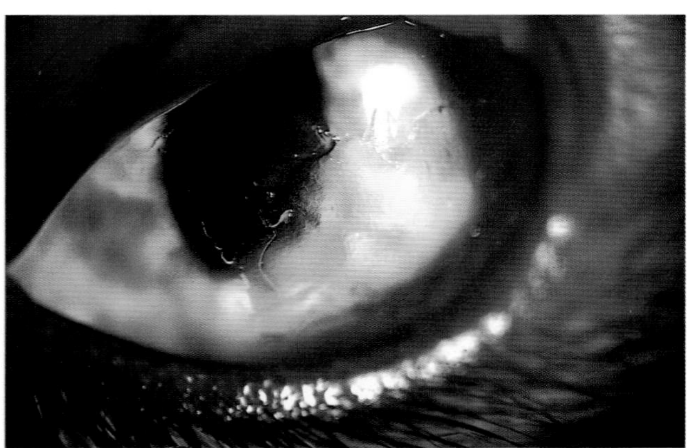

Fig. 9.13 Domestic short hair with epithelial erosions of unknown cause.

nonadherent epithelium. Sequential examination confirms the indolent nature of this type of superficial ulcer.

All treatment regimes can be carried out under topical local anaesthesia. Initially, the abnormal loose epithelium is removed using, for example, a dry, sterile cotton swab, or cotton wool wound tightly around the tip of fine mosquito forceps. This is sometimes all that is required, but most clinicians would also either support healing by applying a therapeutic soft contact lens (Fig. 9.14), or actively encourage healing with a technique such as punctate keratotomy (punctate or grid pattern) using a 22 gauge neeedle held perpendicular to the cornea (Champagne and Munger, 1992). Punctate keratotomy appears to offer most promise in terms of reducing healing time (Morgan and Abrams, 1994). Treatment may require repetition if erosions persist. For those cases in which feline herpesvirus is implicated a more radical approach may be required (see below).

Ulcerative keratitis

In all cases of corneal ulceration the underlying cause should be identified and corrected whenever possible. Ulcerative

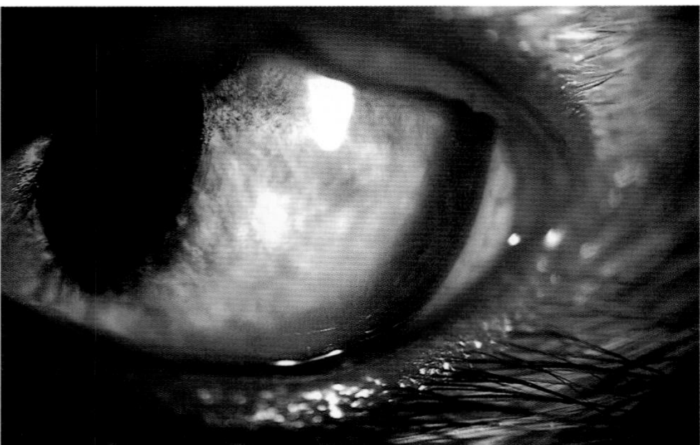

Fig. 9.14 The same cat as shown in Fig. 9.13 with a therapeutic soft contact lens in place.

keratitis is frequently of traumatic origin (see Chapter 3 for Traumatic Ulceration); scratches from other cats are a common cause and infection (e.g. *Pasteurella multocida)* is often introduced at the time of the injury. The physical damage inflicted by other cats ranges from superficial corneal ulceration to full thickness penetration and is usually unilateral, but on rare occasions can be bilateral (see Chapter 3). Feline herpesvirus-1 is a primary corneal pathogen and the most important infectious cause of feline ulceration (see below). Eyelid abnormalities (e.g. colobomatous defects and neoplasms such as squamous cell carcinoma) are less common in predisposing to ulcerative keratitis. Cilia abnormalities which are a common cause of ulcerative keratitis in dogs, are very rare in cats (see Chapter 5). Keratoconjunctivitis sicca and other defects of the pre-ocular tear film are also less common than they are in dogs, but should always be considered at initial assessment (see Chapter 7). Thermal and chemical injuries are unusual causes of corneal ulceration (see Chapter 3) .

Whatever the initiating cause, there is usually an acute onset of pain, blepharospasm and lacrimation. Careful examination with magnification should enable the extent and depth of ulceration to be determined. Superficial lesions are more painful than those more deeply situated because there is a richer nerve supply in the anterior cornea. Deeper lesions have a characteristic crater-like appearance and Descemet's membrane may be exposed when a defect which involves the full thickness of the stroma is present. A descemetocoele can be of spectacular appearance because of the elastic nature of Descemet's membrane.

A Schirmer tear test is usually performed after the initial examination and before anything is applied to the eyes. If infection is likely, scrapes and swabs should be taken into routine bacterial culture media and viral and chlamydial transport medium after applying topical local anaesthetic to the cornea. In the majority of cases oropharyngeal swabs (for virus isolation) should be taken at the same time.

Fluorescein may then be applied topically to the cornea to confirm the extent of the ulceration and excess fluorescein should be flushed away with sterile saline to avoid false positive results. The epithelium and Descemet's membrane do not take up fluorescein, but the stroma does.

Once the cause has been identified and corrected, superficial ulcers should heal quickly and without complication (Figs 1.17, 3.25, 9.15 and 9.16). It is sometimes necessary to excise or debride loose flaps of epithelium to aid healing. For epithelial loss with little stromal involvement a topical broad-spectrum antibiotic applied four times daily for 4–5 days is all that is required unless pain is prominent, in which case a therapeutic soft contact lens should also be inserted. Therapeutic soft contact lenses should not be used when there is active ocular surface infection, or corneal hypoaesthesia, or keratoconjunctivitis sicca. Superficial ulcers heal without scarring if only epithelium is involved. A faint scar will persist if there has been stromal involvement.

For deeper ulcers the antibiotic selected should be based on the results of initial corneal cytology and confirmed by later culture and sensitivity as stromal involvement is suggestive of infection (Figs 9.17–9.19). Protection in the form of a therapeutic soft contact lens, or a third eyelid flap, should be considered for uncomplicated ulcers which do not involve more than half the stromal thickness. If third eyelid flaps are used it is important to ensure that sutures do not penetrate the full thickness of the third eyelid because sutures may exacerbate the problem if they are in contact with the cornea (see Chapter 6).

Ulcers which involve more than half the stromal thickness (Figs 3.26 and 9.19), including those where a descemetocoele is present (Fig. 9.20), should be treated more intensively using topical fortified antibiotic solution or an appropriate proprietary ophthalmic solution (Crispin, 1993a). If there is real risk of perforation fortified antibiotic solutions must be used; cefazolin is effective against Gram-positive bacteria

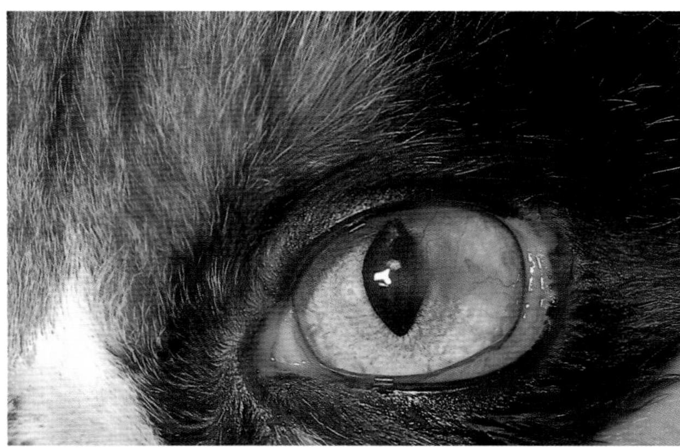

Fig. 9.15 *A 3-year-old British shorthair with multiple ulcers affecting the left eye only. The cat had a nasal squamous cell carcinoma and the ulcers were a possible consequence of reactivation of latent FHV.*

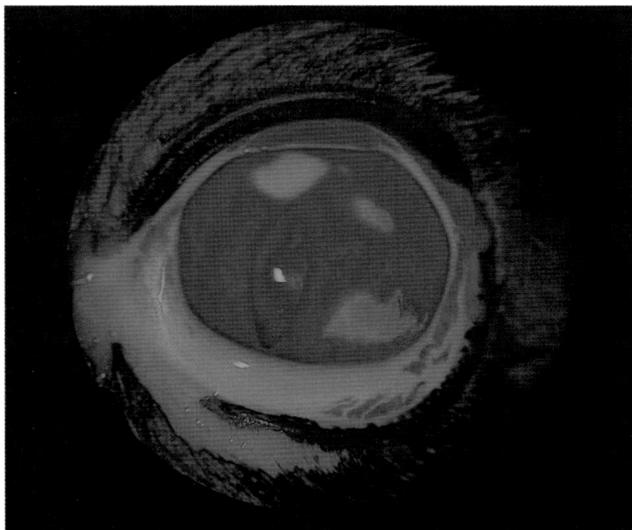

Fig. 9.16 *The same cat as shown in Fig. 9.15. Fluorescein has been applied to the cornea and the ulcers are clearly delineated with blue light. Note the similar appearance of this cat with the cat shown in Fig. 9.9.*

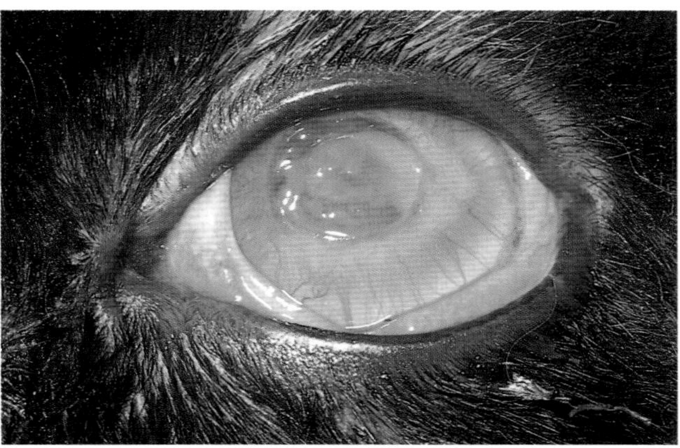

Fig. 9.17 *A 6-year-old Domestic longhair with a central ulcer, possibly as a result of mechanical irritation from sutures which had penetrated the full thickness of the third eyelid on a third eyelid flap. Note the extensive corneal vascularization.*

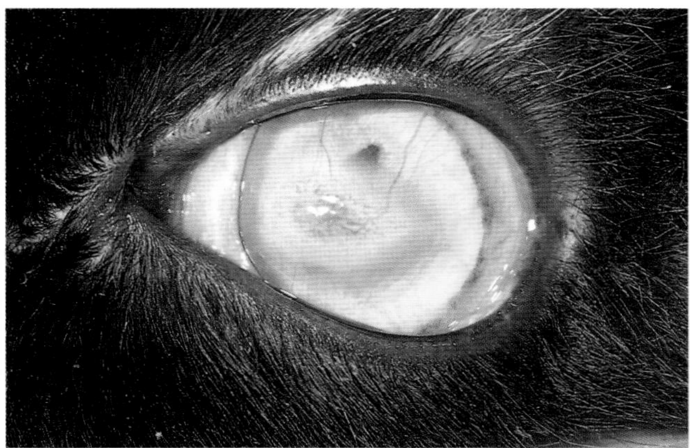

Fig. 9.18 *The same cat as shown in Fig. 9.17 2 weeks later. The ulcer has healed and the calibre of the corneal vessels has decreased, making them much less obvious.*

and gentamicin is effective against Gram-negative bacteria and the two may be used in combination while awaiting the results of culture and sensitivity. Initially, the patient is treated every 1–2 h until there is obvious improvement, then every 4–6 h. Once improvement is maintained an appropriate proprietary antibiotic solution can be substituted for fortified preparations and the selection can include newer generation broad-spectrum antibiotics such as ciprofloxacin hydrochloride (Ciloxan, Alcon) or ofloxacin (Exocin, Allergan) according to the sensitivity results. The course of treatment should be continued for at least 7–10 days or until the ulcer has healed. Topical 1% atropine solution may be required in the early stages if uveitis is present.

Conjunctival pedicle grafts (see Chapter 3) should be used routinely in the treatment of deep, progressive ulcers.

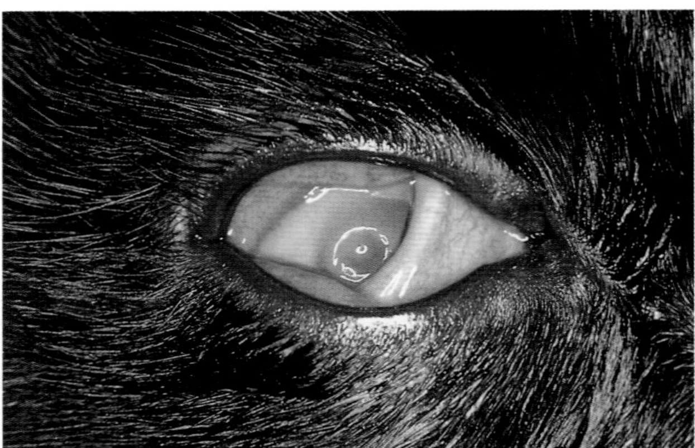

Fig. 9.19 *A 3-year-old Domestic shorthair with a deep ulcer of traumatic origin which had been mistreated with topical corticosteroids. Note the considerable conjunctival hyperaemia and corneal oedema which is also present.*

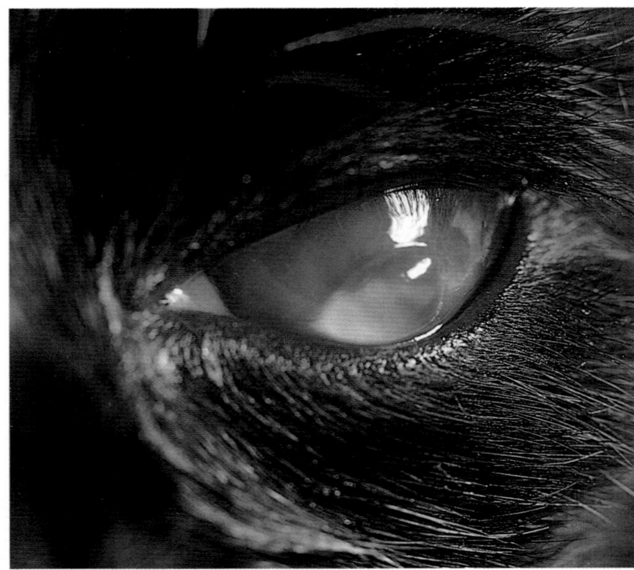

Fig. 9.20 *A 6-year-old Domestic shorthair. A large central descemetocoele is present. The elastic nature of Descemet's membrane allows it to bulge anteriorly.*

Frequent re-examination is necessary for complicated cases to ensure that the ulcer is resolving rather than progressing.

Corneal abscessation (Fig. 9.21) is an unusual complication of feline ulcerative keratitis, most commonly of traumatic origin (Campbell and McCree, 1978; Moore and Jones, 1994). The most effective treatment is probably keratectomy to remove the abscess, support for corneal healing, if necessary, and provision of appropriate topical antibiotic therapy, although the contents of the abscess are often found to be sterile.

If healing is associated with excessive granulation tissue, then topical corticosteroids can be used, but they must only be prescribed when there is no longer any risk of producing iatrogenic complications (Fig. 9.22) and the granulation tissue will become less obvious with time without treatment. If the ulcer has been deeper than pure epithelial loss there will be some degree of corneal scarring (Fig. 9.23) and ghost vessels will persist as the legacy of previous neovascularization.

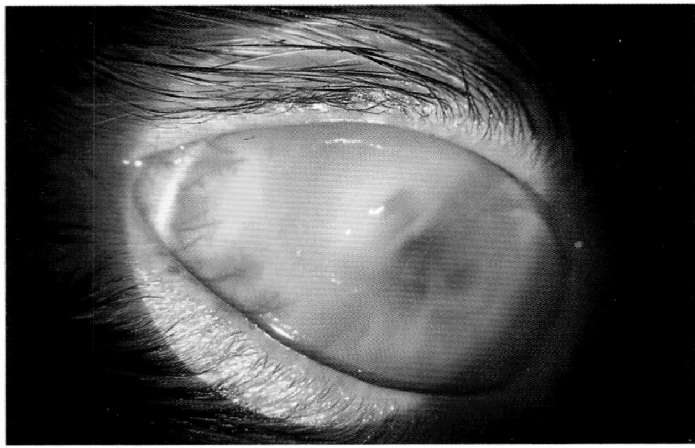

Fig. 9.21 *An 8-year-old Colourpoint. Corneal abscess of unknown cause.*

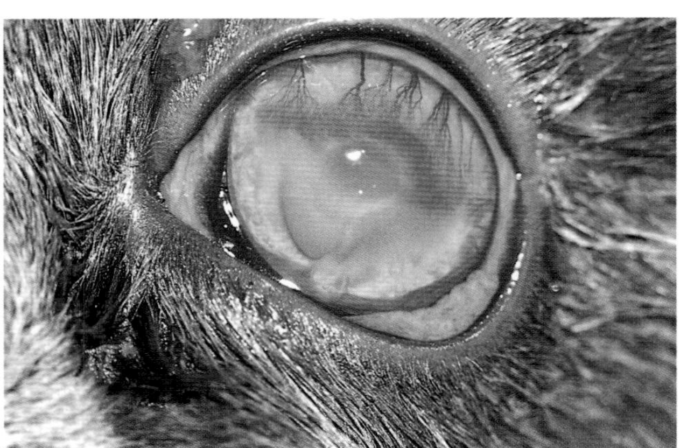

Fig. 9.22 *An 8-month-old Persian with a corneal ulcer which had been treated with topical corticosteroids. Note the vascular response (despite the corticosteroids), the 'mushy' appearance of the central cornea and the sequestrum which is forming.*

Herpetic keratitis

Feline herpesvirus-1 (FHV-1) has already been described as a cause of ophthalmia neonatorum and conjunctivitis (see Chapters 3, 4 and 8); it also has a most important role as a primary corneal pathogen. In adult cats FHV-1 infection is usually a consequence of reactivation of latent virus following primary infection in the past and is not necessarily associated with upper respiratory tract disease (Nasisse, 1990).

The typical clinical presentation is of mild blepharospasm and lacrimation or a serous ocular discharge. The corneal signs are variable (Figs 9.24–9.29). Discrete, superficial punctate corneal opacities form as a result of virus invasion and replication within the corneal epithelial cells which culminates in the death of affected cells. These opacities are not obvious and the eye should be stained with fluorescein or Rose Bengal and then examined with magnification to detect them; however, the stains should not be used until a Schirmer tear test is performed and the relevant samples have been taken. In addition to punctate ulcers, linear branching (dendritic) ulcers, long regarded as pathognomonic of herpetic

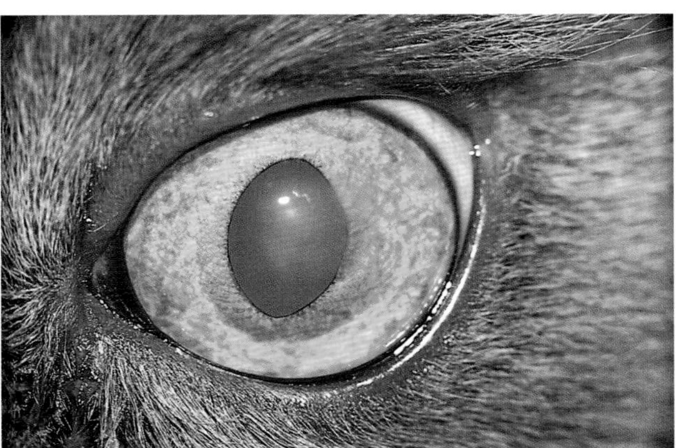

Fig. 9.23 *The same cat as shown in Fig. 9.22 2 months later when the ulcer has healed.*

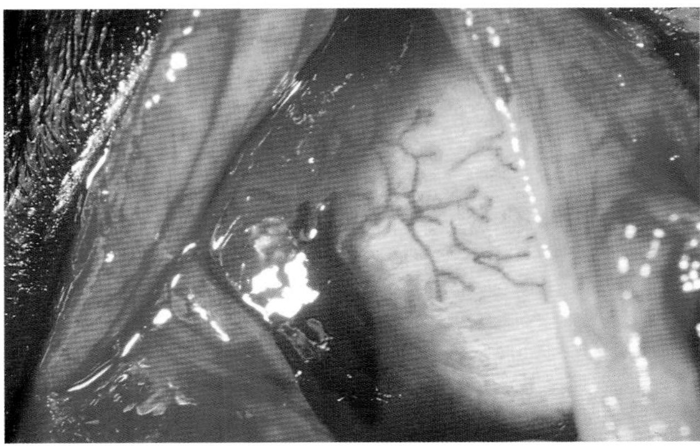

Fig. 9.24 *A 3-year-old Domestic shorthair. Herpetic keratitis associated with acute, primary ocular FHV-1 infection. Dendritic epithelial keratitis stained with Rose Bengal. (Courtesy of J. R. B. Mould.)*

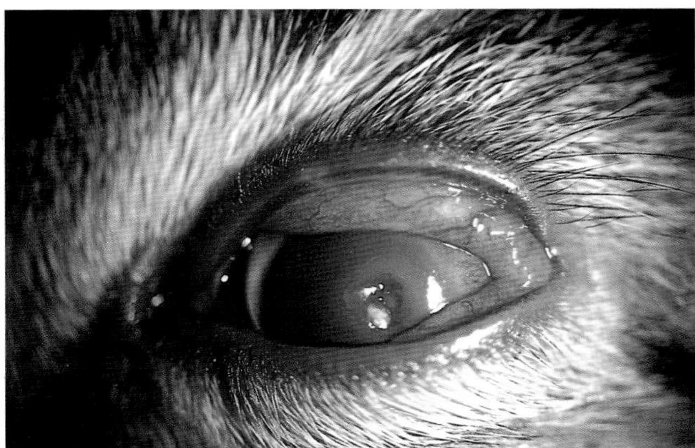

Fig. 9.25 *A 6-week-old Domestic shorthair. Another acute FHV-1 infection with severe conjunctivitis and a deep ulcer (to Descemet's membrane).*

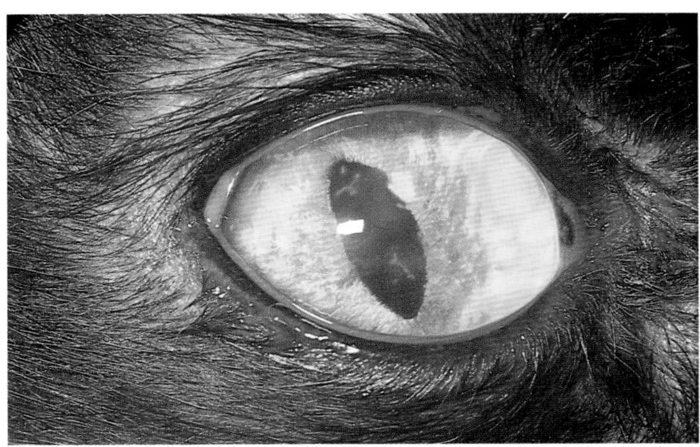

Fig. 9.26 *A 4-year-old Domestic shorthair. Herpetic keratitis associated with recrudescent FHV-1 infection. Characteristic dendritic ulceration stained with fluorescein. The cat also had pemphigus foliaceous.*

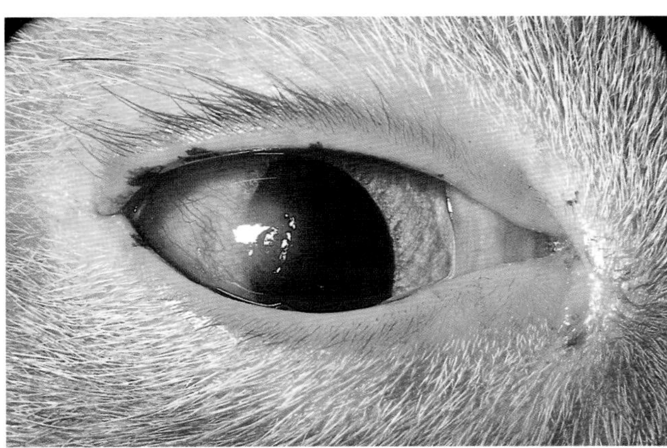

Fig. 9.27 *A 4-year-old Domestic shorthair. FHV-1 infection, geographic epithelial keratitis in a chronic case.*

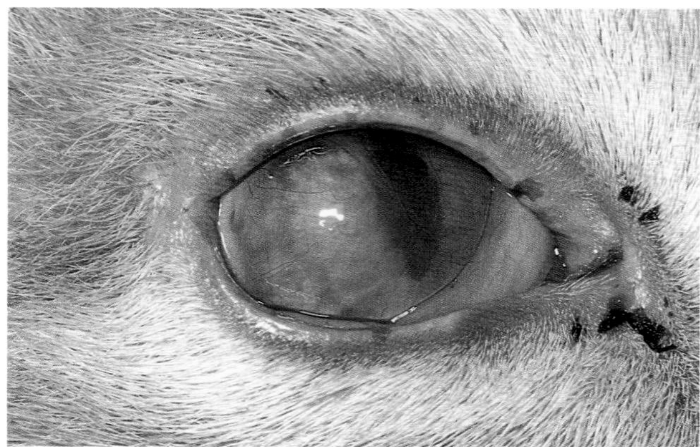

Fig. 9.28 *A 5-year-old Domestic shorthair. Stromal keratitis in chronic FHV-1 infection. Treatment with topical acyclovir produced temporary improvement which was not maintained. The cat was also FIV positive.*

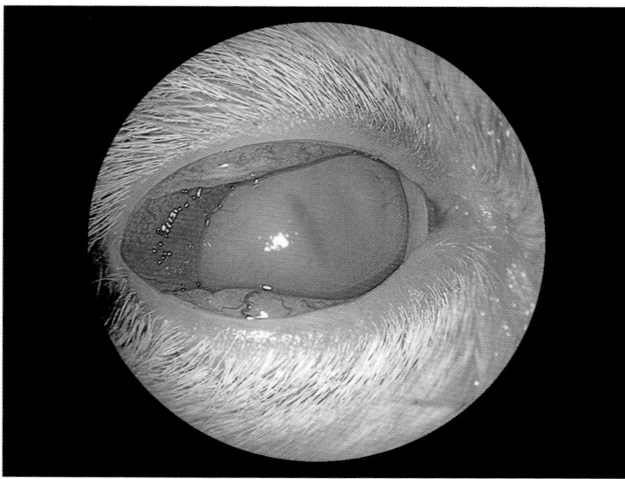

Fig. 9.29 *A 3-year-old Domestic shorthair. Stromal keratitis in chronic FHV-1 infection. The cat was also FeLV positive.*

keratitis, may also be detected. Irregular, but superficial, geographic ulcers are produced when the small ulcers enlarge and coalesce. Deeper corneal involvement is signalled by a circular pattern of oedema known as disciform keratitis and, while the oedema is superficial initially, it may deepen.

Chronic stromal keratitis may result in sight-threatening corneal scarring. Stromal keratitis is usually associated with chronic epithelial ulceration and manifests as stromal oedema, extensive vascularization and stromal cellular infiltration. The pathogenesis of stromal keratitis appears to be a cell-mediated immune response in which CD4+ lymphocytes play a crucial role.

Potential complications of recrudescent herpetic keratitis include bullous keratopathy, deep corneal ulcers, descemetocoele formation, liquefactive stromal necrosis, perforation and endophthalmitis. Secondary bacterial infection of superficial lesions increases the risk of complications.

Cats with feline herpesvirus infection may also be feline leukaemia (FeLV) positive or feline immunodeficiency virus (FIV) positive and, on occasions, intercurrent ocular disease (e.g. *Chlamydia psitacci*) is also present. The prognosis is poor in immunosuppressed animals. Proliferative eosinophilic keratoconjunctivitis and sequestrum formation have also been recorded in FHV-positive cats (Nasisse *et al.*, 1996a), but the significance of these associations is not always clear and they may simply reflect the ability of polymerase chain reaction (PCR) assay to detect FHV-1 DNA in the cornea, a presumed site of latency.

Diagnosis is based on the clinical findings, although these may be so diverse in chronic cases as to be unhelpful. Laboratory tests are also less sensitive in chronic cases (see Chapter 8). FHV-1 DNA seems to be most reliably detected by PCR in corneal scrapes from cats with keratitis (Nasisse *et al.*, 1996b).

Treatment

The condition responds unpredictably to antiviral agents and there is, at present, no drug which can be recommended as the drug of choice. Idoxuridine, vidararabine, trifluorthymidine and acyclovir are the antiviral agents which are used most frequently as topical treatments, but their availability varies in different countries and in the UK, for example, only acyclovir (Zovirax, Glaxo Wellcome) is currently available. Topical treatments require frequent application and lack of compliance (owner and/or animal) may be one reason for failure.

Oral therapy with antiviral agents offers an alternative approach, but toxic side-effects may limit the use of some agents (e.g. valiciclovir). Acyclovir (approximately 200 mg twice daily) is the most commonly used oral antiviral agent. Newer drugs such as famcyclovir await evaluation.

The role of vaccination in the prevention and treatment of FHV-1 infection is equivocal. There is some evidence that vaccine may offer a form of immunotherapy in chronically affected cats (one drop of intranasal vaccine applied to each eye). More recently, oral human interferon-α has been used to limit the severity of FHV-1 infection in experimentally affected cats (Nasisse *et al.*, 1996c). Oral IFN-α and acyclovir may provide an effective synergistic combination in early infections and may be of some benefit in adult cats with chronic ocular infections.

Dietary therapy with L-lysine (200 mg mixed with the food daily) is currently being investigated as a means of suppressing FHV-1 replication in cats (M. P. Nasisse, personal communication).

Surgical treatment by the mechanical removal of affected epithelium may assist in the treatment of epithelial keratitis. Stromal involvement may benefit from lamellar keratectomy as a means of removing antigenic or host proteins and stimulating corneal wound healing; traditional methods of corneal suppport (third eyelid flap or conjunctival graft) will be required while healing occurs. Penetrating keratoplasty and thermokeratoplasty require evaluation as a means of treating chronic stromal keratitis.

Anti-inflammatory drugs have a controversial role in the management of FHV-1 infections. Topical corticosteroids may reduce post-herpetic scarring, but they should only be used in conjunction with antiviral agents to treat chronic cases of stromal keratitis; they will exacerbate active viral infection and are contraindicated in all cases of primary ocular FHV-1 infection. Systemic corticosteroids are contraindicated in FHV-1 infected cats because they will reactivate latent infections.

Eosinophilic (proliferative) keratoconjunctivitis

The cause of this condition is unknown (Paulsen *et al.*, 1987; Pentlarge, 1989; Morgan *et al.*, 1996; Prasse and Winston, 1996) and, unlike corneal sequestrum, there is no breed predilection. While it might be tempting to regard this condition as part of the eosinophilic granuloma complex, most cats have only ocular involvement and skin lesions are absent. In a proportion of cases a circulating eosinophilia is present and the systemic eosinophilic diseases chronic allergic bronchitis and eosinophilic enteritis have been reported in one study (Morgan *et al.*, 1996). Proliferative keratoconjunctivitis is strikingly similar to human vernal disease.

The clinical presentation is quite variable; lesions are initially unilateral, but invariably progress to bilaterality in untreated cases. The clinical signs include ocular discomfort, with mild blepharospasm, a low-grade ocular discharge and involvement of the conjunctiva and cornea (Figs 9.30–9.38). Tear production may be increased as a result of the ocular discomfort but it is occasionally reduced: these may be incidental associations. It is advisable to check for feline herpesvirus as Nasisse *et al.* (1996a) have demonstrated using the polymerase chain reaction (PCR) assay that a high proportion (some 76%) of corneal scrapings are positive for FHV-1 DNA in cats with proliferative keratoconjunctivitis. Given the prevalence of FHV-1 in the feline population and the sensitivity of PCR it is difficult to assess the clinical significance of this observation at present.

The palpebral surface of the upper eyelid is usually affected and there may be more extensive eyelid involvement in established cases. The eyelid margins and third eyelid become thickened and patchy depigmentation may develop. The conjunctiva is often reddened and oedematous and, in untreated cases, conjunctival lesions become more generalized and severe.

Infiltration and vascularization of the cornea are key features of the condition; most commonly the dorsolateral or ventrolateral quadrants of the cornea are affected, but the whole cornea will become involved if the condition is allowed to progress. Corneal oedema and minute erosions may also be part of the clinical presentation; it is important

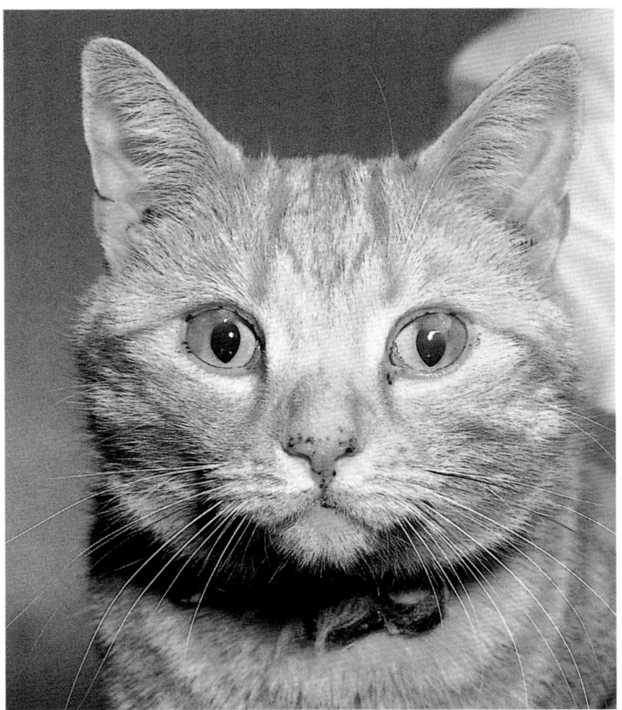

Fig. 9.30 *A 5-year-old Domestic shorthair with bilateral proliferative keratoconjunctivitis.*

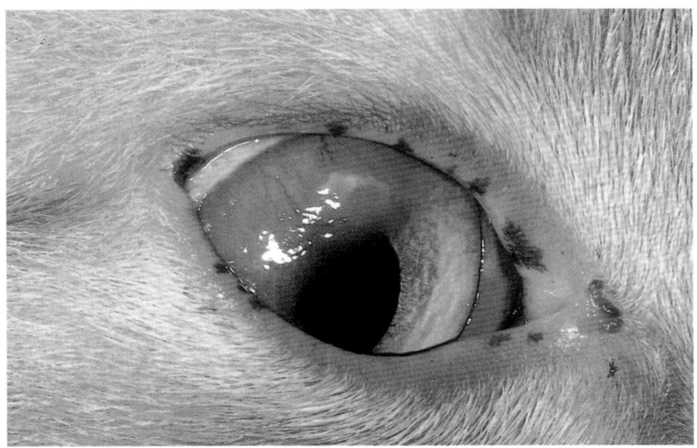

Fig. 9.31 *Close-up of the right eye of the cat shown in Fig. 9.30.*

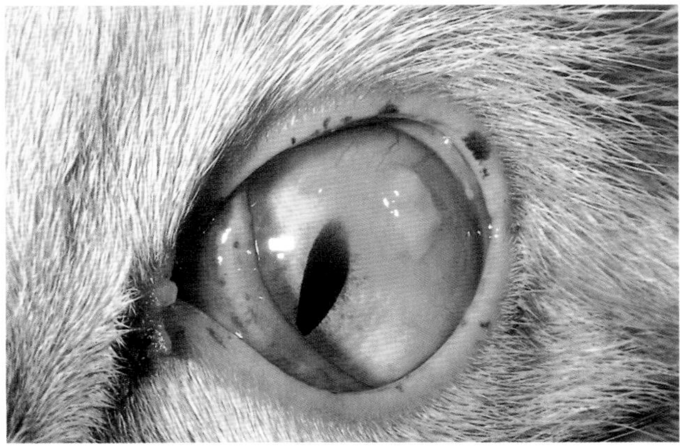

Fig. 9.32 *Close-up of the left eye of the cat shown in Fig. 9.30.*

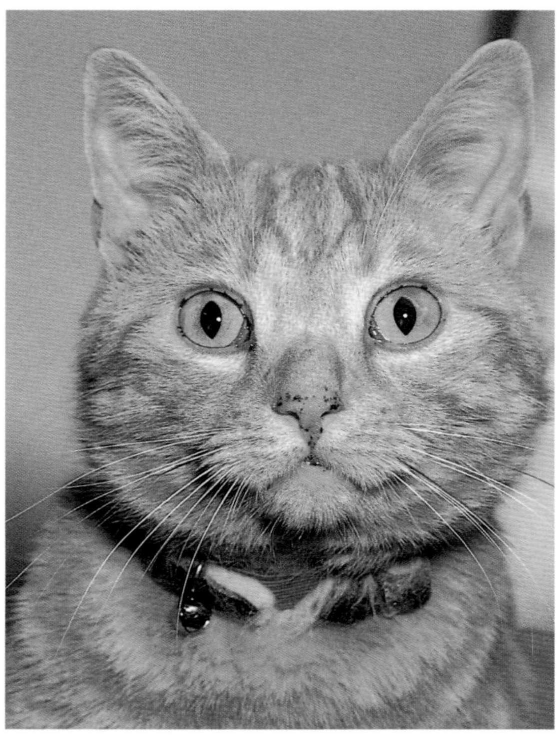

Fig. 9.33 The same cat as shown in Figs 9.30–9.32 after 2 weeks of treatment with topical corticosteroid.

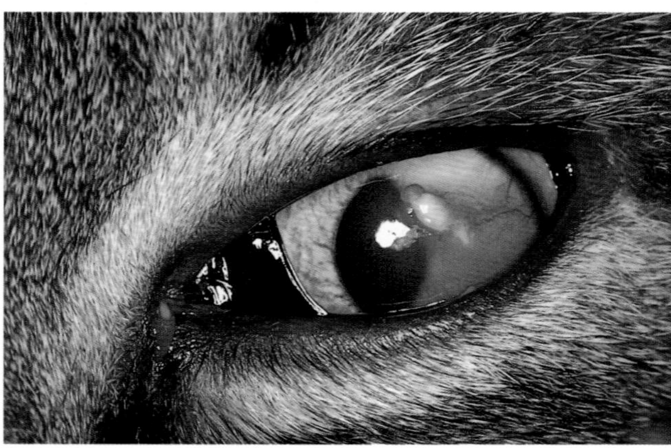

Fig. 9.34 A 4-year-old Domestic shorthair. Unilateral proliferative keratoconjunctivitis affecting the left eye. In addition to the obvious vascularized white plaque on the cornea, note part of a white plaque apparent at the lower eyelid margin. The lesions resolved completely after a 5-day course of megestrol acetate and did not recur in later life. The right eye, however, became affected 4 years later and is illustrated in Fig. 9.35.

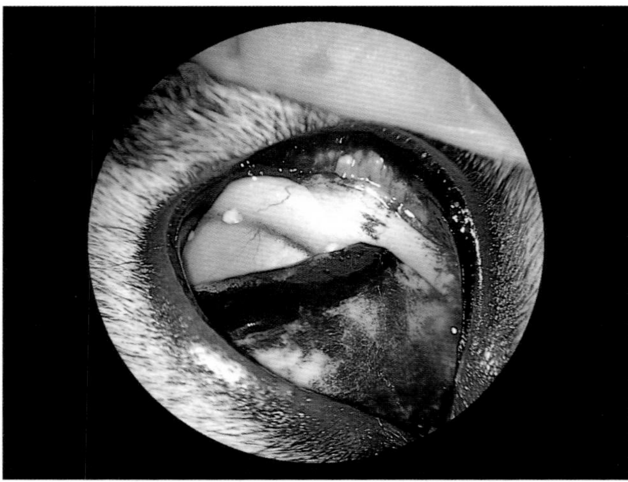

Fig. 9.35 The right eye of the cat shown in Fig. 9.34. The upper eyelid has been everted to show the characteristic white plaques on the palpebral conjunctiva as well as on the limbal conjunctiva and cornea. This eye responded to topical corticosteroid therapy, but had a tendency to episodic recrudescence.

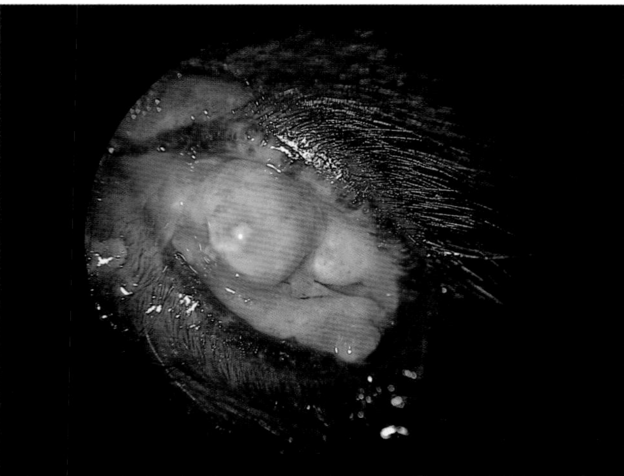

Fig. 9.36 A 9-year-old Burmese cat with bilateral proliferative keratoconjunctivitis. The right eye is illustrated and was the more severely affected. Both eyes responded well to topical corticosteroids.

to flush away excess fluorescein and examine the cornea with blue light to avoid inaccurate interpretation. The pathognomonic feature of proliferative keratoconjunctivitis is a superficial creamy white plaque-like material which has been likened to cottage cheese in appearance and consists of nuclear debris from disrupted cells, eosinophils and eosinophilic granules (Prasse and Winston, 1996). It is possible to confirm the diagnosis by examination of superficial scrapes stained with Wrights or Giemsa reagents to demonstrate epithelial cells, mast cells, eosinophils, neutrophils and lymphocytes.

Management includes the recognition and treatment of any underlying problems like FHV-1 or corneal erosions. The condition itself responds to topical corticosteroid therapy (Figs 9.37 and 9.38) and also to corticosteroids or megestrol acetate given by mouth. All these drugs have potentially undesirable

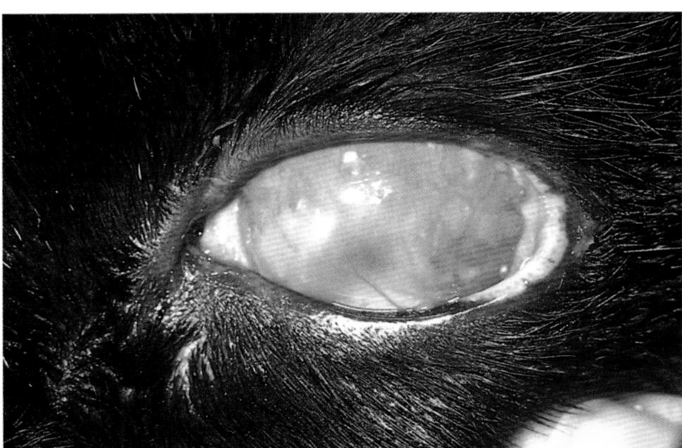

Fig. 9.37 A Domestic shorthair, approximately 8 years old, with bilateral proliferative keratoconjunctivitis; the left eye is illustrated. The cat also had uveitis and was FIV positive. Both eyes were treated with topical corticosteroids (prednisolone acetate).

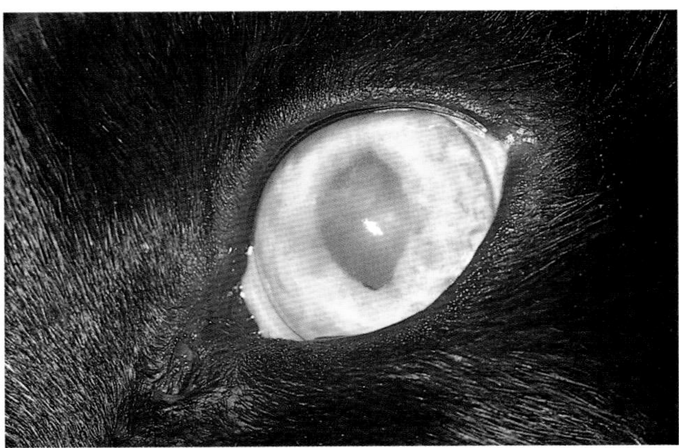

Fig. 9.38 The same eye as illustrated in Fig. 9.37 showing slow improvement after 3 months' treatment.

side-effects, especially in long-term usage; megestrol acetate, in particular, may induce diabetes mellitus and should be used with care. Unfortunately, recurrence is common, so treatment regimes may need to be somewhat flexible with regard to the choice of drug and the length of time for which it is given. Topical cyclosporin, for example, appears less effective than other treatments in the early stages, but may be useful if long-term therapy is thought necessary and once the corneal appearance has returned to normal. The most rational approach to treatment would appear to rest with the induction of localized immunosuppression with either topical corticosteroids (especially initially) or topical cyclosporin (particularly for longer term use) to control a potentially immune-mediated ocular disease (Read *et al.*, 1995).

Corneal sequestrum (sequestration)

This is a condition of unknown cause which is unique to the cat. The many descriptive names (corneal necrosis, corneal

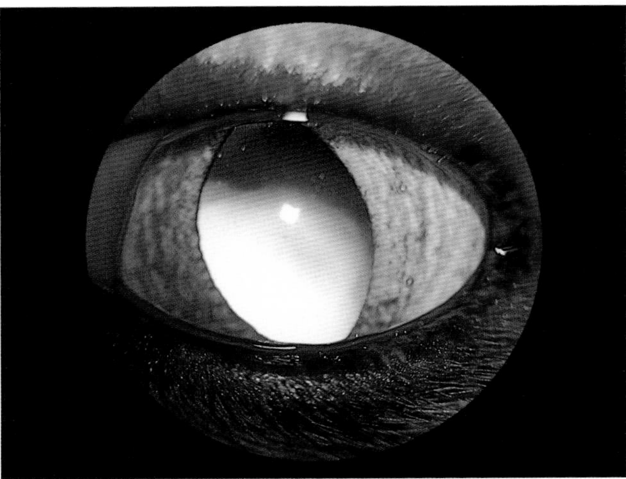

Fig. 9.39 Young adult Domestic shorthair. Unilateral corneal sequestrum. Subtle brown subepithelial corneal staining, not associated with any ocular discomfort or discharge.

sequestration, corneal sequestrum, corneal mummification, corneal nigrum, focal degeneration, keratitis nigrum, primary necrotizing keratitis, isolated black lesion and chronic ulcerative keratitis) emphasize the interest generated in the condition (Startup, 1988; Pentlarge, 1989; Morgan, 1994). There is a breed disposition (e.g. Colourpoint, Persian, Siamese, Birman, Burmese, Himalayan) and breed-related sequestrum might possibly be a type of inherited stromal dystrophy. The condition may also develop in any breed of cat after previous corneal insult (e.g. ulcerative keratitis, herpetic keratitis, keratoconjunctivitis sicca), including those associated with eyelid abnormalities such as absence of the third eyelid, medial canthus trichiasis and entropion. About 55% of affected cats have positive corneal scrapings for FHV-1 DNA as assayed using PCR (Nasisse *et al.*, 1996a) and the clinical significance of this high detection rate is not yet fully understood.

The condition (Figs 9.39–9.51) is usually unilateral, except in those cats with a breed predisposition. The sequestrum is located in the central or paracentral corneal stroma and there is usually ocular discomfort, an ocular discharge, increased blink rate or frank blepharospasm. A comprehensive examination is recommended to exclude complicating factors such as tear film abnormalities, absence of the third eyelid and infection because the appearance of the lesion is often so striking that the necessity for complete examination is forgotten.

In many affected animals the tears and deposits near the eyelid margins, or coating a therapeutic soft contact lens (Fig. 9.52) are of a similar colour to the sequestrum and it seems certain that the characteristic colour of the sequestrum is derived from the pre-ocular tear film, although the dark material which comprises the lesion has not been identified. The most obvious histopathological finding is coagulative necrosis (collagen degeneration) and nonspecific inflammatory cells are also present.

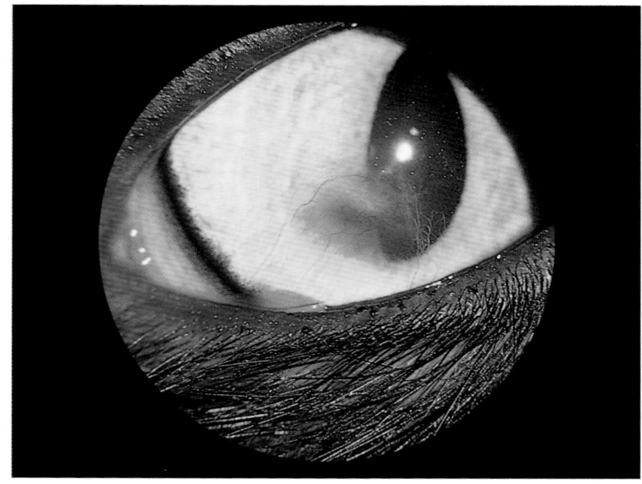

Fig. 9.40 *A 3-year-old Domestic shorthair. Unilateral corneal sequestrum. Discrete lesion with fine vascularization. Slight ocular discharge, but no pain.*

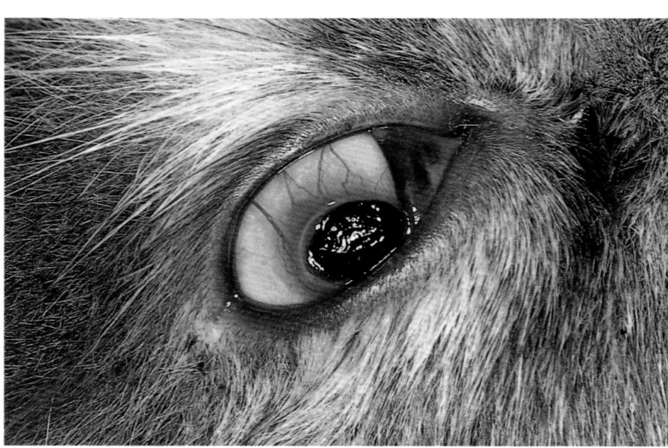

Fig. 9.42 *A 2-year-old Persian female. Bilateral corneal sequestrum, the right eye is shown and was more severely affected than the left eye. A dark serous discharge is present. The sequestrum is beginning to slough and was not associated with any pain. This cat's male littermate was also affected.*

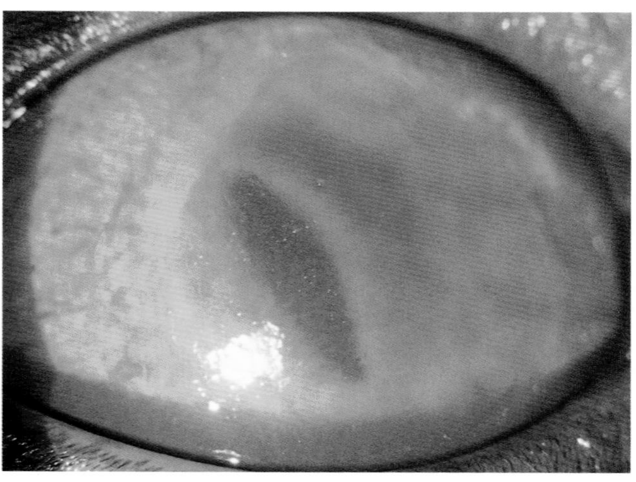

Fig. 9.41 *An 8-month-old Domestic shorthair neutered female. Unilateral corneal sequestrum associated with extensive epithelial erosion. Pain and lacrimation also present.*

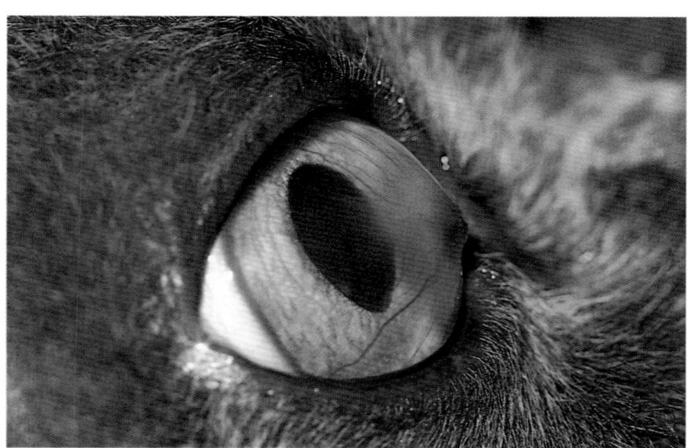

Fig. 9.43 *A 7-year-old Persian neutered male. Unilateral sequestrum formation at the site of previous ulceration.*

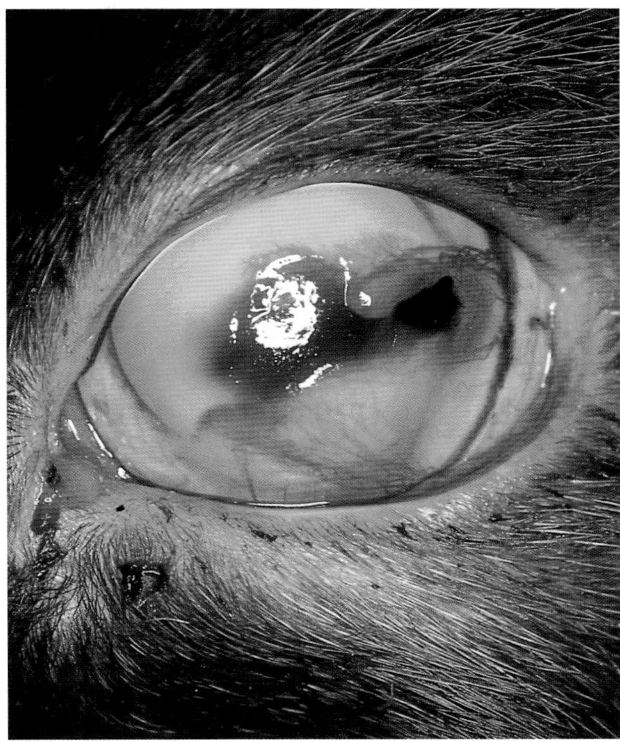

Fig. 9.44 *A 12-year-old Colourpoint Persian. Unilateral corneal sequestrum of the left eye complicating healing after corneal laceration from a cat scratch.*

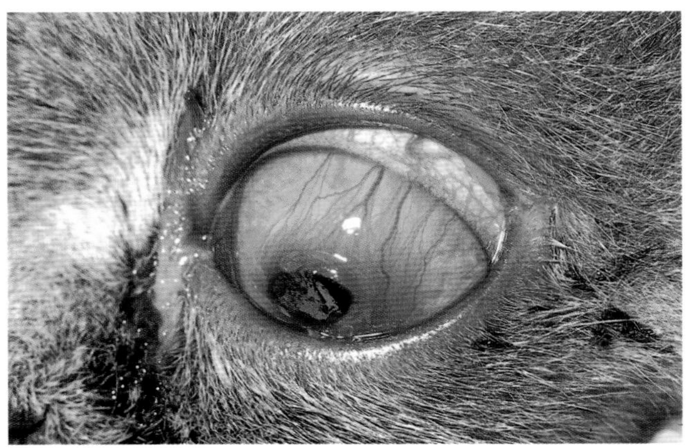

Fig. 9.45 *A 2-year-old Persian cross-bred. Unilateral corneal sequestrum affecting the left eye; Schirmer 1 tear test in the right eye, 1 mm/min and in the left eye, 10 mm/min.*

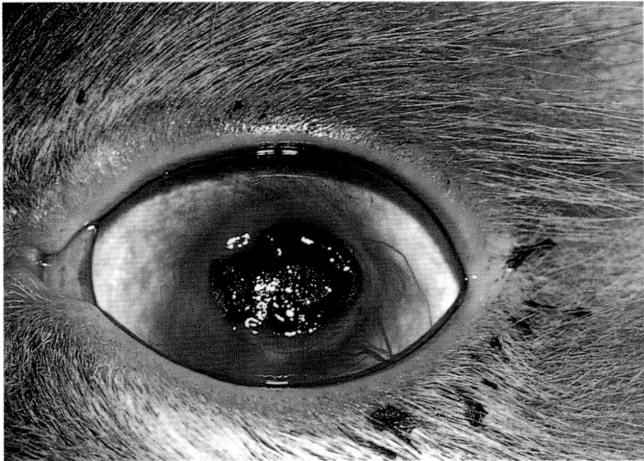

Fig. 9.46 *A 4-year-old Persian. Unilateral corneal sequestrum affecting the left eye. Schirmer 1 tear test readings in both eyes never exceeded 7 mm/min.*

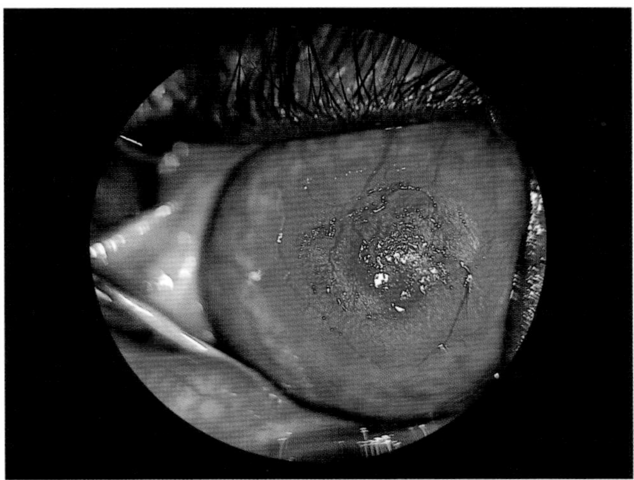

Fig. 9.47 *A 1-year-old Persian. Unilateral corneal sequestrum removed by keratectomy. The immediate postoperative appearance is illustrated. The healing cornea should be protected with a therapeutic soft contact lens or a conjunctival pedicle graft.*

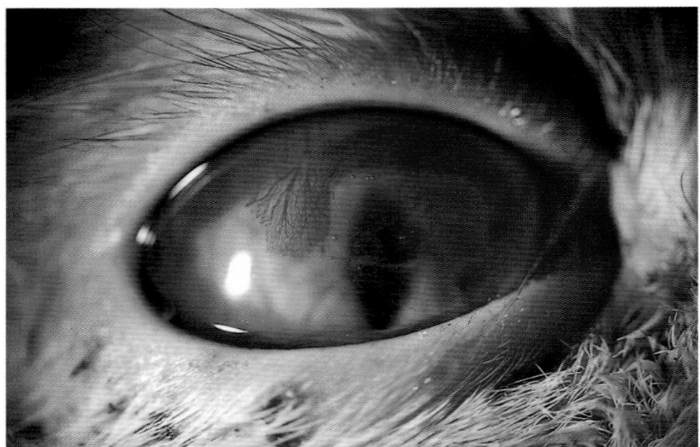

Fig. 9.48 A 2-year-old Persian. Unilateral corneal sequestrum removed by keratectomy, therapeutic soft contact lens in situ.

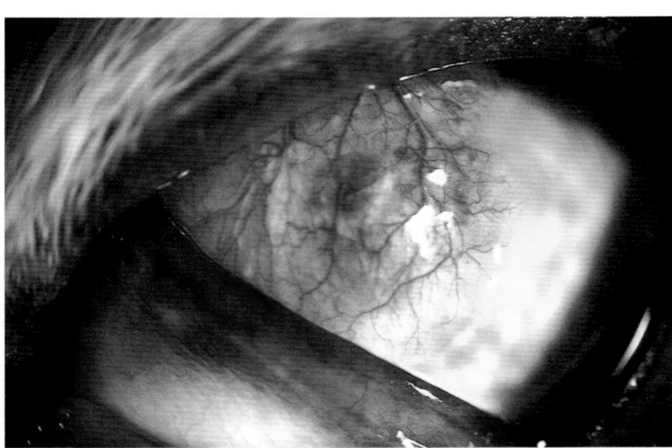

Fig. 9.49 A 6-year-old White Persian neutered female. Unilateral corneal sequestrum removed by keratectomy, a pedicle graft has been used to protect the cornea during healing and the sequestrum is recurring beneath the graft. Excisional surgery had been performed a number of times previously.

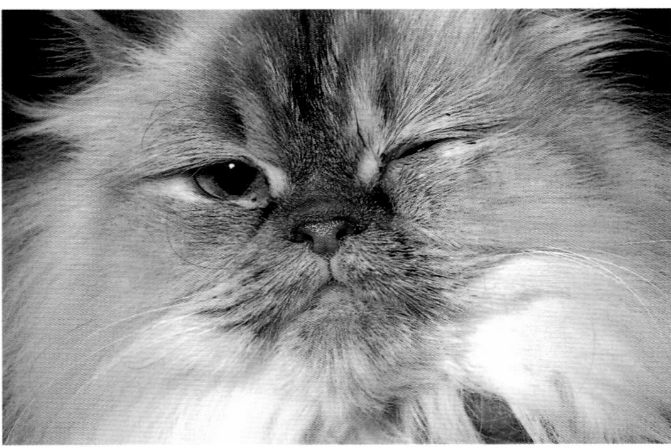

Fig. 9.50 A 2-year-old Persian. Unilateral corneal sequestrum in the process of sloughing, associated with obvious ocular discomfort.

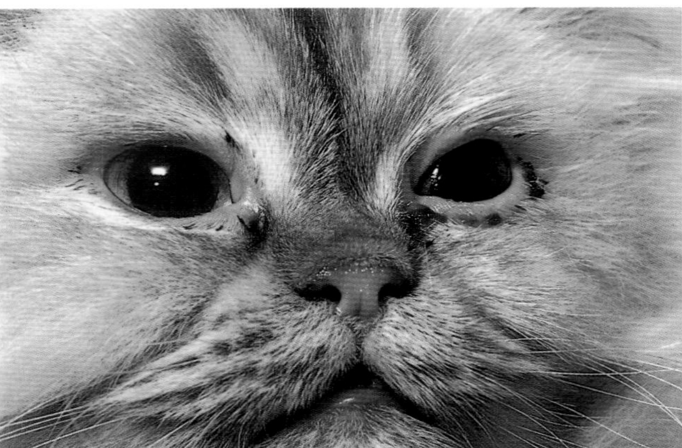

Fig. 9.51 The same cat as shown in Fig. 9.50, with a therapeutic soft contact lens in situ. The pain relief which this treatment has afforded is obvious. Note the dark, coloured ocular discharge.

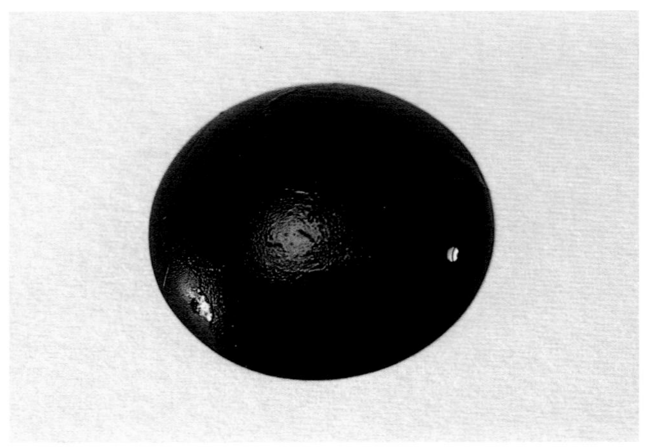

Fig. 9.52 The therapeutic soft contact lens, heavily stained, after removal from the cat illustrated in Figs 9.50 and 9.51.

The lesion is of somewhat variable appearance ranging from an ill-defined golden-brown staining of the corneal stroma covered by an apparently intact epithelium in the early case, to a clearly demarcated dark-brown or black plaque (sequestrum) which is raised above the level of the corneal epithelium later on. The darker lesions usually have an ulcerated peripheral rim and the plaque is often raised above the level of the corneal epithelium with loose oedematous epithelium visible at the edge of the plaque. In chronic cases, corneal neovascularization and perilesional corneal oedema are common. The depth of corneal involvement rarely exceeds mid-stroma, although occasionally a sequestrum may extend to Descemet's membrane. It is likely that the different appearances are in part related to different stages in the evolution of the opacity and to the nature of the initiating insult.

The amount of ocular discomfort exhibited by affected cats varies considerably and, together with the depth of the lesion, determines the management approach adopted; this varies between allowing the lesion to slough naturally and surgical excision. The sequestrum cannot be allowed to slough naturally if there is any possibility of full-thickness corneal penetration (Fig. 9.53). However, it can also be argued that a conservative approach is sometimes warranted as surgery might potentiate FHV-1 infection.

When the sequestrum is not producing any obvious discomfort and provided that it may safely be allowed to slough naturally, the cat can be treated with topical tear replacement solution (e.g. 0.2% polyacrylic acid; 0.2% w/w Carbomer 940) during the intervening period. With this conservative approach corneal healing usually takes between 1 to 6 months.

If the sequestrum is superficial and producing mild ocular discomfort then a therapeutic soft contact lens should be inserted. Provided that there are no signs of ocular discomfort the lens may be left *in situ* for up to 3 months; corneal healing should occur within this period.

If there is marked discomfort keratectomy should be performed and corneal protection (e.g. conjunctival pedicle graft, lamellar corneoscleral transposition) will be required if the sequestrum approaches half the corneal thickness or more. Alternatively penetrating keratoplasty can be used for deep lesions. A therapeutic soft contact lens or, less commonly, a third eyelid flap can be used after more superficial surgery. There will be some scarring, but keratectomy greatly reduces the time course of the disease; healing is usually complete within 1 month of surgery. Following surgery the patient is given topical antibiotic until epithelialization occurs, after which corticosteroids can be used. Recurrence must be expected in predisposed breeds, especially if surgery has been incomplete, but is unusual without breed predisposition.

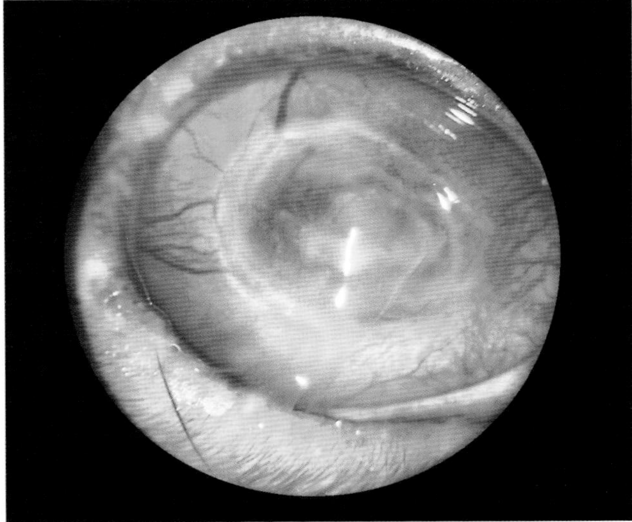

Fig. 9.53 *A 10-year-old Burmese with corneal rupture associated with sloughing of a deep sequestrum.*

Mycotic keratitis

Mycotic keratitis can be connected with long-term corticosteroid therapy or other types of immunosuppression, and is unlikely to be seen in the UK unless the animal has been imported from countries where such problems are endemic. *Aspergillus* (Ketring and Glaze, 1994), *Candida albicans* (Gerding *et al.*, 1994; Ketring and Glaze, 1994), *Cladosporidium* (Miller *et al.*, 1983), *Drechslera spicifera* (Zapater *et al.*, 1975) and *Rhinosporidium* (Peiffer and Jackson, 1979) have been reported as causes of feline keratomycosis in the USA.

Parasitic keratitis

There is a single case report from North America of protozoal keratitis caused by *Encephalitozoon* infection (Buyukmihci *et al.*, 1977).

Mycobacterial keratitis

Mycobacterial keratitis (Fig 9.54) as a manifestation of ocular tuberculosis is very rare (Veenendaal, 1928); tubercular choroiditis is a slightly commoner ocular manifestation (see Chapter 12). Mycobacterial keratitis is usually confirmed by corneal scrapings, local lymph node biopsy and the demonstration of characteristic granulomatous inflammation and acid-fast bacilli (Dice, 1977), although the precise identification of specific strains is highly specialized (Gunn-Moore *et al.*, 1996). A number of different mycobacterial species can produce infection in cats, resulting in various disease syndromes (Gunn-Moore *et al.*, 1996) which include classical tuberculosis *(Mycobacterium tuberculosis, M. bovis,* and other tubercle group variants), feline leprosy *(M. lepraemurium)* and atypical mycobacteriosis *(M. avium).*

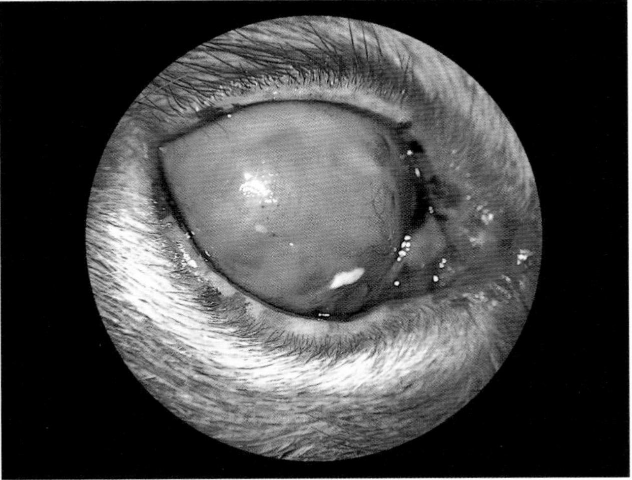

Fig. 9.54 *A 20-year-old Domestic shorthair neutered male. The history was of weight loss despite a ravenous appetite. Both eyes were affected, with both intraocular and ocular surface changes; there was also submandibular lymphadenopathy. The right eye is shown here; the left eye is illustrated in Chapter 12 (Fig. 12.51). The diagnosis (confirmed post mortem) was of mycobacterial infection.*

Mycobacterial keratitis should be differentiated from proliferative eosinophilic keratoconjunctivitis and neoplastic infiltration, notably squamous cell carcinoma and lymphosarcoma, all of which can be confirmed by scrapings or biopsy.

Iatrogenic complications

Topical and systemic corticosteroids may complicate keratitis if they are used incorrectly; in such cases there is little sign of active healing and the cornea has a characteristic 'mushy' appearance (Fig. 9.55). In most situations where there is uptake of fluorescein by the corneal stroma the use of corticosteroids by any route is contraindicated.

Immune-mediated keratitis

Little is known of genuine immune-mediated types of feline keratitis. It has been suggested that some types of marginal keratitis which resemble human Terrien's marginal degeneration may have an immune-mediated basis and relapsing polychondritis, an immune-mediated systemic connective tissue disorder, has been associated with keratoconjunctivitis sicca and keratitis in the form of superficial stromal opacities and vascularisation (Ketring and Glaze, 1994).

Florida spots

As the name suggests this is a condition which is seen most commonly in the south-eastern states of the USA (Peiffer and Jackson, 1979). It consists of nonprogressive greyish superficial stromal opacities; sometimes discrete spots are present, sometimes the opacities are more diffuse (Fig. 9.56). The condition is usually bilateral and does not appear to be associated with any kind of ocular discomfort. The cause is unknown, but they have been linked to an outdoor lifestyle and can resolve if the cat is kept indoors.

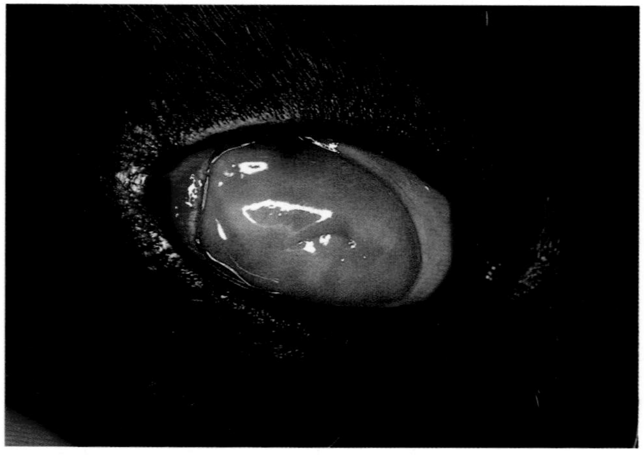

Fig. 9.55 *An 8-year-old Domestic shorthair with liquefactive stromal necrosis as a complication of inappropriate corticosteroid therapy for ulcerative keratitis.*

Exposure keratopathy

Exposure keratopathy (Fig. 9.57) may occur because of inadequate eyelid function (e.g. colobomatous lid defects, facial nerve damage, symblepharon formation), or loss of eyelid function (e.g. extensive symblepharon formation, following eyelid surgery, especially after removal of the third eyelid), because of damage to the trigeminal nerve or facial nerve (e.g. following orbital or facial trauma), or because the eyeball is proptosed (e.g. space-occupying orbital lesion or orbital trauma) or enlarged (e.g. hydrophthalmos associated with glaucoma). The underlying cause should be addressed in the management of exposure keratopathy. See also Chapters 3–6, 10 and 15.

Corneal lipid deposition

Lipid keratopathy (Figs 9.58–9.60) is the deposition of lipid within the cornea and is always associated with vascularization (Carrington, 1983; Crispin, 1993a). In cats, the condi-

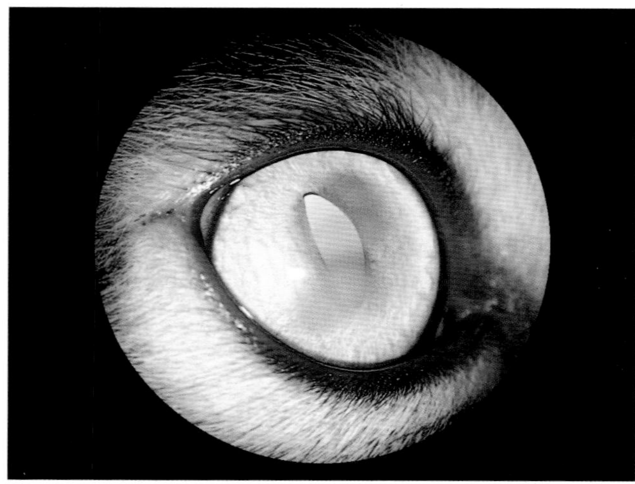

Fig. 9.56 *A Domestic shorthair with Florida spots (courtesy of M. P. Nasisse).*

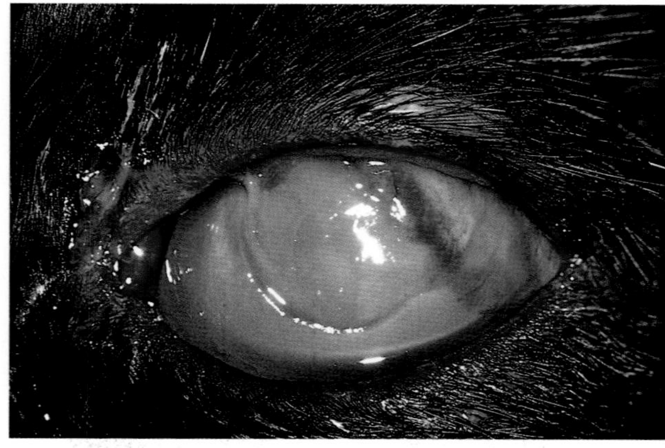

Fig. 9.57 *A 12-year-old Domestic shorthair with hydrophthalmos associated with chronic glaucoma. Extensive exposure keratopathy because of lagophthalmos.*

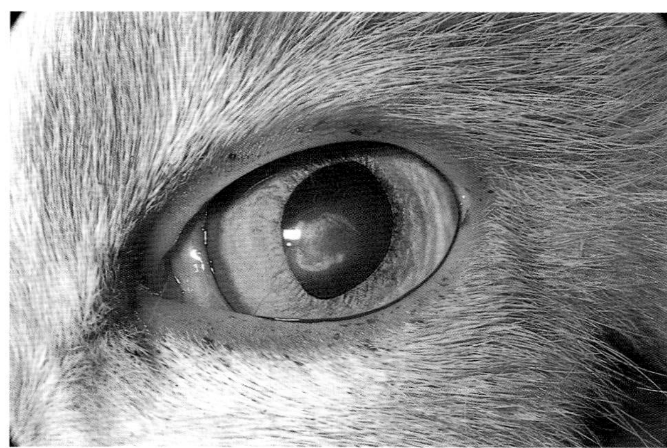

Fig. 9.58 *An 8-year-old Domestic shorthair. Lipid keratopathy associated with traumatic injury some months earlier. The cat was normolipoproteinaemic (serum cholesterol 3.54 mmol/l, serum triglyceride 0.62 mmol/l).*

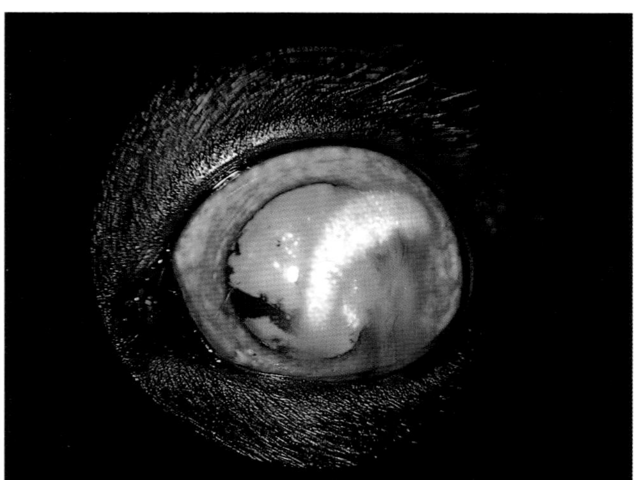

Fig. 9.59 *A 5-year-old Domestic shorthair with lipid keratopathy. The arcuate lipid deposition lies dorsal to the site of original corneal penetration. Lens material is adherent to the posterior cornea as the cat claw injury had also damaged the lens. This eye is at risk of subsequent post-traumatic sarcoma. The cat was normolipoproteinaemic (serum cholesterol 4.28 mmol/l, serum triglyceride 0.57 mmol/l).*

tion is rare, usually unilateral and often associated with some form of anterior segment inflammation. Lipid keratopathy may be found in animals with normolipoproteinaemia as well as in those with hyperlipoproteinaemia. Its form and distribution vary according to the precipitating cause and management is centred around establishing that the systemic lipoprotein profile is normal or treating any underlying dyslipoproteinaemia (e.g. primary chylomicronaemia) if it is not (see Chapter 14). The cause of any anterior segment inflammation should be diagnosed and treated, but there is no need to treat the lipid keratopathy.

Bilateral peripheral corneal lipid deposition (corneal arcus, arcus lipoides corneae) associated with hyperlipoproteinaemia (Fig. 9.61) is limited to a single case report in the cat and in this case the increase of serum lipid was a consequence of endotoxaemia associated with Gram-negative pyelonephritis (Crispin, 1993b).

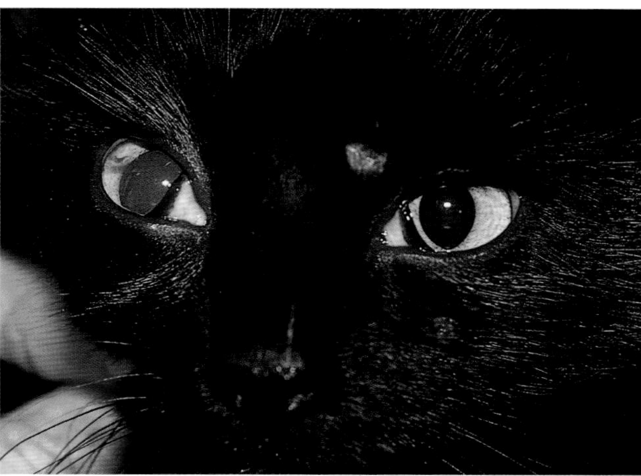

Fig. 9.60 *A 4-year-old Domestic shorthair with lipid keratopathy. An adult cat with chylomicronaemia diagnosed because lipid keratopathy developed precipitously at the site of a cat claw injury. Note the skin xanthomata above and below the left eye. The diagnosis was confirmed by examination of the fundus which revealed lipaemia retinalis (see Fig. 14.39) and from visual inspection of a blood sample and lipoprotein analysis.*

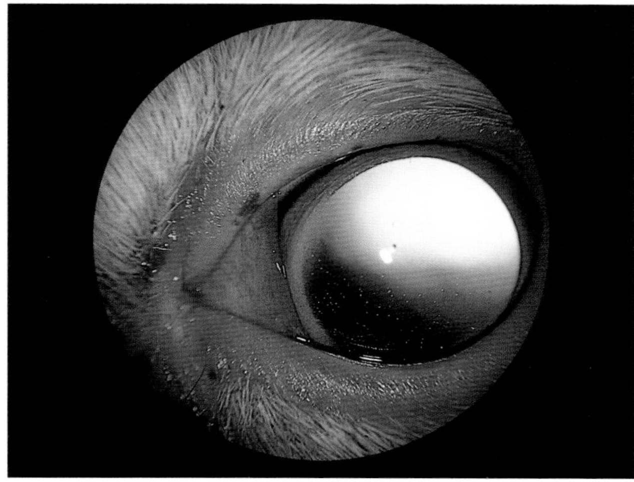

Fig. 9.61 *An 18-month-old Persian with bilateral corneal arcus (left eye shown) as a consequence of hyperlipoproteinaemia associated with endotoxaemia. Serum lipid levels returned to normal after treatment of the endotoxaemia.*

CORNEAL CALCIFICATION

Calcification is an unusual corneal response (Figs 9.62 and 9.63) which may either be a consequence of local corneal degeneration because of chronic inflammatory insult, or associated with any systemic disorder which produces

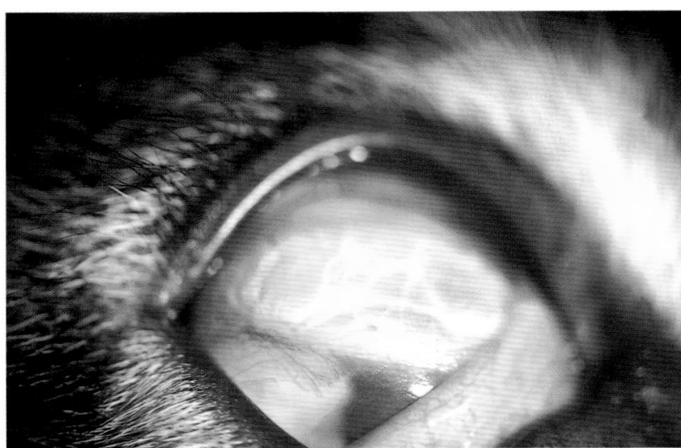

Fig. 9.62 *A 1-year-old Domestic shorthair with calcium keratopathy of unknown cause. Note the superficial nature of the calcium plaque. Treatment consists of surgical removal of the plaque and application of ethylene diaminetetraacetic acid (EDTA).*

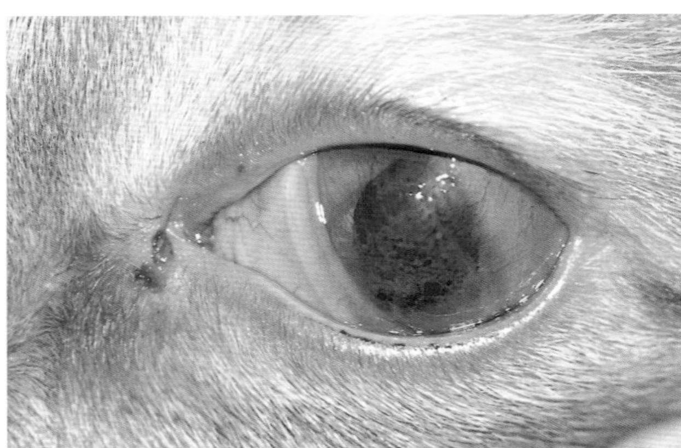

Fig. 9.63 *A 7-month-old Domestic shorthair with calcium keratopathy of unknown cause.*

hypercalcaemia (e.g. hyperparathyroidism, excessive ingestion of vitamin D).

References

Adam SM, Crispin SM (1995) Differential diagnosis of keratitis in cats. *In Practice* **17**, 355–363.

Bahn CF, Meyer RG, MacCallum DK, Lillie JH, Lovett EJ, Sugar A, Martonyi CL (1982) Penetrating keratoplasty in the cat. *Ophthalmology* **89**: 687–699.

Bistner SI, Aguirre G, Shively JN (1976) Hereditary corneal dystrophy in the Manx cat: A preliminary report. *Investigative Ophthalmology and Visual Science* **15**: 15–26.

Buyukmihci N, Bellhorn RRW, Hunziker J, Clinton J (1977) Encephalitozoon (Nosema) infection of the cornea in a cat. *Journal of the American Veterinary Medical Association* **171**: 355–357.

Campbell LH and McCree AV (1978) Corneal abscess in a cat: Treatment by subconjunctival antibiotics. *Feline Practice* **8**: 30–31.

Carrington SD (1983) Lipid keratopathy in a cat. *Journal of Small Animal Practice* **24**: 495–505.

Carrington SD (1985) Observations on the structure and function of the feline cornea. PhD thesis, University of Liverpool, UK.

Carrington SD, Woodward EG (1986) Corneal thickness and diameter in the domestic cat. *Ophthalmic and Physiological Optics* **3**: 823–826.

Carrington SD, Crispin SM, Williams DL (1992) Characteristic conditions of the feline cornea. In Raw ME, Parkinson TJ (eds), *The Veterinary Annual*, 32nd Issue, pp. 83–96. Blackwell Scientific Publications, Oxford.

Champagne ES, Munger RJ (1992) Multiple punctate keratotomy for the treatment of recurrent epithelial erosions in dogs. *Journal of the American Animal Hospital Association* **28**: 213–216.

Crispin SM (1982) Corneal dystrophies in small animals In Raw ME, Parkinson TJ (eds) *The Veterinary Annual. 22nd Issue*, pp. 198–310. Blackwell Scientific Publications, Oxford.

Crispin SM (1993a) The pre-ocular tear film and conditions of the conjunctiva and cornea. In *Manual of Small Animal Ophthalmology*. Eds SM Petersen-Jones and SM Crispin. British Small Animal Veterinary Association, pp. 137–171.

Crispin SM (1993b) Ocular manifestations of hyperlipoproteinaemia. *Journal of Small Animal Practice* **34**: 500–506.

Dice P (1977) Intracorneal acid-fast granuloma. *Proceedings of the American College of Veterinary Ophthalmologists* **8**: 91.

Gerding PA, Morton LD, Dye JA (1994) Ocular and disseminated candidiasis in an immunosuppressed cat. *Journal of the American Veterinary Medical Association* **204**: 10, 1635–1638.

Glover TL, Nasisse MP, Davidson, MG (1994) Acute bullous keratopathy in the cat. *Veterinary and Comparative Ophthalmology* **4**: 2, 66–70.

Gunn-Moore DA, Jenkins PA, Lucke VM (1996) Feline tuberculosis; a literature review and discussion of 19 cases caused by an unusual mycobacterial variant. *Veterinary Record* **138**: 53–58.

Haskins ME and Patterson DF (1987) Inherited metabolic diseases. In J Holzworth (ed.) *Diseases of the Cat*. WB Saunders, Philadelphia. pp. 808–819.

Kern TJ (1990) Ulcerative keratitis. In NJ Millichamp, JD Dziezyc (eds) *Veterinary Clinics of North America: Small Animal Practice*. Philadelphia, W. B. Saunders, **20**: 643–666.

Ketring KL, Glaze MB (1994) *Atlas of Feline Ophthalmology*. Veterinary Learning Systems, USA.

Kirschner SE (1990) Persistent corneal ulcers. In NJ Millichamp, JD Dziezyc (eds) *Veterinary Clinics of North America: Small Animal Practice*. Philadelphia, W. B. Saunders, **20**: 627–642.

Miller DM, Blue JL, Winston SM (1983) Keratomycosis caused by *Cladosporidium* sp in a cat. *Journal of the American Veterinary Medical Association* **182**: 1121–1122.

Moore DL and Jones RG (1994) Corneal stromal abscess in a cat. *Journal of Small Animal Practice* **35**: 432–434.

Morgan RV (1994) Feline corneal sequestration: A retrospective study of 42 cases (1987–1991). *Journal of the American Animal Hospital Association* **30**: 24–28.

Morgan RV, Abrams KL (1994) A comparison of six different therapies for persistent corneal erosions in dogs and cats. *Progress in Veterinary and Comparative Ophthalmology* **4**: 38–43.

Morgan RV, Abrams KL, Kern TJ (1996) Feline eosinophilic keratitis: A retrospective study of 54 cases (1989–1994). *Progress in Veterinary and Comparative Ophthalmology* **6**: 131–134.

Nasisse MP (1990) Feline herpesvirus ocular disease. In NJ Millichamp, JD Dziezyc (eds) *Veterinary Clinics of North*

America: Small Animal Practice. Philadelphia, W. B. Saunders, **20**: 667–680.

Nasisse MP, Luo H, Wang YJ, Glover TL, Weigler BJ (1996a) The role of feline herpesvirus-1 (FHV-1) in the pathogenesis of corneal sequestration and eosinophilic keratitis *Proceedings of the American College of Veterinary Ophthalmologists* **27**: 80.

Nasisse MP, Luo H, Wang YJ, Boland L, Weigler BJ (1996b) The diagnosis of ocular feline herpesvirus-1 (FHV-1) infections by polymerase chain reaction. *Proceedings of the American College of Veterinary Ophthalmologists* **27**: 83.

Nasisse MP, Halenda RM, Luo H (1996c) Efficacy of low dose oral, natural human interferon alpha (nHuIFN'') in acute feline herpesvirus infection: A preliminary dose determination trial. *Proceedings of the American College of Veterinary Ophthalmologists* **27**: 79.

Paulsen ME, Lavach JD, Severin GA, Eichenbaun JD (1987) Feline eosinophilic keratitis: A review of 15 clinical cases. *Journal of the American Animal Hospital Association* **23**: 63–69.

Peiffer RL, Jackson WF (1979) Mycotic keratopathy of the dog and cat in the southeastern United States: A preliminary report. *Journal of the American Animal Hospital Association* **15**: 93–97.

Pentlarge VW (1989) Corneal sequestration in cats. *Compendium on Continuing Education for the Practicing Veterinarian* **11**: 24–29.

Prasse KW, Winston SM (1996) Cytology and histopathology of feline eosinophilic keratitis. *Veterinary and Comparative Ophthalmology* **6**: 74–81.

Read A, Barnett KC, Sansom J (1995) Cyclosporin-responsive keratoconjunctivitis in the cat and horse. *Veterinary Record* **137**: 170–171.

Schoster JV, Wickman L, Stuhr C (1995) The use of ulrasonic pachymetry and computer enhancement to illustrate the collective corneal thickness profile of 25 cats. *Veterinary and Comparative Ophthalmology* **5**: 68–73.

Startup FG (1988) Corneal necrosis and sequestration in the cat: A review and record of 100 cases. *Journal of Small Animal Practice* **29**: 476–486.

Veenendaal H (1928) Tuberculoom op de cornea bij een kat. *Tijd Diergeneeskd* **55**: 607–611.

Zapater RC, Albesi EJ, Garcia GH (1975) Mycotic keratitis by *Drechslera spicifera*. *Sabouraudia* **13**: 295–298.

10 Aqueous and glaucoma

Introduction

The cat has a deep anterior chamber despite the marked curvature of the anterior face of the lens. The cornea is large and the irido-corneal angle wide (Fig. 10.1). Gonioscopy, examination of the angle of filtration, is possible in this species without the use of a goniolens due to the deep anterior chamber and large cornea. It reveals the slender, more widely separated and unbranching fibres of the pectinate ligament with numerous fibres behind in the trabecular meshwork (Figs 10.2 and 10.3). The colour of the pectinate ligament varies with the iris from gold to blue and almost white.

The normal intraocular pressure of the cat is quoted as 22.2 ± 5.2 (Miller and Picket, 1992).

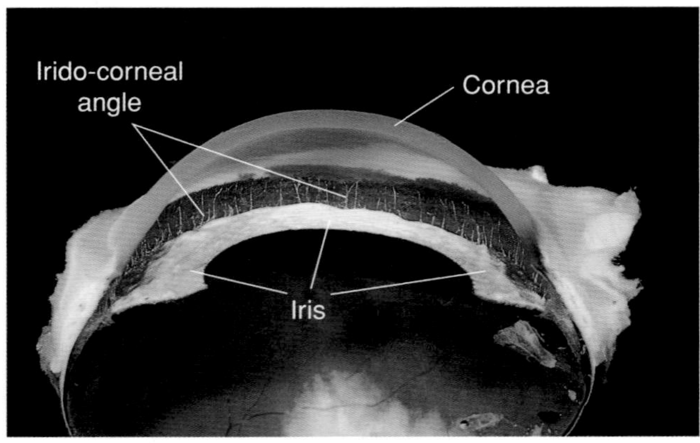

Fig. 10.1 *Anterior segment, feline eye (lens removed). Note wide angle, pectinate ligament, deep anterior chamber and large cornea.*

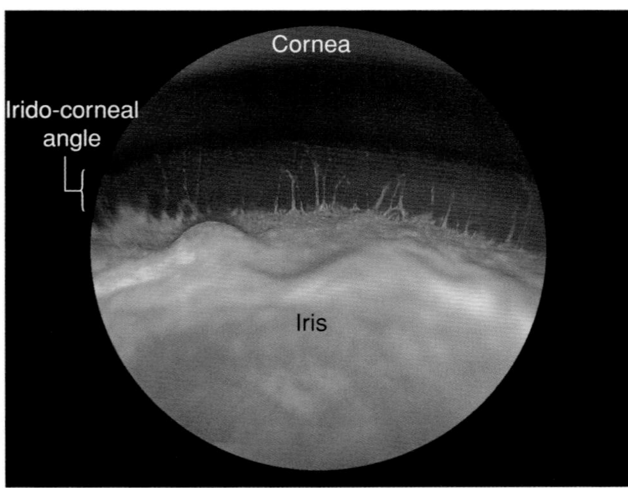

Fig. 10.2 *Gonio-photograph showing the normal feline drainage angle.*

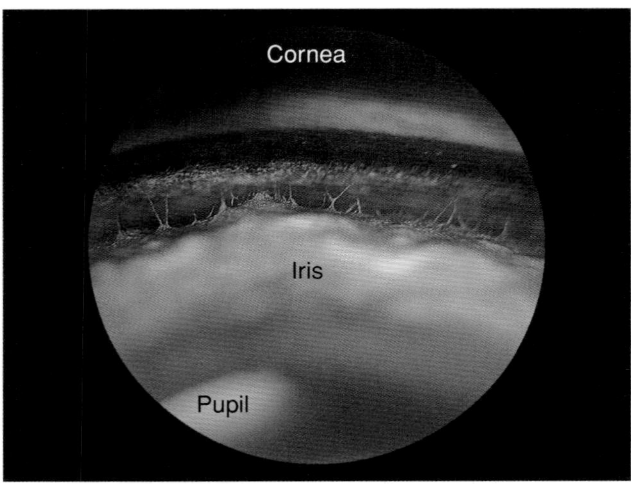

Fig. 10.3 *Gonio-photograph showing the normal feline drainage angle.*

Congenital anomalies

Congenital glaucoma, or buphthalmos, has been recorded on a number of occasions in the kitten as both unilateral and bilateral cases. It presents as a grossly enlarged globe(s) sometimes with intense corneal oedema (Fig. 10.4). The cause is unknown but presumably is due to a developmental abnormality preventing adequate drainage. It is known that scleral stretching, with consequent globe enlargement, occurs more readily in young animals. A single case of congenital glaucoma in a Siamese kitten caused by iridoschisis (cleavage of the iris layers) has been reported (Brown *et al.*, 1994).

Glaucoma

Glaucoma is defined as an increase in the intraocular pressure with resultant damage to the retina and optic nerve causing total and irreversible blindness (Fig. 14.76). It is not a simple condition but a complex of several separate entities and would be better described as 'the glaucomas'. Glaucoma may be subdivided into primary glaucoma, with no antecedent ocular disease (Fig. 10.5); or secondary, following some other ocular disease (Fig. 10.6). The canine primary glaucomas are considered to be hereditary and a number of breeds are affected. In the cat a breed predisposition in the Siamese and Persian has been noted (Brooks, 1990) but no proven primary hereditary glaucoma has yet been recorded and cases of glaucoma occur in all breeds of cat. There have been pathological reports of glaucoma in the cat in which no other ocular disease was apparent (Wilcock *et al.*, 1990) but, to date, the glaucomas in the cat can be considered almost invariably as secondary and associated with inflammation, in particular uveitis (Fig. 10.6) and neoplasia, especially uveal melanoma (Fig. 10.7) and lymphosarcoma (Fig. 10.8).

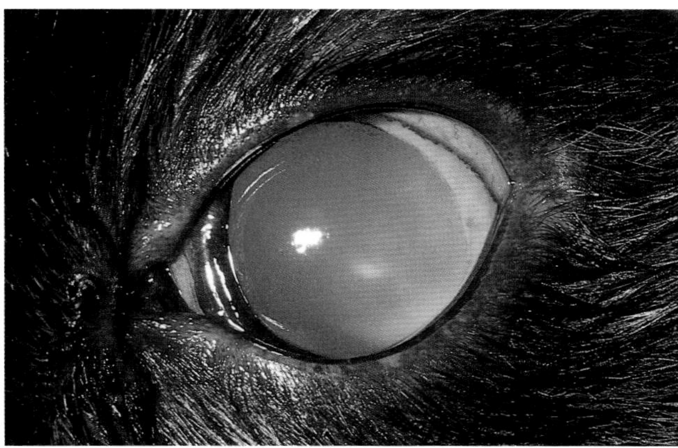

Fig. 10.6 *Secondary glaucoma following uveitis associated with toxoplasmosis. Note inflammatory material posterior cornea and anterior vitreous and dilated pupil.*

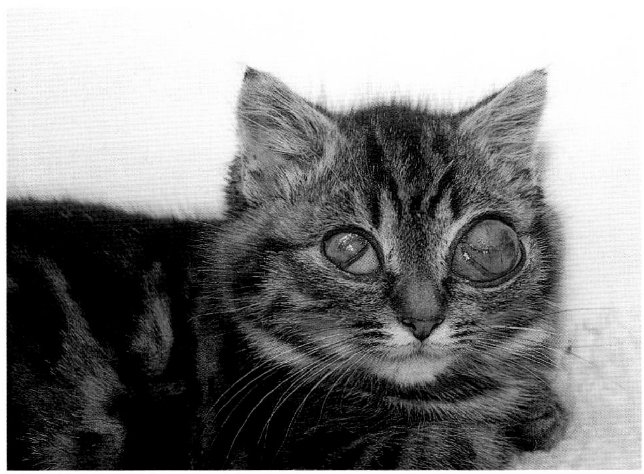

Fig. 10.4 *Tabby kitten with bilateral buphthalmos of differing degrees. Note both eyes wide open with no apparent sign of pain.*

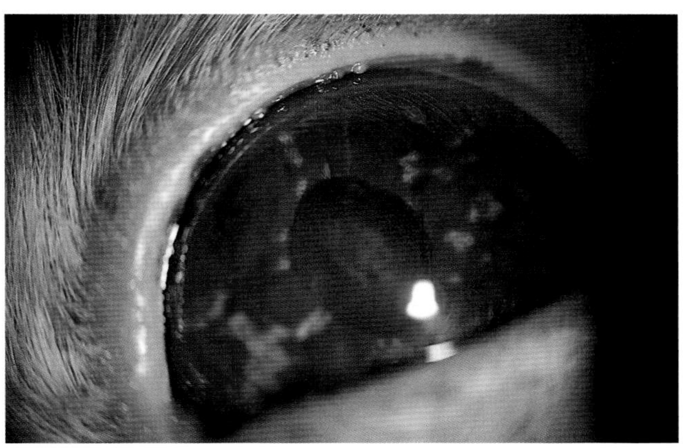

Fig. 10.7 *Domestic shorthaired cat with secondary glaucoma caused by extensive uveal melanoma.*

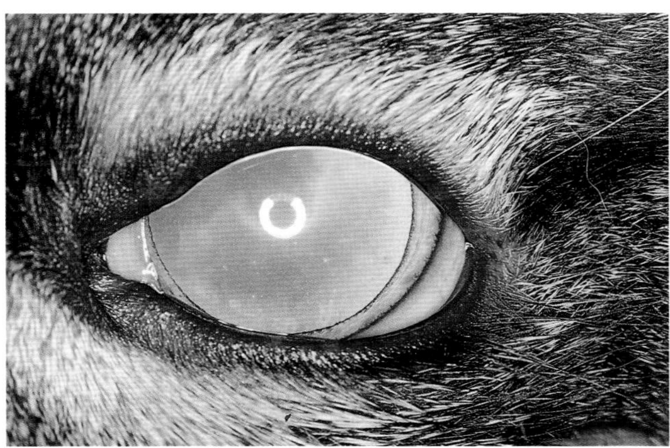

Fig. 10.5 *Domestic shorthaired cat with primary glaucoma and dilated pupil. Note no signs of uveitis, neoplasia or other antecedent ocular disease.*

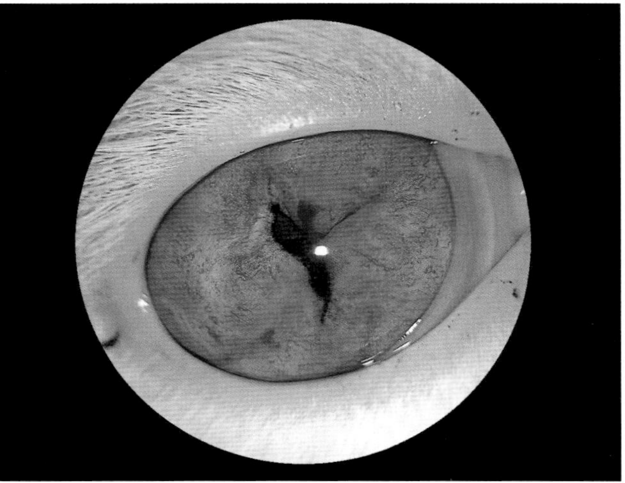

Fig. 10.8 *Domestic shorthaired cat with secondary glaucoma caused by uveal lymphosarcoma. Note distortion of pupil and obliteration of the angle of filtration.*

Trauma, lens rupture (anterior capsule) and lens luxation are other known causes although in the last instance it can be difficult to decide whether the lens luxation was the cause of the glaucoma or whether the glaucoma, with subsequent hydrophthalmos and zonular rupture (Fig. 10.9), resulted in lens luxation. With the absence in the cat of primary hereditary glaucoma and primary hereditary lens luxation as causes of glaucoma, it is not surprising that this condition is much rarer than in the dog. However, uveitis and uveal neoplasia are probably more frequent causes of glaucoma in the cat than in the dog. Nevertheless, feline glaucoma can be described as an uncommon condition.

The glaucomas can also be subdivided into acute and chronic, but in the cat acute glaucoma is rare and the hyperacute and painful congestive glaucoma, which occurs in the dog, has not been seen. In the cat, glaucoma is usually insidious in onset and blepharospasm and lacrimation may be noted in the early stages although ocular pain is rarely exhibited. Conjunctival and episcleral congestion, classic signs of 'the red eye', occur (Figs 10.10 and 10.11), but to a much lesser extent than in the dog; occasionally chemosis is seen (Fig. 10.12). Corneal opacity (oedema) is usually mild (Fig. 10.13) but in longstanding cases bullous keratopathy may occur (Fig. 10.14). Peripheral corneal vascularization (Fig. 10.15) also occurs in feline glaucoma but again does not show the intensity seen in the canine glaucomas. Fractures in Descemet's membrane (corneal striae) in cases of hydrophthalmos have not been seen in the cat. Opinions would appear to differ on the incidence of corneal oedema, Ridgway and Brightman (1989) found it to be the most frequent clinical sign but Wilcock *et al.* (1990), in a pathological study of 131 eyes, did not find diffuse corneal oedema but did record two cases of Descemet's fractures. With the rise in intraocular pressure due to a reduced aqueous outflow facility the pupil of an affected eye will be dilated (Figs 10.5 and 10.6) in comparison to the other eye and it is this anisocoria (Fig. 10.16) which may be the first obvious ocular sign. The

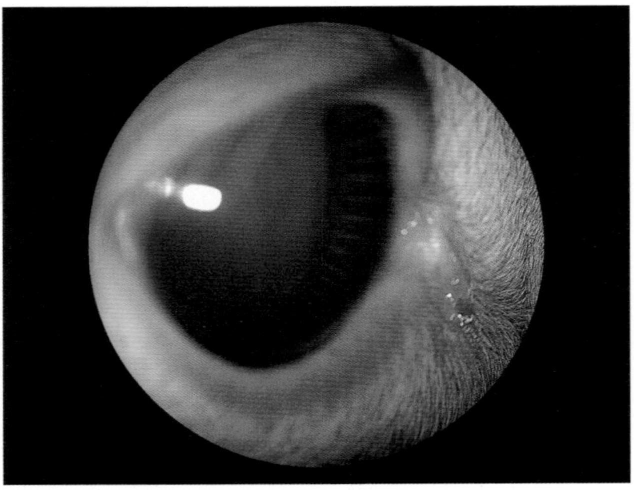

Fig. 10.9 *Stretching and rupture of zonular fibres caused by glaucoma.*

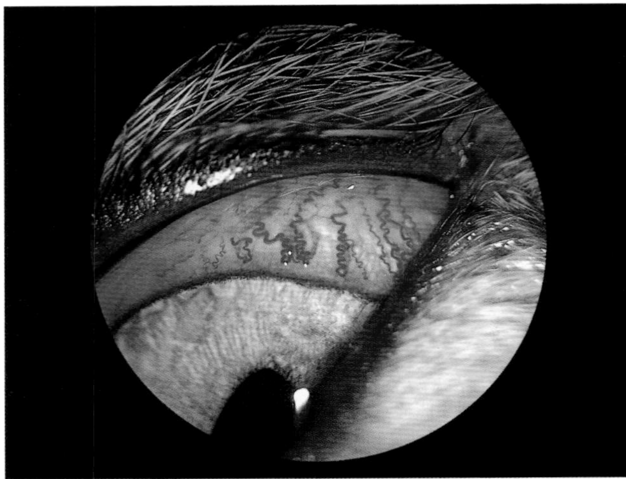

Fig. 10.10 *A 12-year-old Domestic shorthaired male with conjunctival and episcleral congestion. Note clear cornea.*

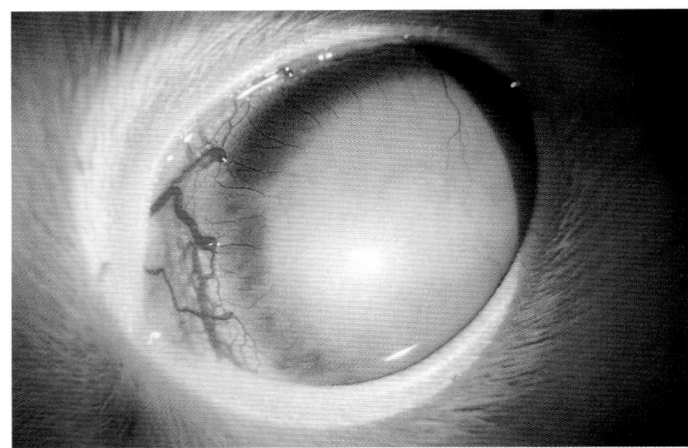

Fig. 10.11 *Conjunctival and episcleral congestion, broad but fine corneal vascular fringe and central corneal oedema. Note absence of corneal striae.*

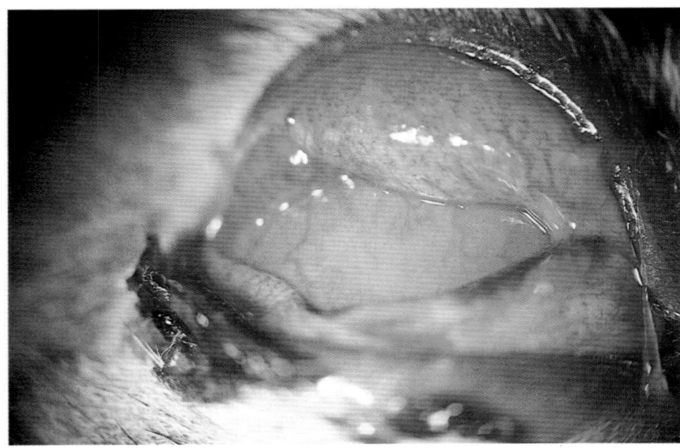

Fig. 10.12 *Domestic shorthaired cat showing severe glaucoma (secondary to uveitis) with conjunctival chemosis and corneal oedema and vascularization.*

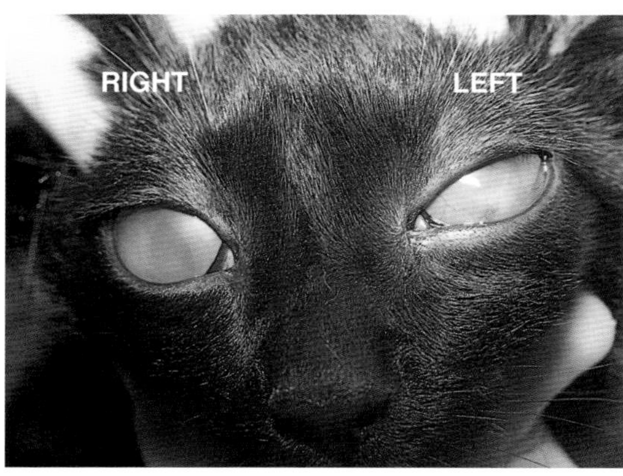

Fig. 10.13 *Burmese cat with bilateral hydrophthalmos and corneal opacity. Note absence of corneal striae and undilated pupil in right eye.*

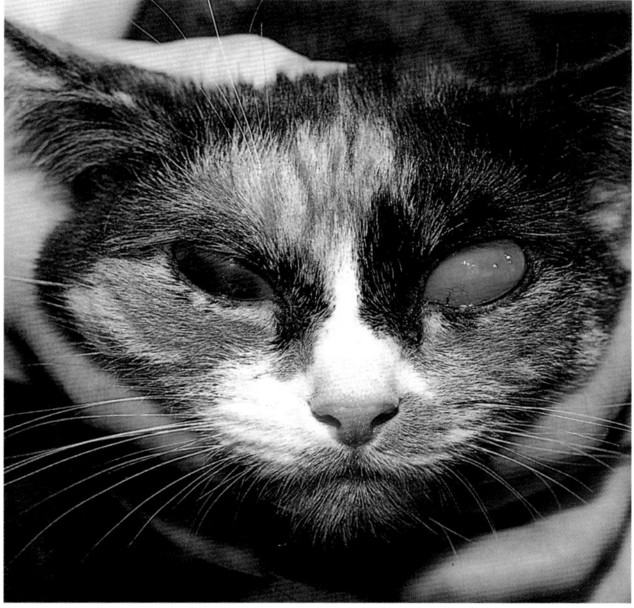

Fig. 10.14 *Domestic shorthaired cat with chronic glaucoma showing hydrophthalmos and bullous keratopathy.*

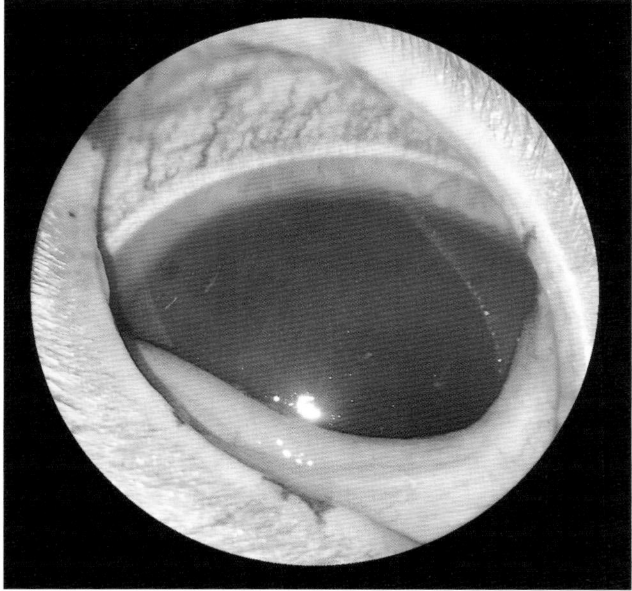

Fig. 10.15 *Domestic shorthaired cat with secondary glaucoma resulting from intraocular haemorrhage (hypertension); note the conjunctival congestion and early fine corneal vascular fringe.*

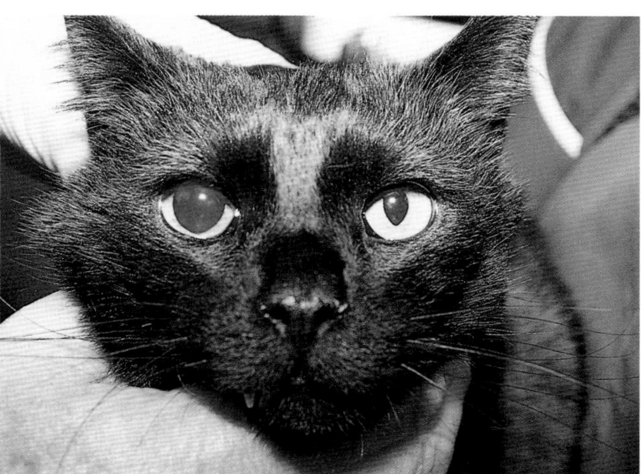

Fig. 10.16 *Anisocoria. Note dilated pupil in the right eye in a case of early glaucoma.*

globe of the cat stretches fairly easily and thus hydrophthalmos (megaloglobus) (Fig 10.17) is common and may lead to an exposure keratopathy (Figs 10.18 and 10.19) and resultant ulceration. The hydrophthalmos is not always obvious and minor degrees of globe enlargement occur. Cataract and lens luxation due to stretching (Fig. 10.9) and breakdown of the zonular fibres (see also Chapter 11) may occur and ultimately retinal degeneration and optic atrophy with cupping of the disc (Fig. 14.76) – more difficult to recognize in this species – also occur as a result of the increased intraocular pressure.

Glaucoma in the cat may be unilateral or bilateral, whatever the cause, and gonioscopy reveals an open angle in the apparently primary cases.

Treatment of glaucoma in the cat is difficult and often unsuccessful in either restoring or saving vision for a number of reasons. The feline glaucomas are usually insidious in onset and ocular signs much less marked than in the dog and, consequently, cases are usually presented late and with advanced and irreversible vision loss. However, of greater importance is the fact that the majority of cases in this species are secondary to another eye condition and therefore the primary condition should be treated wherever possible. The cause of most glaucoma cases in the cat is an anterior uveitis (Wilcock *et al.*, 1990). The use of corticosteroids and other anti-inflammatory agents may therefore be of value, although some uveitis cases are poorly responsive to medical therapy (see also Chapter 12). The use of miotics, such as pilocarpine, has proved to be of little or no value and might be contraindicated in cases of uveitis. Carbonic anhydrase inhibitors, which decrease aqueous production, can be of some value although dichlorphenamide (5 mg/kg twice daily, per os) is less well tolerated in this species and dosage may have to be reduced (unfortunately dichlorphenamide has recently been withdrawn in the UK). Acetazolamide (10 mg/kg twice daily, per os) may also be used. β-Adrenergic blockers (Timolol 0.5%, 1 drop once to twice daily) can be used topically in combination with a carbonic anhydrase inhibitor. Unfortunately, enucleation is often the only possible treatment and may be indicated in certain cases, particularly the buphthalmic or hydrophthalmic eye, in cases of uveal neoplasia, except perhaps the aged cat with a slow-growing tumour, and in trauma cases, especially where there may be lens rupture and the danger of the subsequent development of intraocular sarcoma.

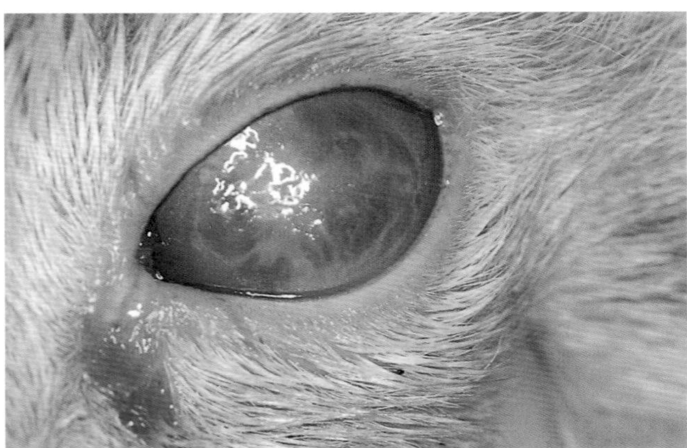

Fig. 10.17 *Hydrophthalmos or megaloglobus. Note disruption of the corneal reflex because of epithelial involvement (bullous keratopathy).*

Other conditions of the aqueous

The aqueous humour may be involved in a number of conditions which are illustrated in the following figures (see also Chapters 9 and 12). Hypopyon (white cells in the anterior

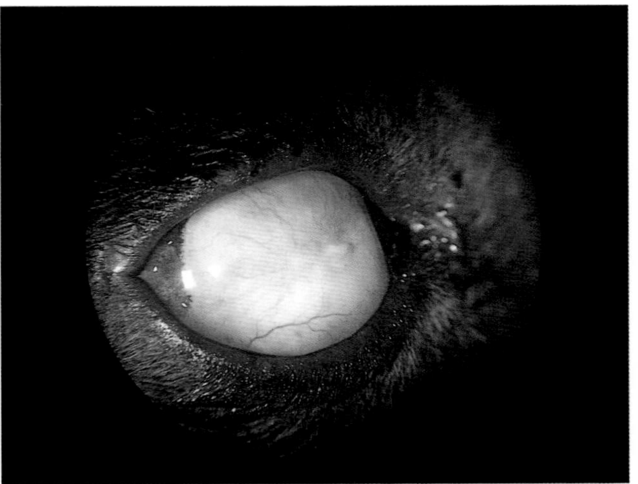

Fig. 10.18 *Chronic glaucoma with hydrophthalmos and early exposure keratopathy.*

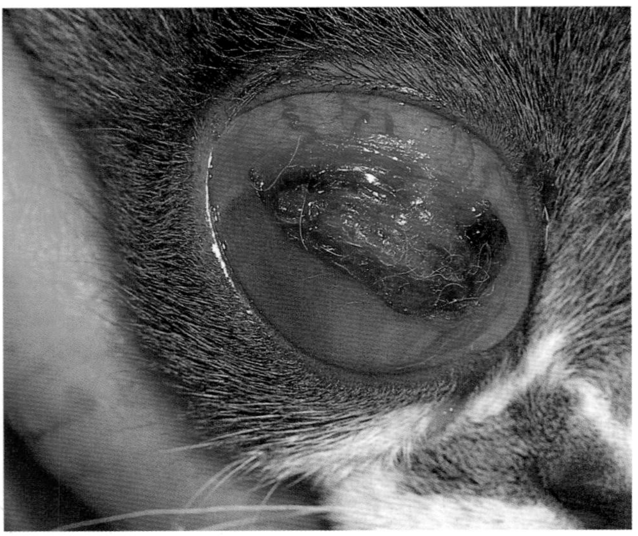

Fig. 10.19 *Severe hydrophthalmos, complication of endophthalmitis, and advanced exposure keratopathy.*

chamber) and hyphaema (red cells in the anterior chamber) accompany severe iritis (Fig. 10.20) which may often be a sign of systemic disease. Hypopyon may also indicate lymphosarcoma (Figs 10.21–10.23). Hyphaema may be present in severe iritis (Fig. 10.20); following trauma (Fig. 10.24); associated with infections such as FIP and FeLV (Fig. 10.25); with anaemia and thrombocytopenia (Fig. 10.26); in cases of hypertension (Figs 10.15, 10.27 and 10.28); and with blood dyscrasias (Martin, 1982). Hyphaema rarely requires treatment as the blood is readily cleared and a secondary glaucoma is unusual. Complete turbidity of the aqueous due to lipaemia is shown in Figs 10.29–10.31). Rare cases of larvae in the anterior chamber do occur (Fig. 10.32).

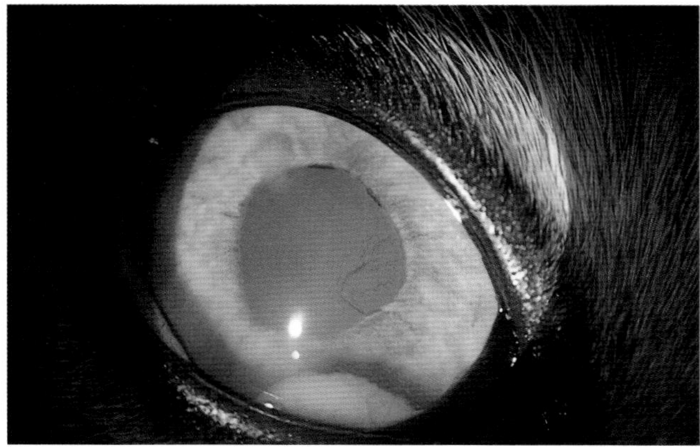

Fig. 10.22 *Dense hypopyon in iritis. Note extensive posterior synechiae around the pupil margin and vascularization of the anterior lens capsule.*

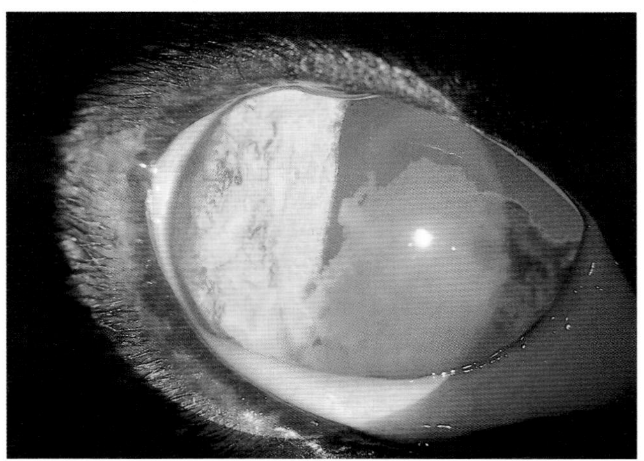

Fig. 10.20 *Hypopyon and hyphaema in a case of severe iritis. Note the vascular congestion of the iris.*

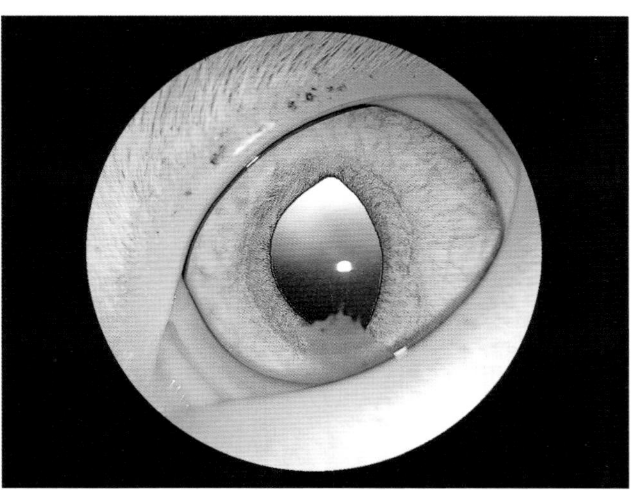

Fig. 10.23 *Neoplastic white cells in the aqueous in a case of generalized lymphosarcoma. The other eye of this cat is shown in Fig. 10.8.*

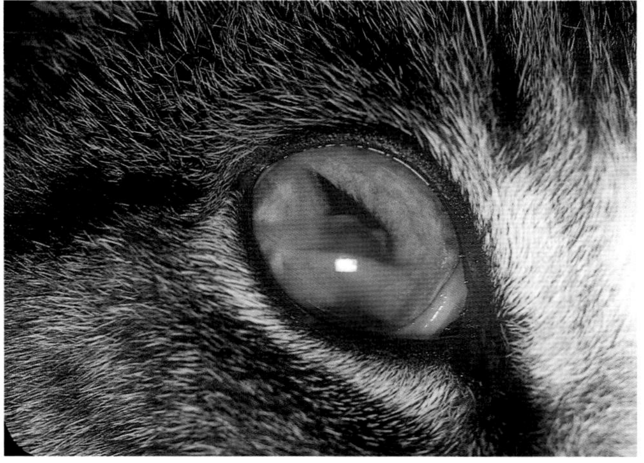

Fig. 10.21 *Hypopyon and hyphaema in a case of lymphosarcoma. Note swollen iris and pupil distortion.*

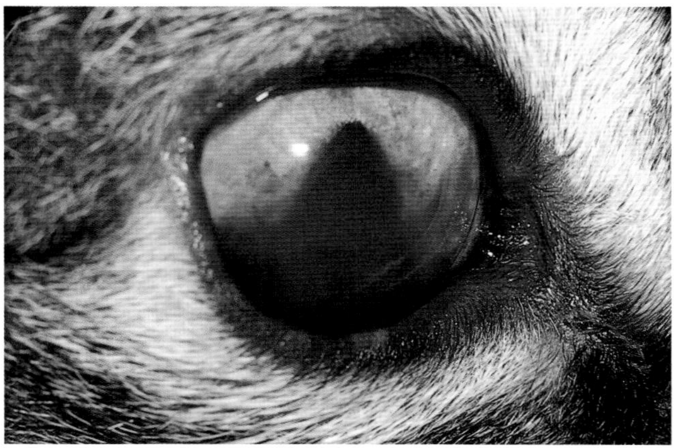

Fig. 10.24 *Hyphaema due to trauma.*

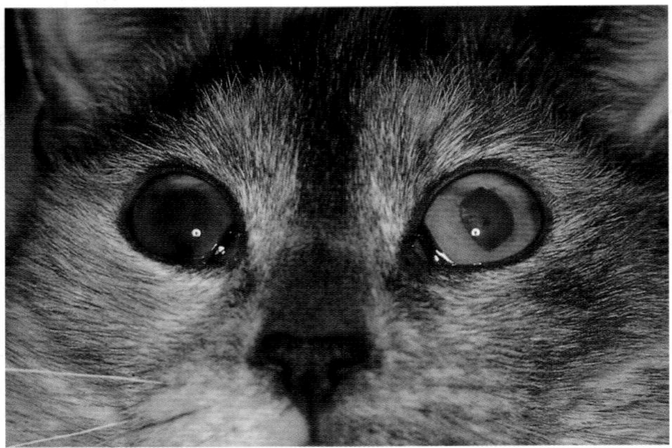

Fig. 10.25 Bilateral hyphaema in an FeLV positive cat.

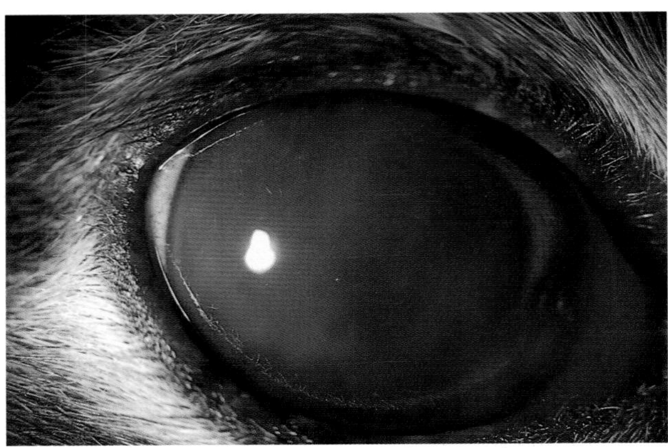

Fig. 10.28 Hyphaema in a case of hypertension. Fundus changes were present in the other eye.

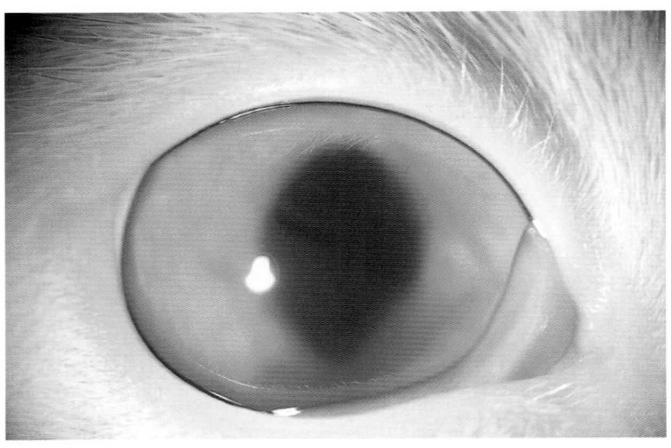

Fig. 10.26 Hyphaema associated with severe anaemia and thrombocytopenia.

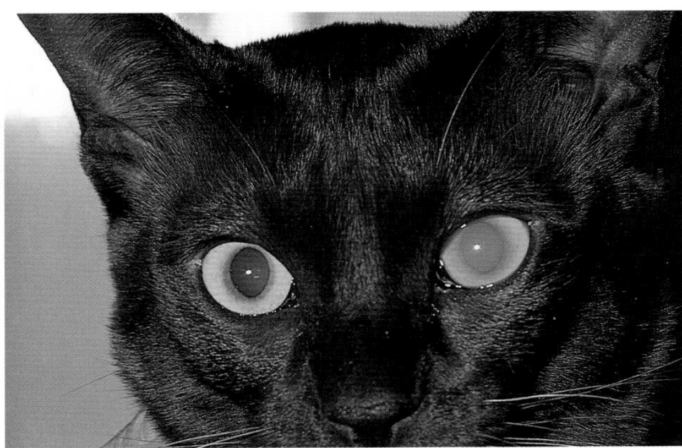

Fig. 10.29 Lipaemic aqueous (triglyceride rich) no apparent uveitis.

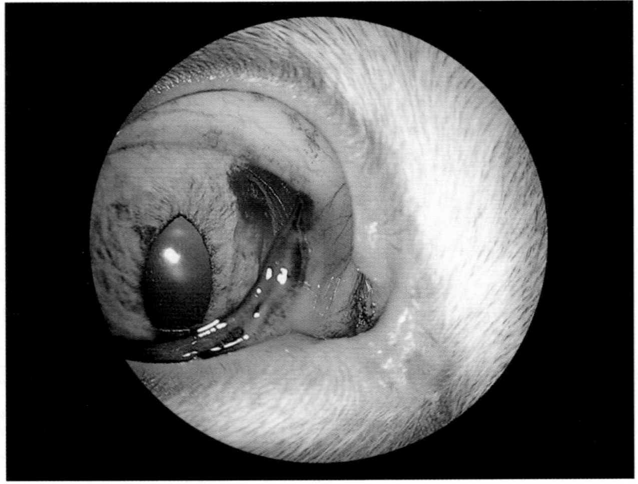

Fig. 10.27 Hyphaema in a case of hypertension. Fundus changes were present in both eyes.

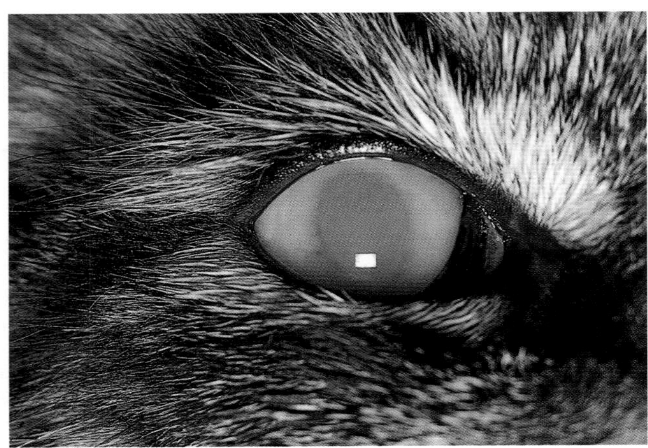

Fig. 10.30 Lipaemic aqueous (triglyceride rich) associated with uveitis.

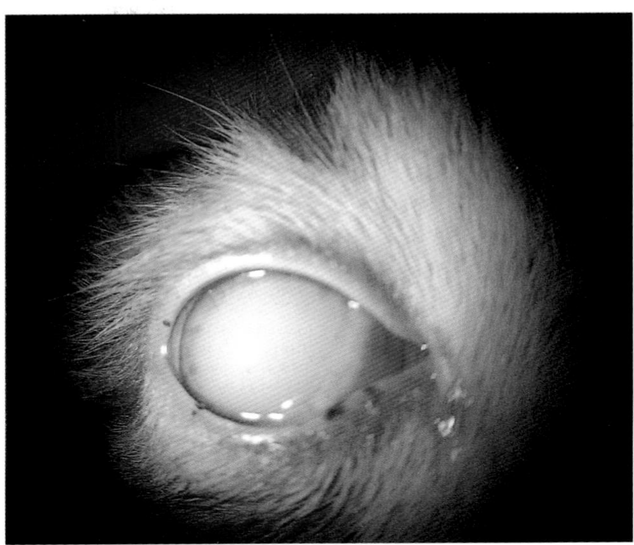

Fig. 10.31 *Severe case of lipaemic aqueous (serum triglyceridaemia and chylomicronaemia) with secondary glaucoma and vascular fringe following trauma.*

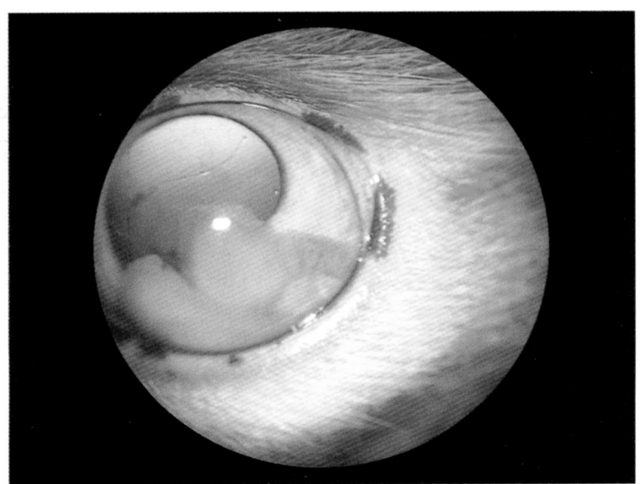

Fig. 10.32 *Ophthalmomyiasis interna of the anterior chamber, species unknown (courtesy of J. Wolfer).*

References

Brooks DE (1990) Glaucoma in the dog and cat. *The Veterinary Clinics of North America* **20**: 775–797.

Brown A, Munger R, Peiffer RL (1994) Congenital glaucoma and iridoschisis in a Siamese cat. *Veterinary and Comparative Ophthalmology* **4**: 121–123.

Martin CL (1982) Feline Ophthalmologic Diseases. *Modern Veterinary Practice* **63**: 209–213.

Miller PE, Pickett JP (1992) Comparison of human and canine tonometry conversion tables in clinically normal cats. *Journal of the American Veterinary Medical Association* **201**: 1017–1020.

Ridgway MD, Brightman AH (1989) Feline glaucoma: a retrospective study of 29 clinical cases. *Journal of the American Animal Hospital Association* **25**: 485–490.

Wilcock BP, Peiffer RL, Davidson MG (1990) The causes of glaucoma in cats. *Veterinary Pathology* **27**: 35–40.

Lens

Introduction

The lens is a biconvex, transparent and refractive structure suspended by zonular fibres, situated behind the iris (which it supports) and posterior chamber, and arbitrarily dividing the anterior and posterior segments of the eye (Fig. 11.1). The lens consists of a capsule, lens epithelium lying beneath the capsule of the anterior face and at the equator, and lens fibres which form throughout life; the lens fibres are partially responsible for the normal ageing change of senile nuclear sclerosis. Sclerosis of the lens occurs in the older cat, as in all animals, but is not as obvious as in the dog. The lens is subdivided into a nucleus (embryonic, foetal and adult), cortex and capsule and these can be further subdivided clinically into anterior and posterior portions.

The lens of the cat is large with a volume quoted as 0.5 ml and a diameter of 9–12 mm and with an anterior surface that has a steeper curvature than the posterior surface. The lens is therefore relatively larger than in most dogs. Dynamic accommodation in the cat is poor.

The lens is derived from surface ectoderm, the lens vesicle initially separating and remaining at the opening into the optic cup. The cavity of the vesicle is then obliterated by elongation of the primary lens fibres (future embryonic nucleus). Secondary lens fibres grow from the equatorial region and form the pattern of the anterior and posterior lens sutures (Fig. 11.2). Nutrition of the developing lens is via the hyaloid artery (see also Chapter 13) and tunica vasculosa lentis, a form of perilenticular vascular network of mesenchymal origin; remnants of the latter forming the persistent pupillary membrane (see also Chapters 2 and 12). Lens development is rapid and occurs early in embryogenesis.

Disorders of the lens can be classified into congenital anomalies and cataract (simply defined as an opacity of the lens and/or its capsule) and luxation or subluxation of the lens (abnormal position due to partial or complete rupture of the zonular fibres).

Congenital anomalies

Aphakia (absence of the lens) is rare; microphakia (small lens) and lenticonus (abnormally shaped lens) have all been

Fig. 11.1 *Section of feline eye showing shape, position and size of the lens.*

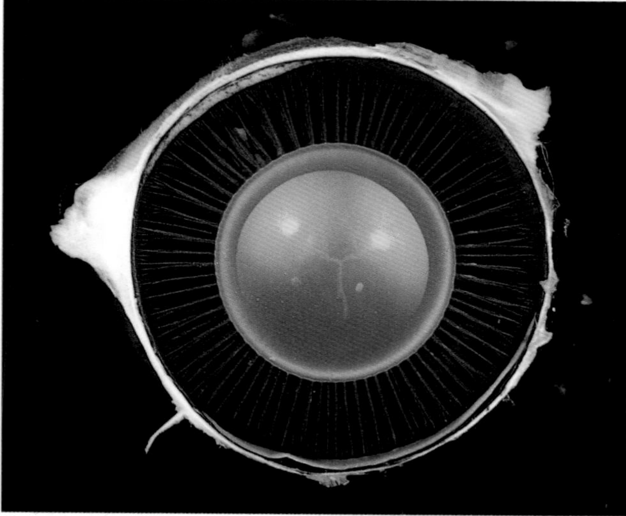

Fig. 11.2 *Anterior segment as viewed from behind showing posterior suture lines of lens and encircling ciliary processes of ciliary body.*

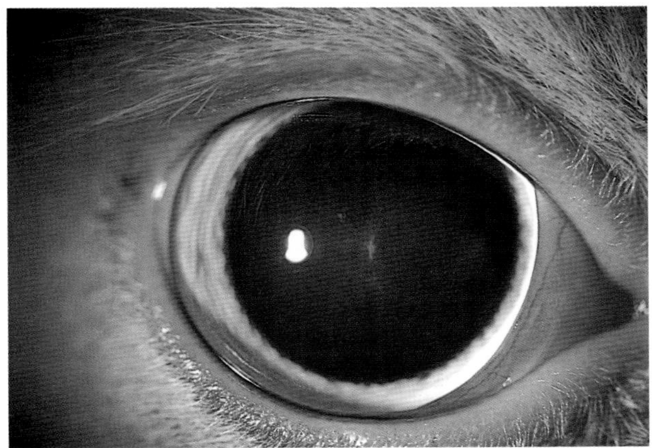

Fig. 11.3 Congenital cataract in a 6-month-old Persian female.

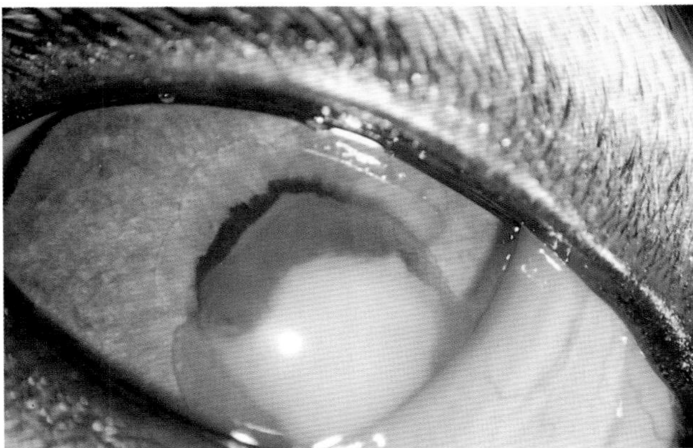

Fig. 11.5 Dislocated cataract and microphakia in a 17-week-old Tabby/white Domestic shorthaired female.

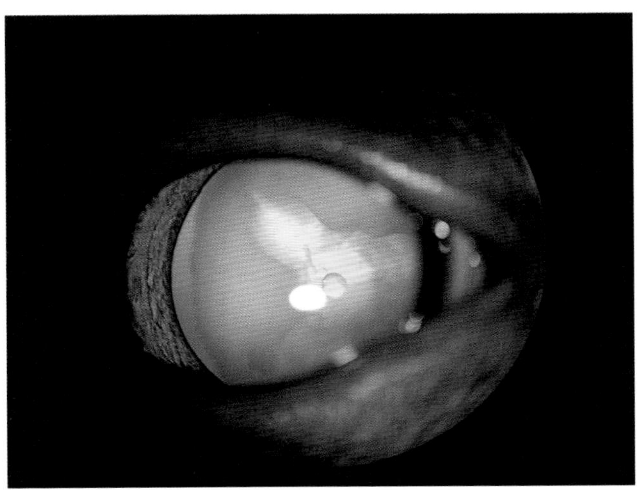

Fig. 11.4 Congenital cataract in a 7-week-old Tabby Domestic shorthaired female.

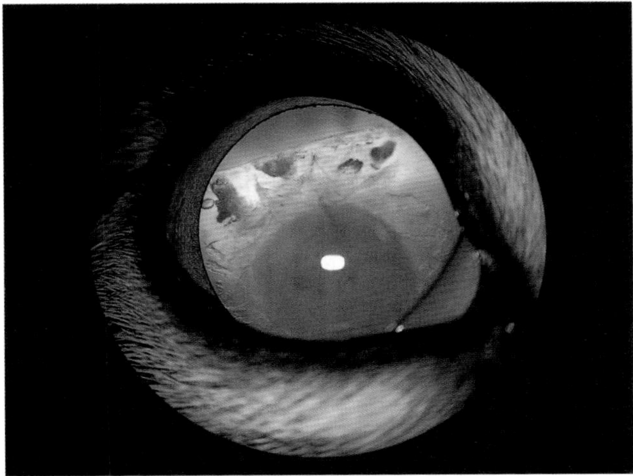

Fig. 11.6 Lens coloboma with mainly nuclear cataract in a 7-month-old Domestic longhaired male.

reported as isolated cases in the cat and are all associated with other ocular abnormalities (Aguirre and Bistner, 1973; Peiffer, 1982; Peiffer and Belkin, 1983). Multiple congenital ocular defects usually include cataract (Figs 4.5–4.8) but are rare in this species.

Congenital cataract may be unilateral or bilateral and has been reported in the Persian (Peiffer and Gelatt, 1975) and in the British shorthaired cat, nuclear in type and with a presumed autosomal recessive mode of inheritance (Irby, 1983).

Isolated cases of congenital cataract also occur with no apparent breed incidence or aetiology. Examples are shown in Figures 11.3 and 11.4. Figure 11.5 depicts one eye of a kitten with an anteriorly dislocated total cataract which also exhibits degrees of microphakia; both eyes were affected.

A rare case of uniocular lens coloboma is depicted in Figure 11.6, together with nuclear and complicated cataract.

CATARACT

Cataract in the cat is uncommon and, whereas in the dog many cases of cataract are presented to the veterinary ophthalmologist, opacity of the lens in the cat is a rare presenting sign. This difference in incidence is partially due to the fact that many cataracts in the dog have been proven to be primarily hereditary, as for example in the Golden Retriever, American Cocker Spaniel and Miniature Schnauzer, etc. However, there are only occasional reports of feline breed-related cataract. In addition, cataract secondary to the generalized form of progressive retinal atrophy does not occur in the cat, although in the dog this form of cataract is a common, if not invariable, sequel in such breeds as the Irish Setter, Miniature Poodle, Cocker Spaniel and Labrador Retriever, for example. Cases of advanced hereditary retinal degeneration in the Abyssinian cat have been examined over several years and the lens has always remained entirely free from any opacity (see also Chapter 14).

To date, there are no proven reports of primary, hereditary, noncongenital cataract in the cat. However, Rubin (1986) reported three cases in related Himalayan cats in which the condition was bilateral and present as early as 12 weeks and with variable expression from posterior polar through posterior subcapsular to total; progression was recorded in one case. The relationship of the cats indicated simple autosomal recessive inheritance. Figures 11.7 and 11.8 illustrate possible cases of primary hereditary cataract in related British blue-cream cats in which the condition was bilateral and similar in the two eyes, affecting the anterior and posterior poles and suture lines.

The Chédiak–Higashi syndrome has been recorded in blue-smoke Persian cats as an autosomal recessive condition and includes cataract in addition to thin pale irises and fundic hypopigmentation (Collier *et al.*, 1979; see also Chapter 12).

Feline cataract is, therefore, almost always secondary in form and can be classified under the following headings:

(1) Post-inflammatory (uveitis) – probably the most frequent and often associated with posterior synechiae; Figures 11.9–11.15 illustrate several cases.
(2) Traumatic – particularly following penetrating corneal injuries involving the anterior lens capsule. These cataracts, as with the previous type, may be partial or total. Note that lens resorption does occur, particularly in young cats, both with and without damage to the anterior capsule and may itself lead to uveitis. Examples are shown in Figures 11.16–11.19. The extent and progression of traumatic cataract in the cat is variable and adhesions to the iris are usually present.
(3) Metabolic – diabetic cataract has been described as rare in the cat and is certainly much less common than in the dog and of slower onset; Figures 11.20 and 11.21 show two cases, the latter occurring in a very young animal.
(4) Secondary to another eye disease – examples in this category include glaucoma and following lens luxation (see Chapter 10 and the following section).

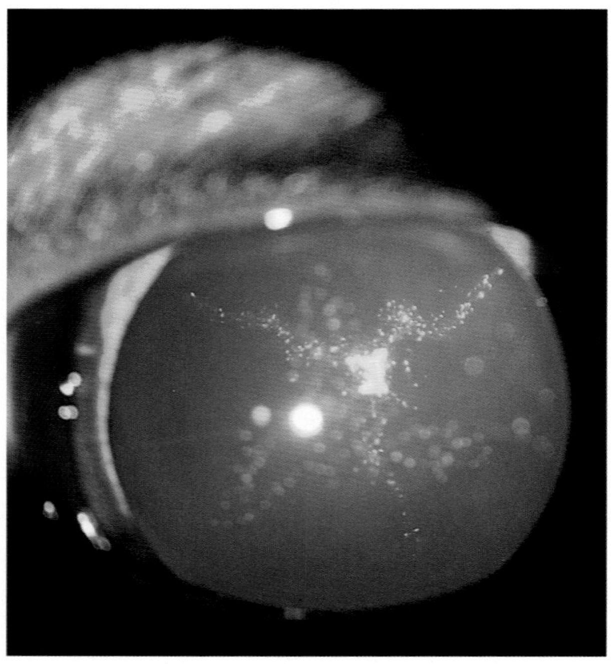

Fig. 11.7 *Primary cataract, anterior polar and posterior suture line in a British Blue-cream.*

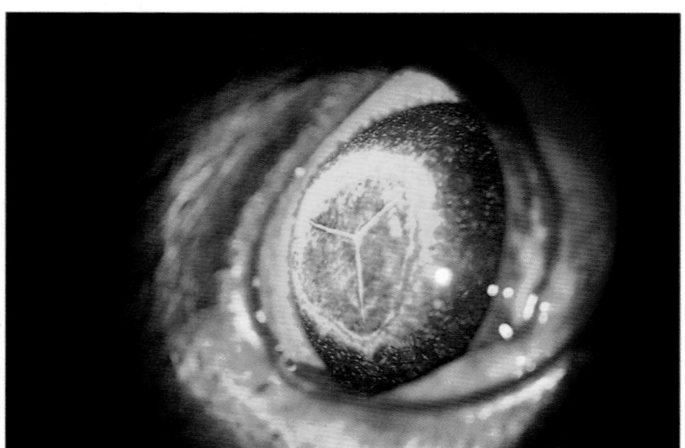

Fig. 11.8 *Primary cataract, suture line and subcapsular in a British Blue-cream.*

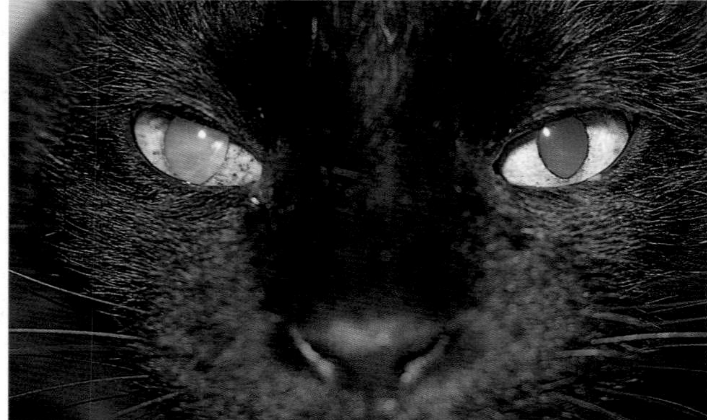

Fig. 11.9 *Uniocular cataract secondary to uveitis. Note the pigmentary changes in the iris of the right eye.*

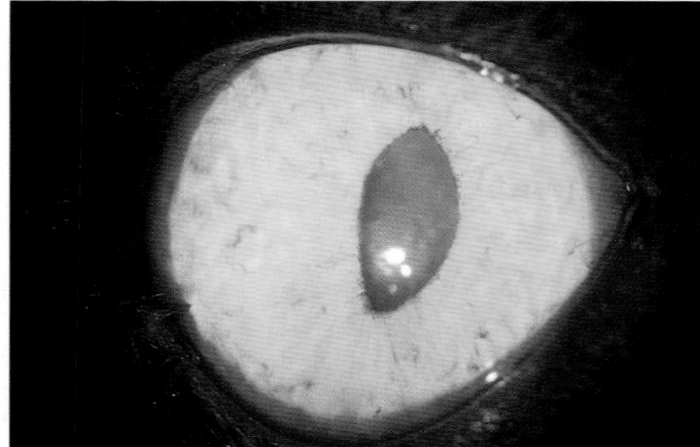

Fig. 11.10 *Cataract secondary to uveitis. Note the hyperaemic blood vessels on the iris.*

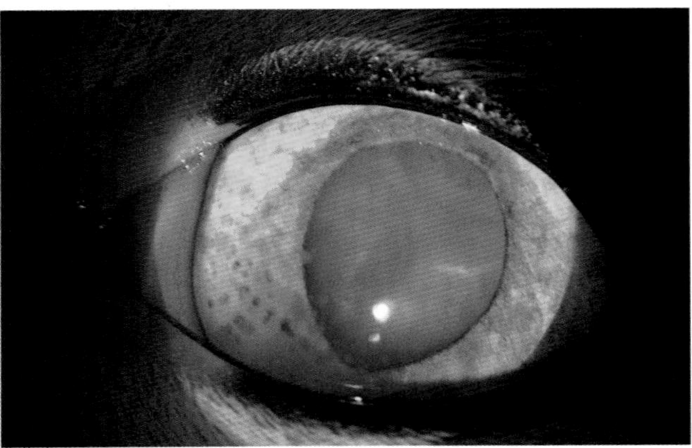

Fig. 11.11 *Cataract secondary to uveitis. Note the keratic precipitates on the corneal endothelium ventrally.*

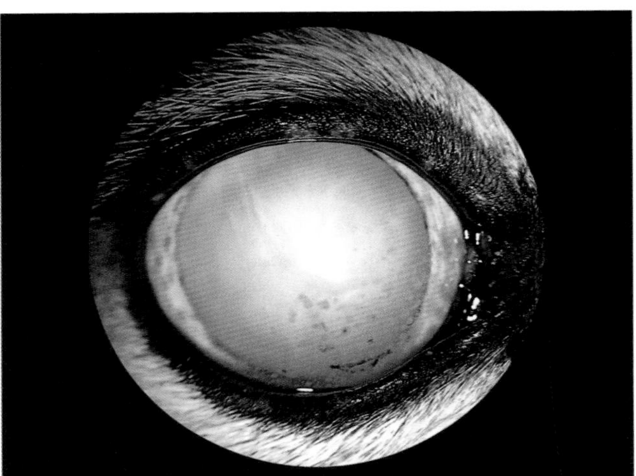

Fig. 11.12 *Total cataract secondary to uveitis. Again, note keratic precipitates and iris changes.*

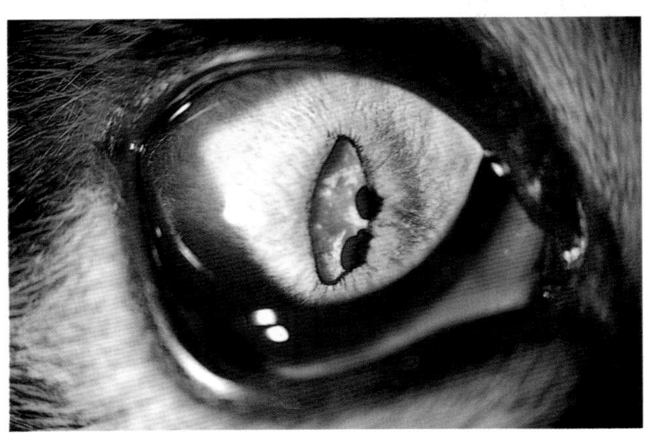

Fig. 11.13 *Cataract and lens resorption with low-grade iritis and associated uveal cysts.*

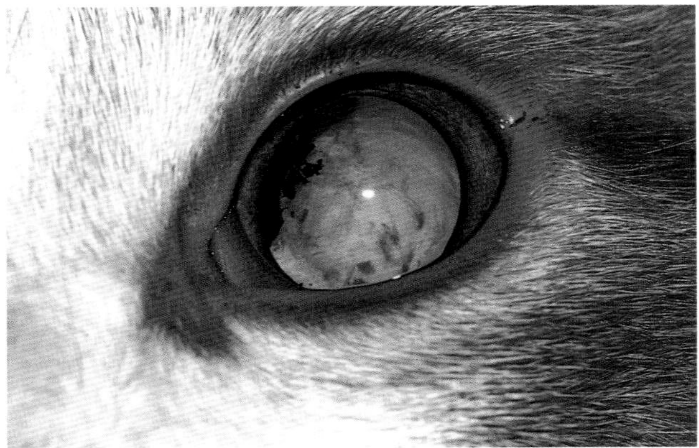

Fig. 11.14 *Secondary cataract and posterior synechiae. Note colour change in iris.*

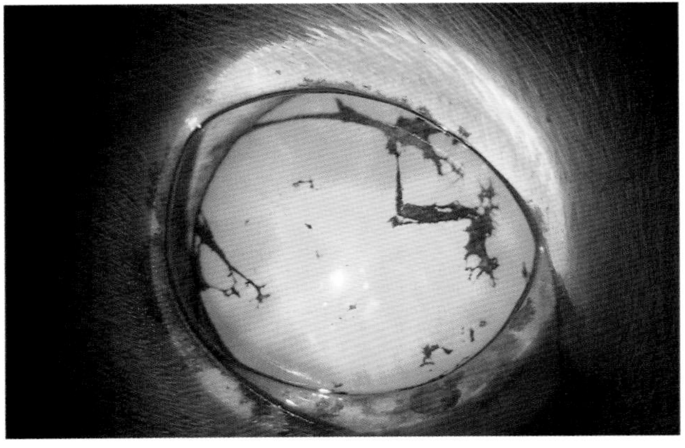

Fig. 11.15 *Cataract and extensive posterior synechiae.*

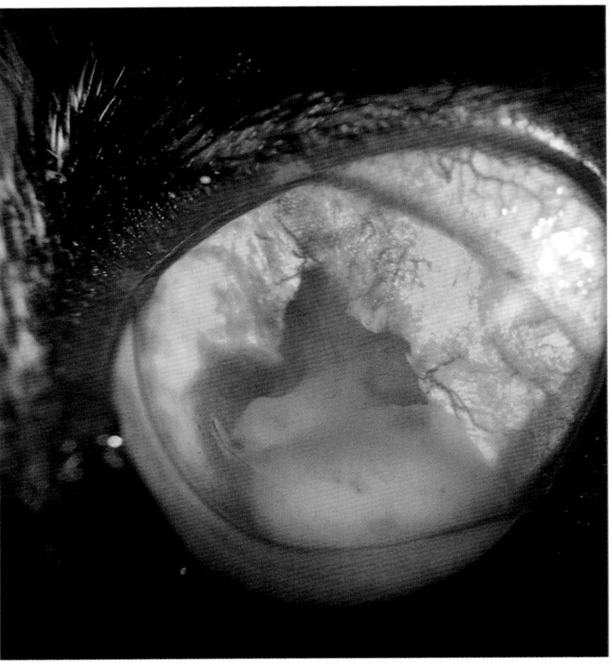

Fig. 11.16 *Penetrating corneal injury with uveitis, cataract and escape of lens material into the anterior chamber.*

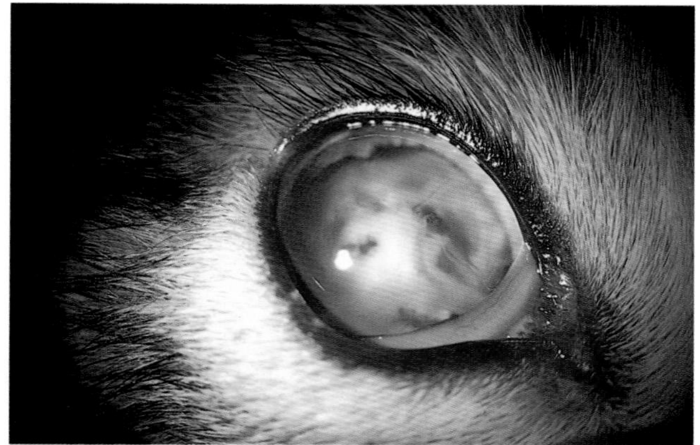

Fig. 11.17 *Traumatic cataract with rupture of anterior lens capsule and escape of lens material.*

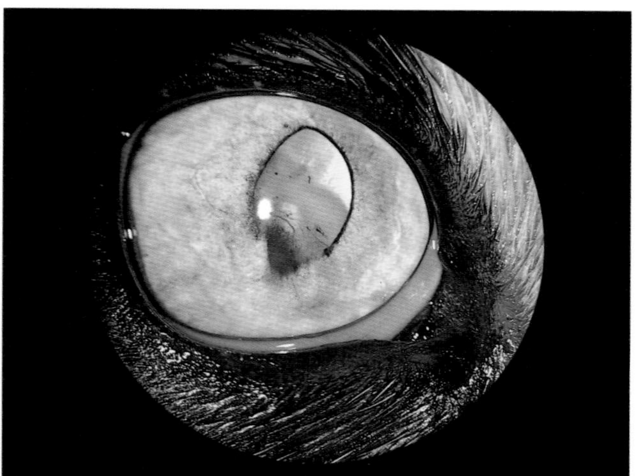

Fig. 11.18 *Partial traumatic cataract following penetrating claw injury. Note posterior synechiae and blood vessel on lens capsule. This progressed to become total within 12 months and was subsequently resorbed.*

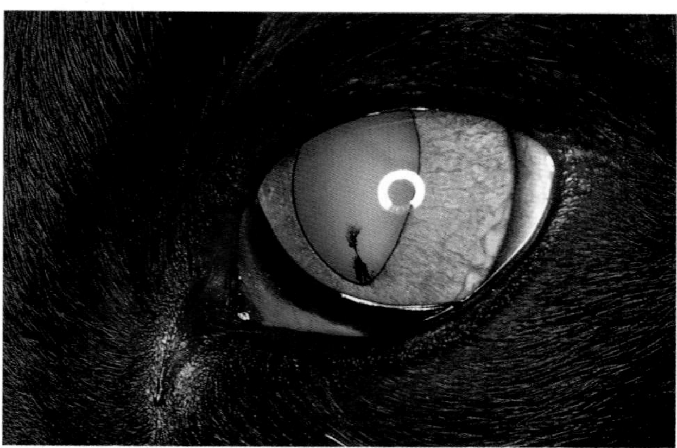

Fig. 11.19 *Traumatic cataract developing some months after blunt ocular trauma.*

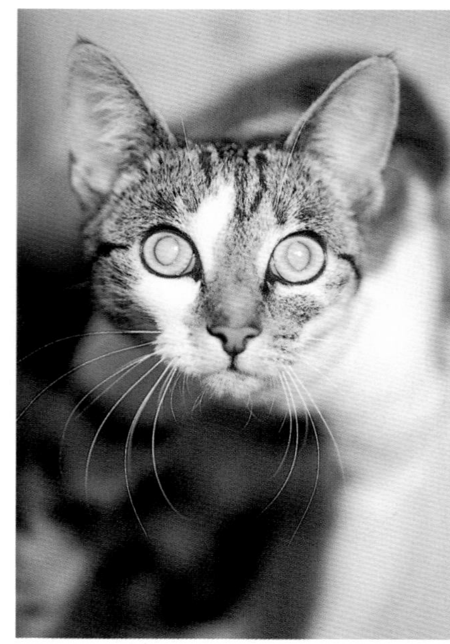

Fig. 11.20 *Bilateral and symmetrical diabetic cataract in a 2½-year-old Domestic shorthaired female.*

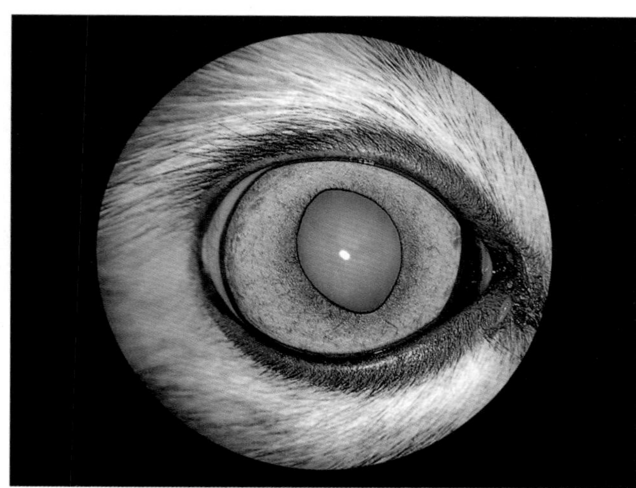

Fig. 11.21 *Diabetic cataract in a 22-week-old Chinchilla cross Persian male kitten. Note the typical 'Y' shaped water cleft.*

Nutritional cataracts have been described in the feline, including a deficiency of arginine occurring in young kittens (Remillard *et al.*, 1993). Bilateral cataract has also been seen in several of the big cats, e.g. tiger, cheetah, leopard and black leopard, and always in animals hand-reared from birth and frequently given a variety of supplements in addition to various milk substitutes (Figs 11.22 and 11.23).

Senile nuclear sclerosis occurs in the cat but usually only becomes evident at a more advanced age than in the dog, where it may first become noticeable as early as 6 or 7 years; in the cat it is not apparent until 10 years and older (Fig. 11.24).

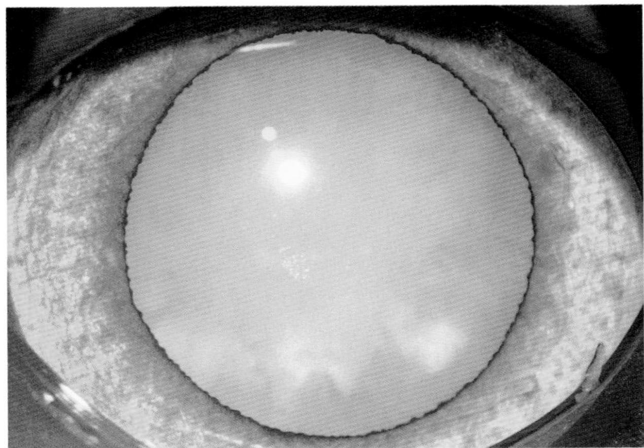

Fig. 11.22 *Total cataract in a leopard cub.*

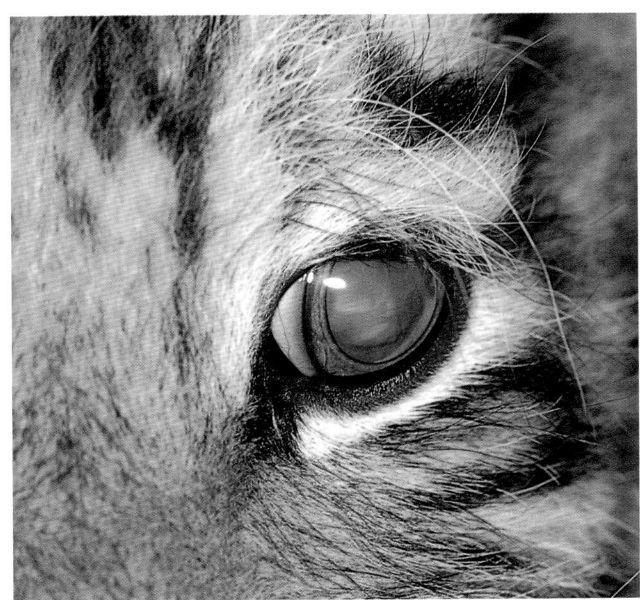

Fig. 11.23 *Cataract in a tiger cub.*

Cataract may also be classified according to the position of the opacity within the lens, e.g. nuclear, cortical, capsular, etc. Figures 11.25 to 11.32 show examples including nuclear, perinuclear, suture line, posterior polar, capsular, equatorial, cortical and focal, i.e. small and well demarcated.

The management of cataract in the cat is similar to that in the dog in that surgery is the only possible treatment. Although cataract in the cat is commonly secondary to another eye disease, although rarely to a retinal disorder, cataract surgery seldom results in severe intraocular inflammation, as is so often the case in the dog; despite the fact that cataract is often secondary to uveitis. The cause of the uveitis should, if possible, be ascertained prior to surgery and any active cases of uveitis treated. A cat blind with

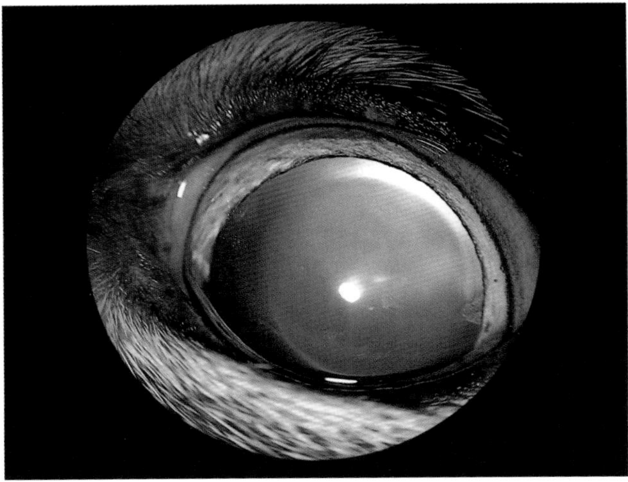

Fig. 11.24 *Senile nuclear sclerosis and small wedge of cortical cataract at '3 o'clock' in a 17-year-old Domestic shorthaired neutered male.*

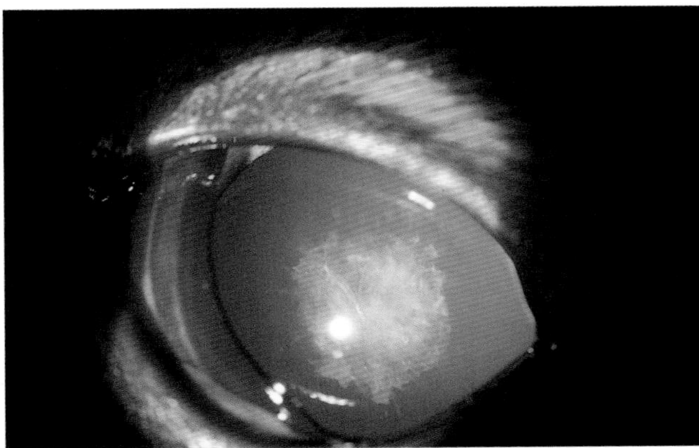

Fig. 11.25 *Nuclear cataract in a Burmese female kitten.*

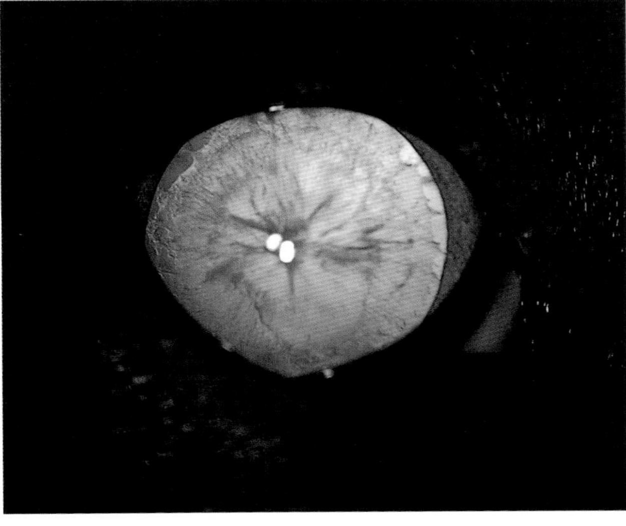

Fig. 11.26 *Nuclear and perinuclear and suture line cataract in a 6-month-old Domestic shorthair.*

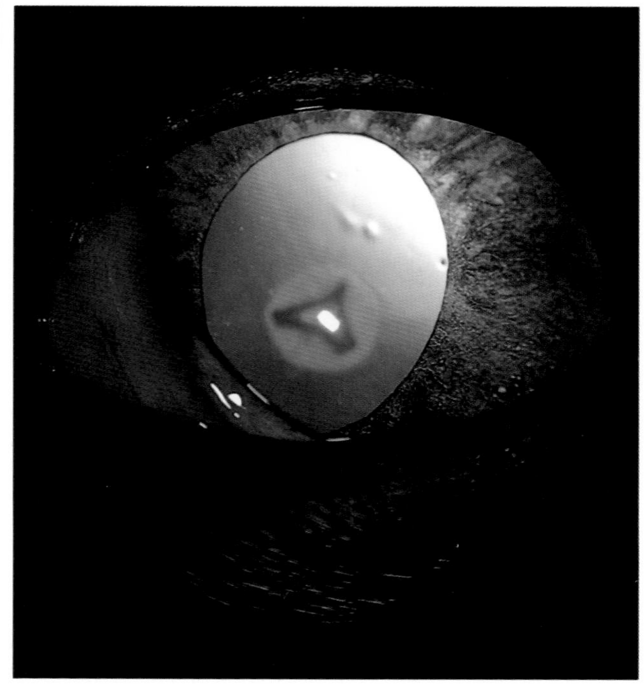

Fig. 11.27 Posterior polar capsular cataract in a 3-year-old Siamese.

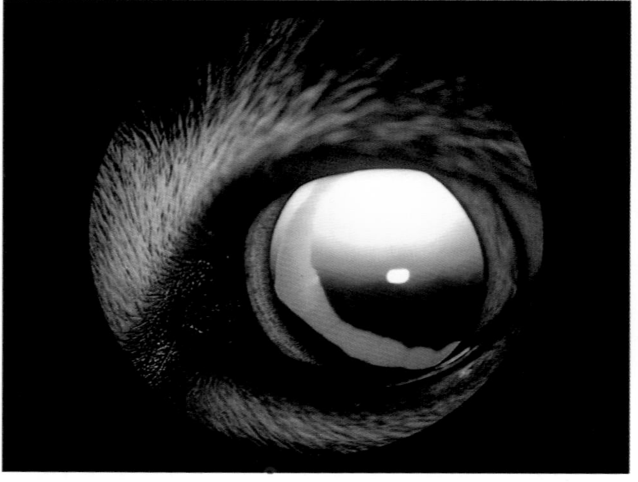

Fig. 11.28 Equatorial cataract (bilateral case) in a 16-week-old Domestic shorthaired female.

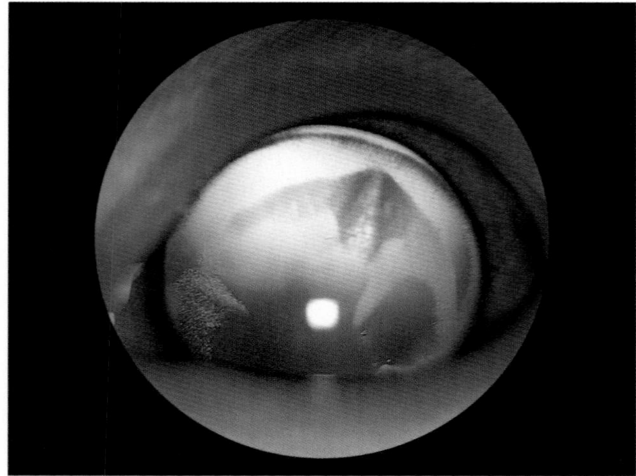

Fig. 11.29 Equatorial cataract and opacities at the ends of the posterior suture lines in a young Domestic shorthaired male kitten.

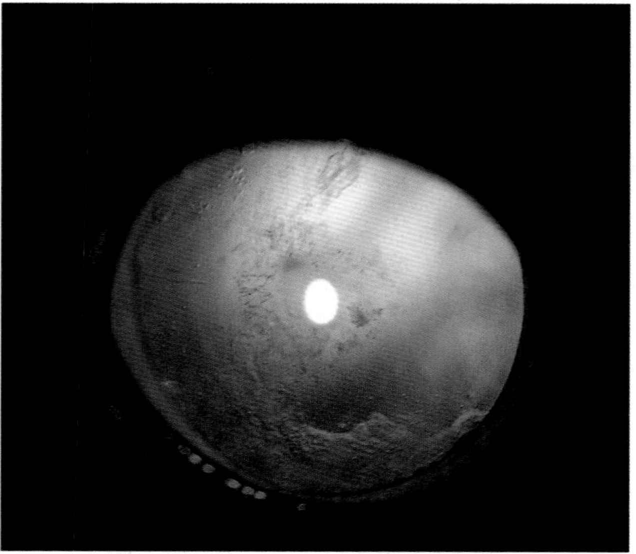

Fig. 11.30 Cortical cataract in an adult Domestic shorthair.

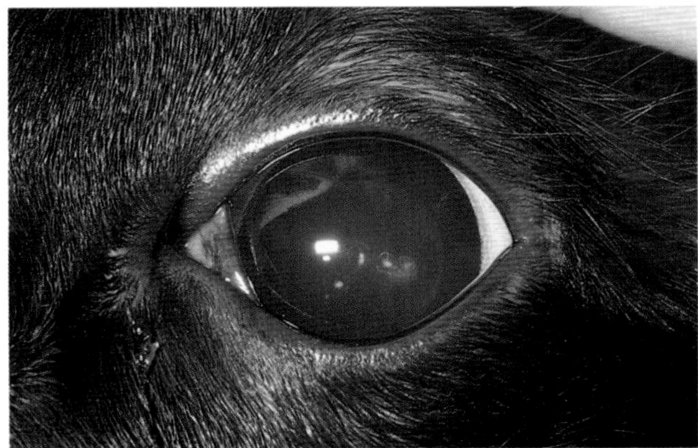

Fig. 11.31 *Focal cataracts in a 5-year-old Burmese neutered female.*

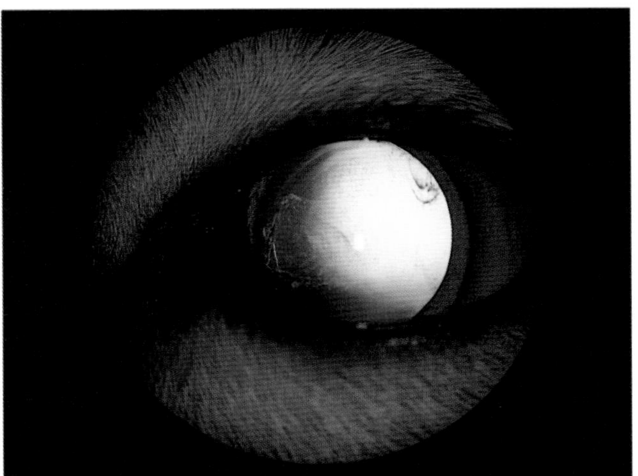

Fig. 11.32 *Focal cataracts in a 6-month-old Bengal female.*

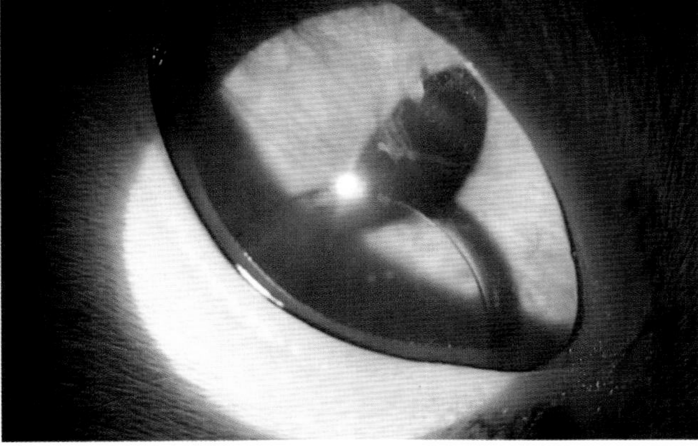

Fig. 11.33 *Anterior luxation of a clear microphakic lens in a 6-month-old Domestic shorthaired kitten.*

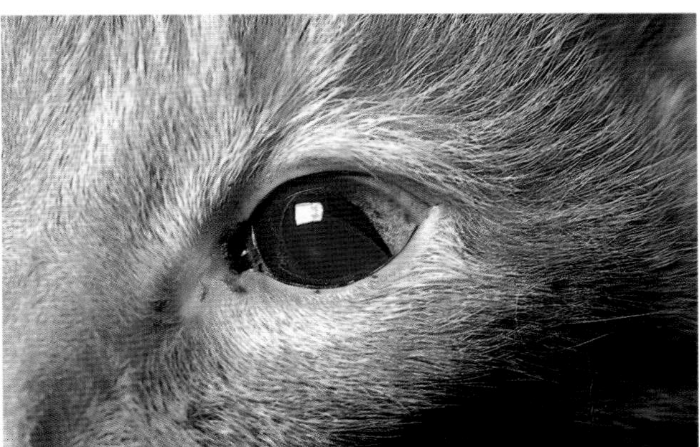

Fig. 11.34 *Posterior luxation with aphakic crescent.*

bilateral cataract does not always adapt well and cataract surgery in this species can be particularly rewarding.

Lens luxation

In the cat, lens luxation, both unilateral and bilateral, occurs less frequently than in the dog and primary hereditary lens luxation has not been reported in the cat, although a breed predisposition in the Siamese has been noted (Olivero *et al.*, 1991). Congenital lens luxation (with microphakia) is rare but Fig. 11.33 illustrates a single case in a kitten in which the lens was clear (see also Fig. 11.5). Wilkie (1994) also records familial lens luxation with congenital microphakia.

Feline secondary lens luxation may follow trauma, anterior uveitis and glaucoma, particularly the latter when the zonular fibres have been stretched by the increased intraocular pressure, and in hydrophthalmos by globe enlargement.

Lens luxation is more commonly seen in aged cats in which it presumably follows a degree of zonular degeneration. Probably, for a similar reason, lens luxation of a total cataractous lens is not of rare occurrence and neither are secondary cataractous changes in an originally clear and dislocated lens. Olivero *et al.* (1991), in an analysis of 345 cases, gave 7–9 years as the most common age at presentation.

In the cat anterior luxation is the rule and posterior luxation (Fig. 11.34) is unusual. Glaucoma secondary to anterior lens luxation can occur, although not of the acute and severe type that is so often seen in the terrier breeds of dog. The removal of a dislocated lens is a rewarding surgical procedure in the cat and is indicated when secondary glaucoma is present or when cataract formation affects vision, provided always that underlying predisposing factors such as uveitis are also addressed (Figs 11.33–42).

References

Aguirre GD, Bistner SI (1973) Microphakia with lenticular luxation and subluxation in cats. *Veterinary Medicine (Small Animal Clinician)* **68**: 498.

Collier LD, Bryan GM, Prieur DJ (1979) Ocular manifestations of the Chédiak-Higashi Syndrome in Four Species of Animals. *Journal of the American Veterinary Medical Association* **175**: 587–595.

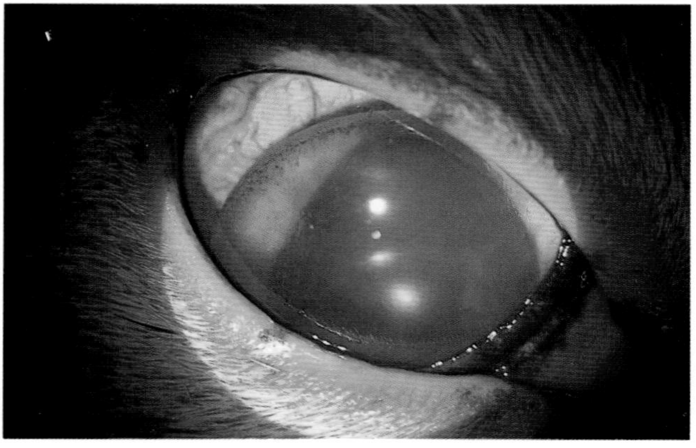

Fig. 11.35 Anterior luxation in a 10-year-old Domestic shorthair. Note associated uveitis.

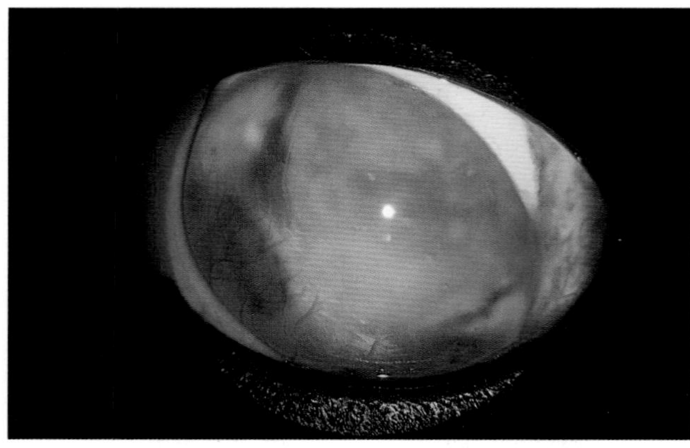

Fig. 11.38 Anterior luxation. Note corneal vascularization and opacity caused by pressure from the lens in the ventral cornea.

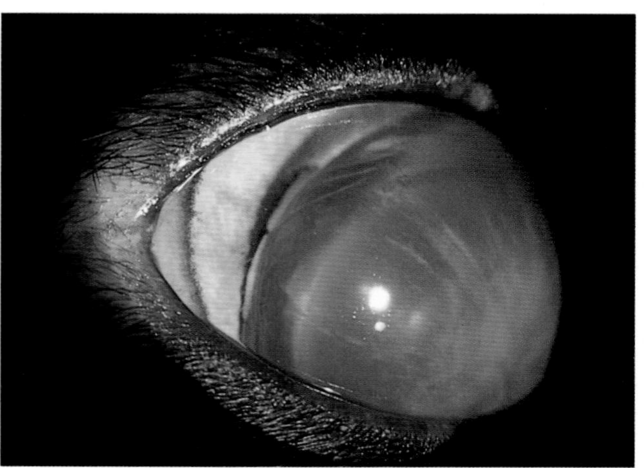

Fig. 11.36 Anterior luxation in a 10-year-old Domestic shorthair. Note very large size of normal lens and compare with microphakic lens in Fig. 11.33.

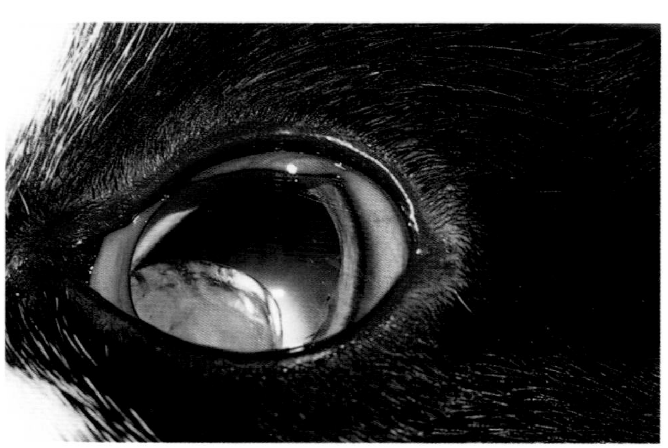

Fig. 11.37 Posterior luxation of congenitally abnormal lens, uniocular condition in a 15-month-old Domestic shorthaired female.

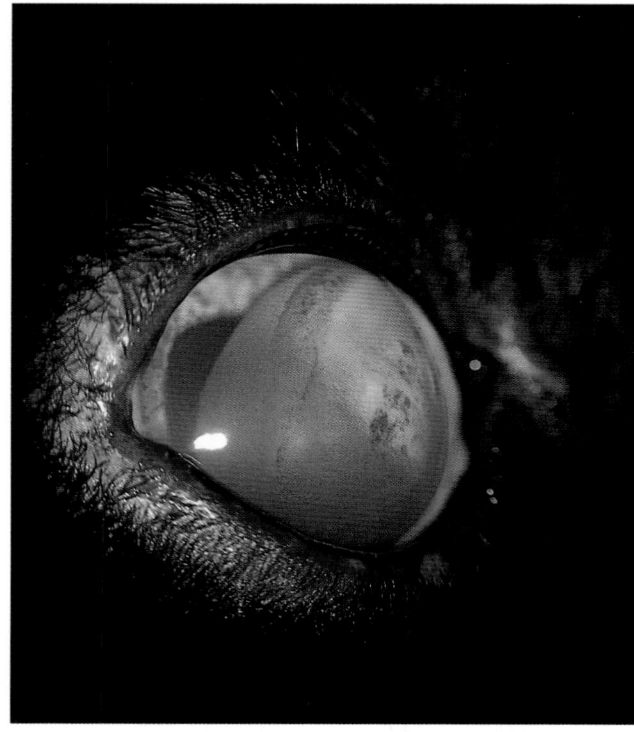

Fig. 11.39 Anterior luxation and early cataract in a 16-year-old neutered Domestic shorthaired male. Note the obvious uveitis.

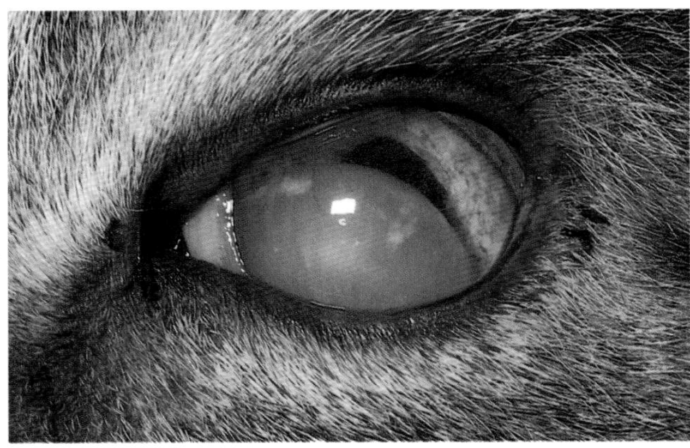

Fig. 11.40 *Luxation of cataractous lens secondary to uveitis in a 10-year-old Domestic shorthaired male. The other eye of this cat showed evidence of uveitis but the lens was clear indicating that this cataract followed the lens luxation.*

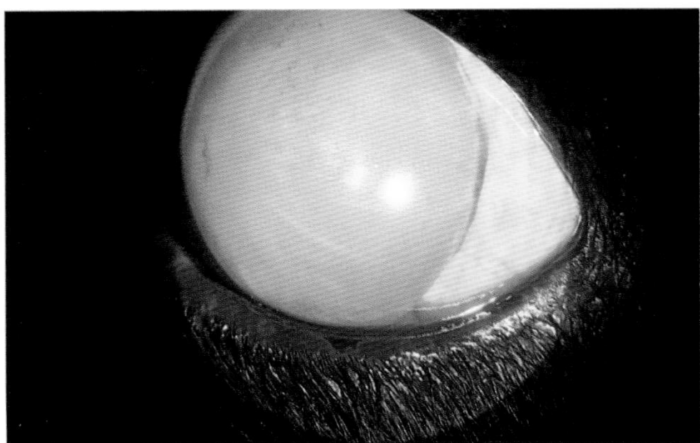

Fig. 11.41 *Anterior luxation of primary cataractous lens in a 10-year-old Domestic shorthaired male. Note no evidence of uveitis.*

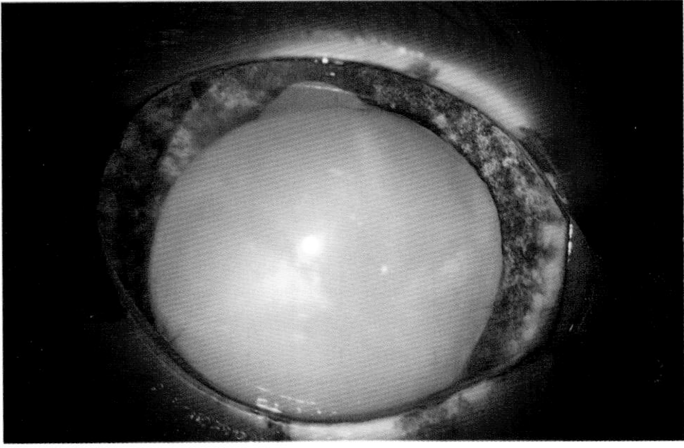

Fig. 11.42 *Anterior luxation of cataractous lens in a 3-year-old Domestic shorthaired female. Note abnormal iris pigmentation (see Chapter 12).*

Irby NI (1983) Hereditary cataracts in the British Shorthair Cat. In *American College of Veterinary Ophthalmology Genetics Workshop.*

Olivero DK, Riis RC, Dutton AG, Murphy CJ, Nasisse MP and Davidson MG (1991) Feline Lens Displacement. A Retrospective Analysis of 345 Cases. *Progress in Veterinary and Comparative Ophthalmology* 1 (No. 4): 239–244.

Peiffer RL (1982) Bilateral Congenital Aphakia and Retinal Detachment in a Cat. *Journal of the American Animal Hospital Association* **18**: 128–130.

Peiffer RL and Belkin PV (1983) Keratolenticular Dysgenesis in a kitten. *Journal of the American Veterinary Medical Association* **182**: 1242–1243.

Peiffer RL and Gelatt KN (1975) Congenital cataracts in a Persian kitten. *Veterinary Medicine (Small Animal Clinician)* **70**: 1334–1335.

Remillard RL, Pickett JP, Thatcher CD, Davenport DJ (1993) Comparison of kittens fed queen's milk with those fed milk replacers. *American Journal of Veterinary Research* **54**: 901–907.

Rubin LF (1986) Hereditary Cataract in Himalayan Cats. *Feline Practice* **16**(1): 14–15.

Wilkie DA (1994) In Sherding RD (ed.) *The Cat Diseases and Clinical Management*, 2nd edn, RG Sherding, Churchill Livingstone, New York, p. 2029.

12 UVEAL TRACT

INTRODUCTION

The uveal tract consists of the iris, ciliary body and choroid (Fig 12.1). It is derived from both neuroectoderm and mesenchyme. Mesenchyme is the term used to describe all the embryonic tissue between the epithelial layers; mesenchymal cells may be derived from several sources, notably mesoderm or neural crest. Melanocytes of neural crest origin are scattered throughout the uveal tract and produce the characteristic pigment. In addition to the specialized muscular functions of the iris and ciliary body the uveal tract is concerned with the nutrition of the eye.

The iris is the most anterior part of the uveal tract and functions as a movable diaphragm in front of the lens. It consists of a cellular anterior border layer which is a modification of the loosely arranged stroma that lies beneath it. The iris sphincter muscle is located in the pupillary portion of the stroma. Two layers of epithelial cells form the posterior part of the iris. The anterior epithelium consists of an epithelial apical portion and a muscular basal portion, the iris dilator muscle, which projects into the iris stroma. The posterior surface of the iris consists of very heavily pigmented epithelial cells. Iris musculature and the epithelial layers are of neuroectodermal origin, whereas the stroma is of mesenchymal origin.

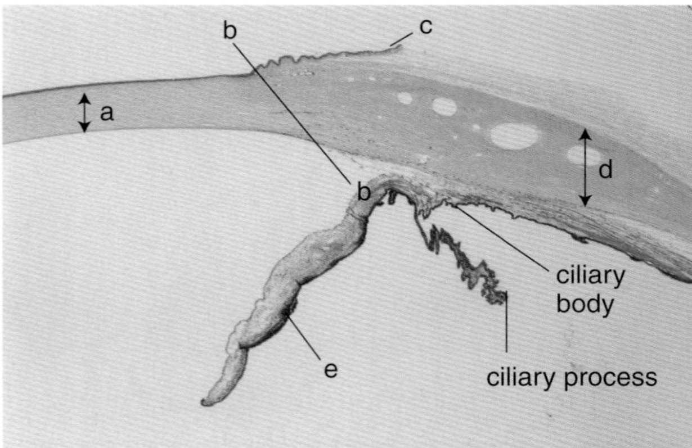

Fig. 12.1 Histological section of the cornea, limbus and anterior uveal tract (stained with haematoxylin and eosin). The lens has been removed prior to processing. (a) cornea; (b) limbus; (c) conjunctiva; (d) episclera and sclera – note the large vessels of the intrascleral venous plexus; (e) iris.

Iris colour depends on the number of melanocytes in the stroma and the thickness of the anterior border layer. The iris of young kittens is grey to slate-blue in colour (see Chapter 2). In most adult cats the iris is yellow to gold in colour (Figs 1.1–1.3), but other variations include shades of green and blue (Fig. 12.2 and other examples throughout the Chapter). Rarely, in complete albinos, the iris is pink (Fig. 12.3). Occasionally, especially in oriental and white cats, each iris is of different colour with one eye blue and the other yellow to green (Fig. 12.4).

The anterior surface of the iris is grossly divisible into a central (pupillary) zone and a peripheral (ciliary) zone separated by the collarette; the pupillary zone is slightly darker than the ciliary zone, but this distinction is much less clear in cats than dogs and may not be apparent in some animals.

The sphincter muscle (sphincter pupillae), which controls pupil size under different lighting conditions, circles the iris at the pupillary zone and also contains fibres which intersect dorsally and ventrally. This arrangement effectively produces a scissor-like action so that the constricted pupil forms a vertical slit. Constriction is mediated by parasympathetic (cholinergic) branches of the oculomotor nerve; the medial short ciliary nerve innervates the medial half of the iris sphincter and the lateral short ciliary nerve innervates the lateral half of the iris sphincter. There are also sparse sympathetic (adrenergic) fibres supplying the pupil sphincter muscle.

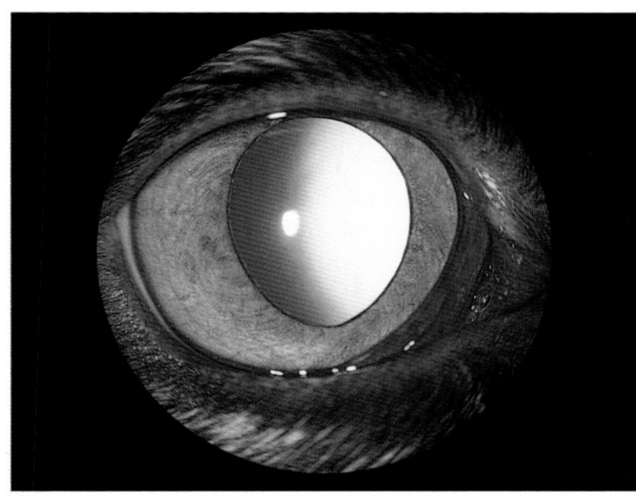

Fig. 12.2 A 2-year-old Siamese with blue iris.

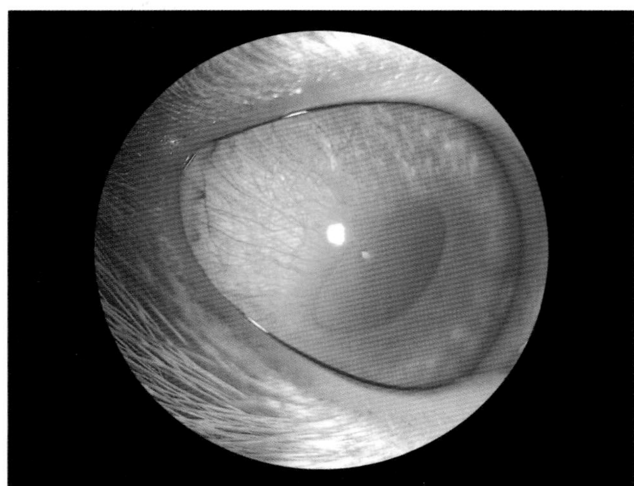

Fig. 12.3 *White Domestic shorthair with subalbinotic eye. Note that the iris lacks pigment and is almost translucent. The pink fundus reflex indicates a similar lack of pigment and also absence of tapetum in the fundus.*

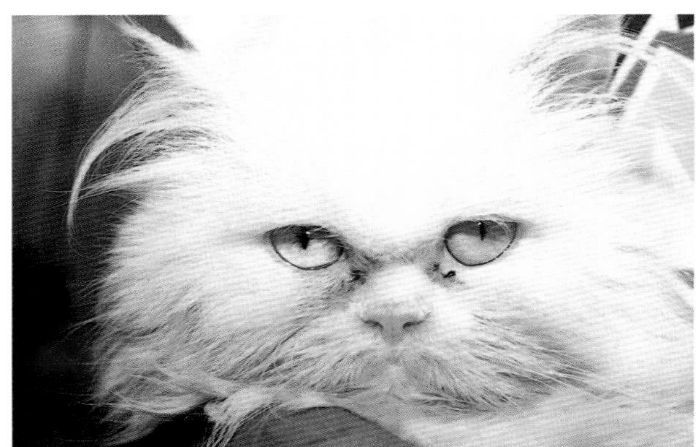

Fig. 12.4 *Persian with heterochromia iridum.*

The dilator muscle (dilator pupillae), which controls pupillary dilation, consists of radially orientated fibres which pass from close to the pupil towards the root of the iris. There is dual innervation of the dilator muscle, from both sympathetic nerve fibres, which predominate, and from parasympathetic nerve fibres.

The ciliary body is located posterior to the iris and anterior to the choroid (Fig. 11.2). The stroma, ciliary muscles and blood vessels are of mesenchymal origin, the pigmented and nonpigmented epithelium are derived from neuroectoderm. The ciliary body has an approximately triangular outline; it is bounded by the vitreous, the sclera, the base of the iris and the iridocorneal angle. Two portions are usually defined; the pars plicata and the pars plana, the latter extends to the edge of the retina, a junctional zone known as the ora ciliaris retinae. Histologically the ciliary body can be divided into ciliary epithelium, ciliary body stroma and ciliary muscle.

Ciliary body functions in the cat include the production and removal (uveoscleral outflow) of aqueous humour, replenishment of vitreous glycosaminoglycans, provision of anchoring points for the lens zonular fibres and rather limited dynamic accommodation of the lens (the ciliary muscle is poorly developed). The tight junctions between nonpigmented ciliary epithelial cells constitute the major site of the blood aqueous barrier. Most of the aqueous is produced by the pars plicata of the ciliary body, mainly by active secretion from the ciliary epithelium; aqueous humour is a source of nutrients for the cornea, lens and other adjacent tissues. The rate of aqueous production is 15 μl/min (Bill, 1966) and is normally equalled by aqueous outflow, thus maintaining a relatively constant intraocular pressure. The outflow is regulated by several different mechanisms: notably the trabecular meshwork of the iridocorneal angle (conventional outflow) and the uveoscleral pathway (unconventional outflow).

The choroid is situated between the retina and the sclera. It is highly vascularized and in most cats the stroma contains many melanocytes. Melanocytes are reduced in number or absent in cats with blue or pink irides.

The choroid consists of:

(1) a poorly defined basal complex known as Bruch's membrane adjacent to the retinal pigment epithelium
(2) the choriocapillaris
(3) (in most cats) a cellular tapetum of high riboflavin content located as an almost triangular area in the dorsal choroid; this increases visual sensitivity, at some cost to visual acuity, by reflecting light back through the photoreceptors
(4) the stroma containing large vessels
(5) the suprachoroid.

The retina depends on both choroidal and retinal vessels for nutrition. There is a very high rate of blood flow through the uvea so that oxygen extraction for each millilitre of blood is very low (oxygen extraction fom retinal blood is much higher). The high uveal blood flow protects the eye from thermal damage and produces a high arterial oxygen tension in the uvea which facilitates the diffusion of oxygen into the retina.

Congenital and Early Onset Anomalies and Abnormalities

Heterochromia

Heterochromia is a difference in colour between the two irides (heterochromia iridum) (Fig. 12.4) or between parts of the same iris (heterochromia iridis) (see below) which may be either congenital or acquired; acquired differences are usually the result of previous inflammation. A blue iris lacks pigment in the iris stroma, whereas a gold iris has stromal pigment. Unequal distribution of pigment produces a multicoloured iris.

Albinism

Albinism is an absence of normal pigmentation which can frequently be related to coat colour (Fig. 12.3). White is a common coat colour of cats and partial or complete congenital deafness is not uncommon in white cats, especially when one or both irides are blue (Bergsma and Brown, 1971). Chédiak-Higashi syndrome is a rare type of partial oculocutaneous albinism, which is inherited as an autosomal recessive and abnormalities include cataracts and decreased pigmentation of the iris and fundus.

Coloboma

A coloboma results if a portion of the uvea fails to develop properly (Fig. 5.7). Typical colobomas occur in the region of the foetal (choroidal) fissure at the '6 o'clock' position and are a result of abnormal closure of the embryonic cleft. Colobomas which occur away from the '6 o'clock' position are known as atypical. Both types are rare in cats.

A defect in the iris may be full thickness or partial thickness and colobomatous defects in the cat are most likely to be found in the ventromedial pupillary border. The full-thickness defects produce pseudopolycoria (as distinct from polycoria where there is more than one pupil each with a proper iris sphincter). Other congenital pupil abnormalities such as corectopia (abnormal pupil position) and dyscoria (abnormal pupil shape) are rare in cats (Fig. 5.7).

Colobomas which affect the iris and ciliary body are usually associated with absence of the lens zonule and indentation of the equator of the lens (see Chapter 11).

Iris hypoplasia

Iris hypoplasia (Fig.12.5) may involve the whole iris, or part of the iris and may be partial thickness or full thickness; the latter anomaly is rare.

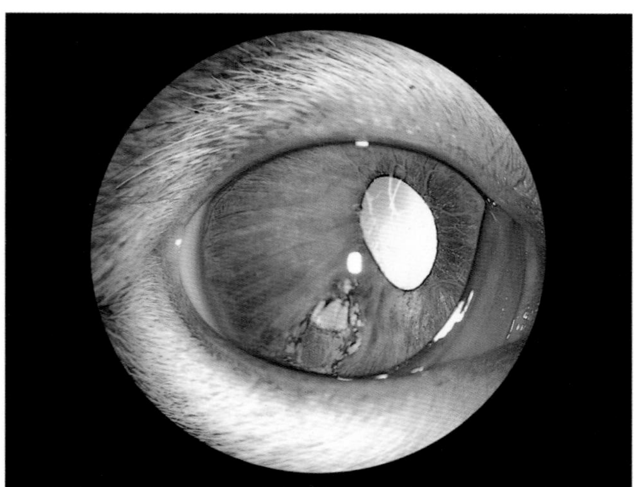

Fig. 12.5 *A 10-month-old Siamese with iris hypoplasia and persistent pupillary membrane. Note that the lens equator is apparent through the full-thickness defect in the iris and that other areas of the iris show less gross hypoplasia.*

Anterior segment dysgenesis

Faulty differentiation of the anterior segment may produce a range of defects, primarily involving the cornea, drainage angle and iris and little information of specific defects is available for the cat (Williams, 1993). It is likely that the most important clinical problem to result from feline anterior segment dysgenesis is congenital glaucoma (see Chapter 10).

Persistent pupillary membrane

Persistence of remnants of the pupillary membrane (ppm) represents a failure of the normal process of atrophy of the anterior component of the tunica vasculosa lentis and, although this developmental anomaly is uncommon in cats, there is a wide range of possible clinical appearances (Figs 12.6–12.9). Ppm remnants are readily distinguished from synechiae (adhesions) as they are congenital, not associated

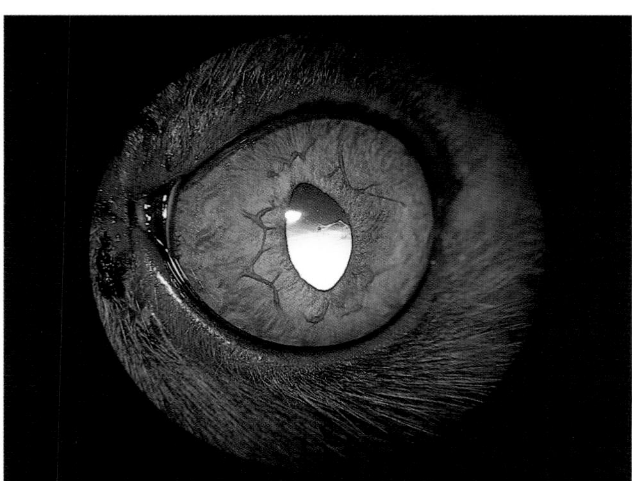

Fig. 12.6 *A 5-month-old Persian. Persistent pupillary membrane (ppm). Most of the ppm remnants arise from the iris collarette and have an annular arrangement, but there are also some fine strands in the pupillary aperture inserting on the lens.*

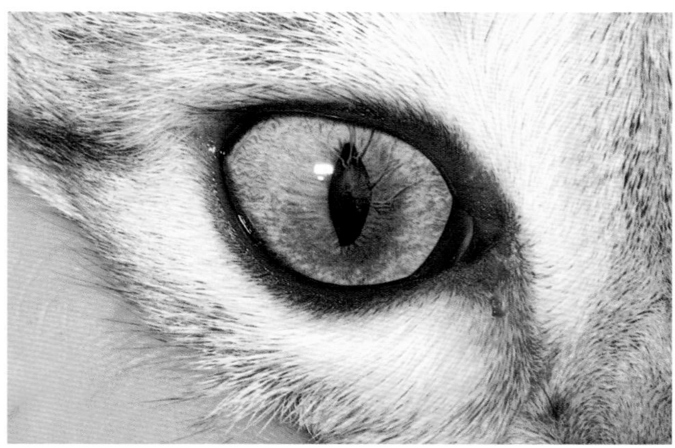

Fig. 12.7 *Domestic shorthaired kitten. Persistent pupillary membrane. The origin of the persistent remnants from the iris collarette is obvious and, in this case, the strands insert on the lens producing an anterior capsular opacity of the lens.*

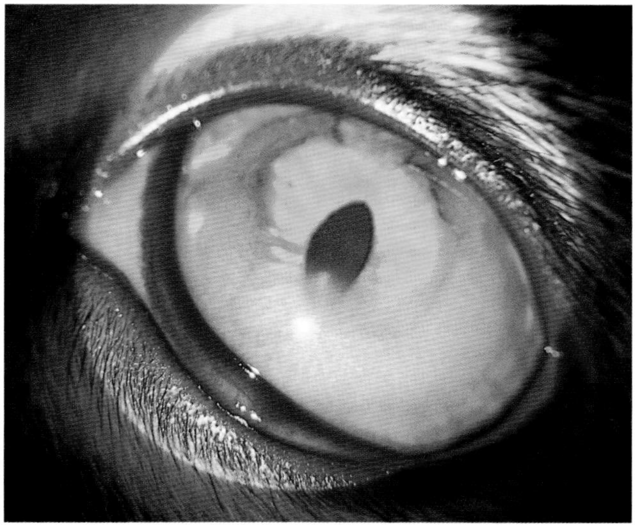

Fig. 12.8 *A 5-month-old British blue. Persistent pupillary membrane arising from the iris collarette and contacting the posterior surface of the cornea to produce an annular area of corneal opacity.*

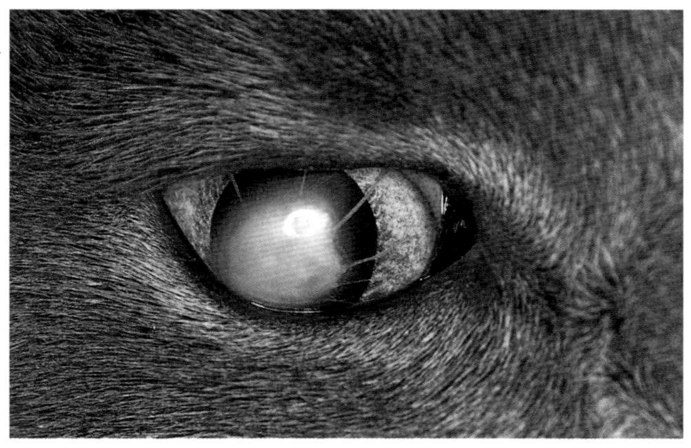

Fig. 12.9 *An 11-month-old Burmese. Persistent pupillary membrane arising from the iris collarette and peripheral iris and attaching to the posterior cornea producing a well-defined area of corneal opacity. Some of the medial ppm are patent and a small amount of intracorneal haemorrhage has originated from the vascular remnants.*

with inflammation or trauma and usually originate from the iris collarette and attach to other sectors of the iris, the lens, or the cornea.

Acquired abnormalities of the iris

Iris pigmentation

Benign Melanosis

Discrete foci of pigment are sometimes observed on the surface of the iris in normal cats (Figs 12.10 and 12.11).

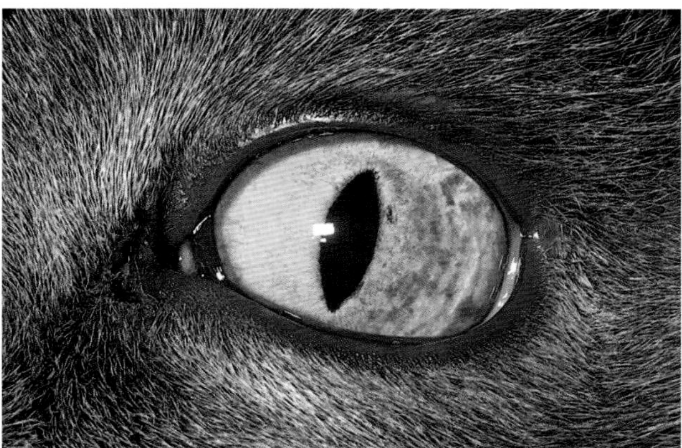

Fig. 12.10 *A 6-year-old Domestic shorthair. A change of iris colour had been noticed by the owner and consists of diffuse pigmentation on the surface of the iris.*

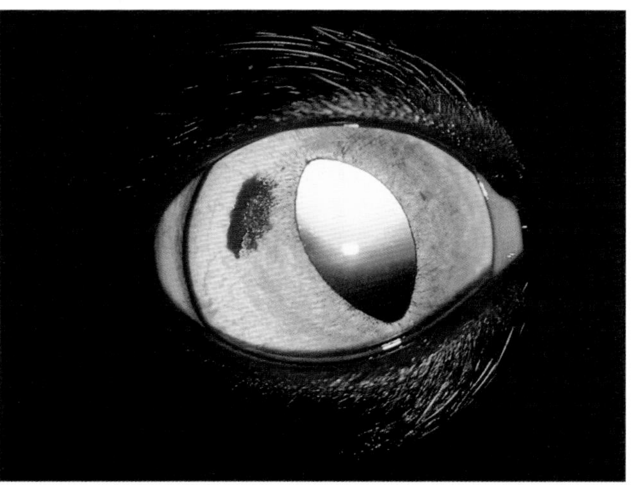

Fig. 12.11 *A 3-year-old Domestic shorthair with benign melanosis. The owner had observed a black mark on the iris laterally. In addition to the obvious lateral pigmentation there is also a small pigmented area medially. (Courtesy of S. R. Ellis.)*

Hyperpigmentation of existing melanocytes in these areas, with consequent increase in size, may occur for reasons unknown or as a phenomenon of ageing. Owners notice the change of appearance and seek veterinary help at this stage, or when the dark areas enlarge and coalesce to produce diffuse pigmentation (Figs 12.11–12.13). They are of no concern when confined to the anterior surface of the iris, but thorough examination is required, especially if there appears to be deeper involvement. Some of these cases have been classified as diffuse iridal melanomas (Acland *et al.*, 1980) but histopathology indicates that not all are neoplastic. The best approach is careful sequential observation and specialist help if there is any doubt about their benign nature – it is important not to remove a visual eye without just cause. If there is deeper stromal involvement, with or without pigment shedding, the approach should be more cautious (see below). Obliteration of the ciliary cleft by abnormal melanocytes is a cause of secondary glaucoma in affected cats and once glaucoma develops the eye is best removed and submitted for histopathology (see Chapter 10).

Iris Neoplasia

Changes of pigmentation not limited to the anterior iris surface, especially when associated with an increase of iris thickness, local vascular response, pupillary distortion or lesion margins which are poorly demarcated, should be regarded with suspicion because they may be indicative of iris melanoma; other primary tumours of the iris are rare (see below).

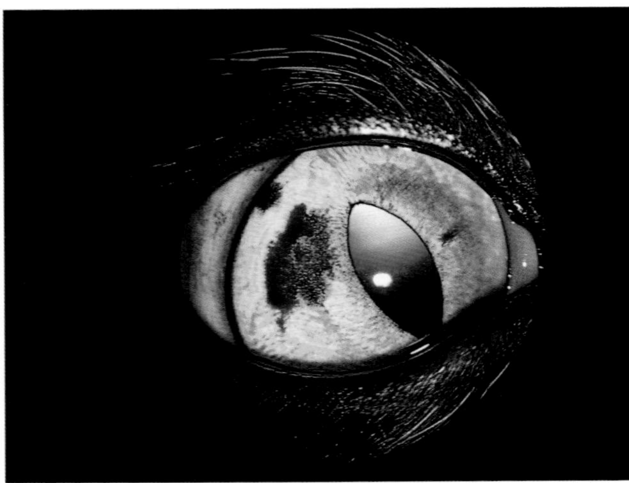

Fig. 12.12 *A 5-year-old Domestic shorthair with benign melanosis. This is the same cat as shown in Figure 12.11 almost 2 years later. Both the areas noted in the previous figure have enlarged and there is another alteration in pigmentation at the iris periphery laterally. (Courtesy of S. R. Ellis.)*

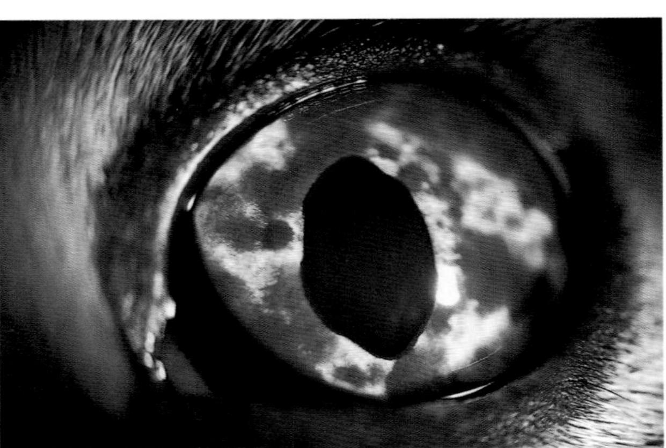

Fig. 12.13 *A 9-year-old Domestic shorthair with benign melanosis. Extensive diffuse iris pigmentation makes the differentiation of this type of lesion particularly difficult. There is also mild ectropion uveae and slight distortion of the pupillary margin. Because an iridal melanoma was suspected the eye was removed. Histopathology confirmed the benign nature of the pigmentary changes.*

Ectropion Uveae

This is not unusual and represents eversion of the posterior pigment epithelium of the iris (Fig. 12.14). Strictly speaking this occurs because shrinkage of the anterior surface of the iris allows the dark posterior pigment to become visible at the pupillary border, but it may also be a manifestation of hyperplasia of the posterior pigment epithelium at the pupillary margin. It can occur in association with iris inflammation, but the cause may not always be obvious and includes congenital derivation (see also iris cysts).

IRIS ATROPHY

Iris atrophy can occur with senility but it can also follow uveitis (Fig. 12.15). The atrophy can be quite extensive so that full-thickness defects result. Loss of the sphincter muscle is associated with poor pupil constriction and photophobia may also be present because of inability to respond appropriately to bright light.

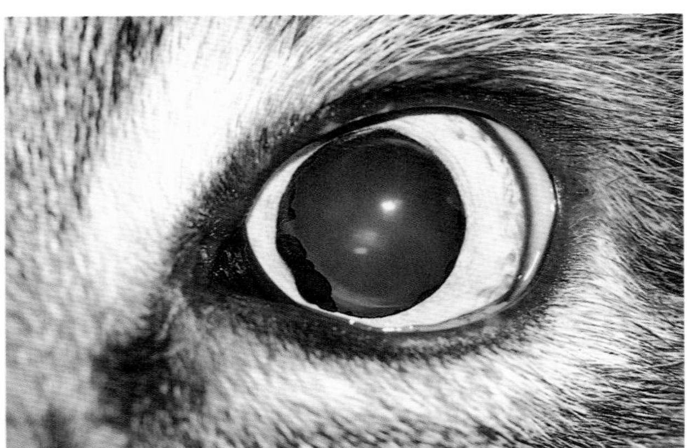

Fig. 12.14 *A 15-year-old Domestic shorthair with ectropion uveae and uveal cysts at the pupillary margin. There is also senile nuclear sclerosis of the lens.*

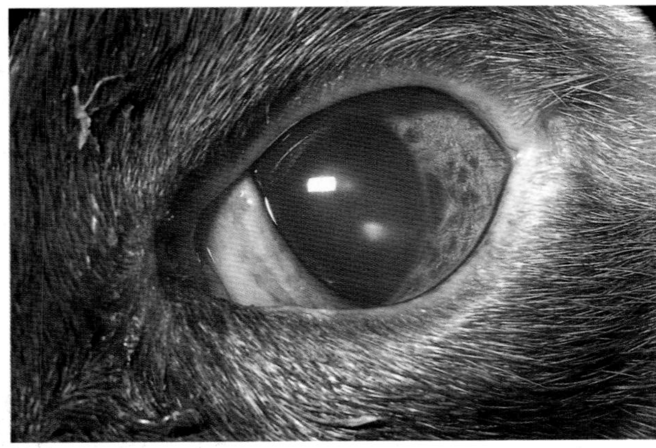

Fig. 12.15 *A 14-year-old Siamese with acquired iris atrophy.*

Iris cysts

Iris cysts probably represent localized dilatations of the marginal sinus and share similarities of origin with ectropion uveae. They are usually an incidental finding of unknown cause, but there is sometimes a history of previous traumatic insult. The cysts may be single or multiple and are visible behind the pupil or free within the anterior chamber (Figs 12.16 and 12.17). Iris cysts are unlikely to cause any problems and treatment (e.g. laser therapy) is only required if they interfere with vision.

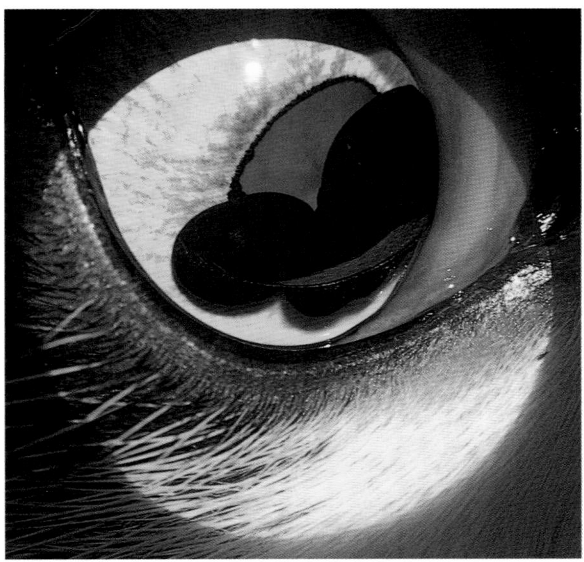

Fig. 12.16 *A 5-year-old Domestic shorthair with three uveal cysts free in the anterior chamber. There was no apparent cause and the cysts were not causing any problems.*

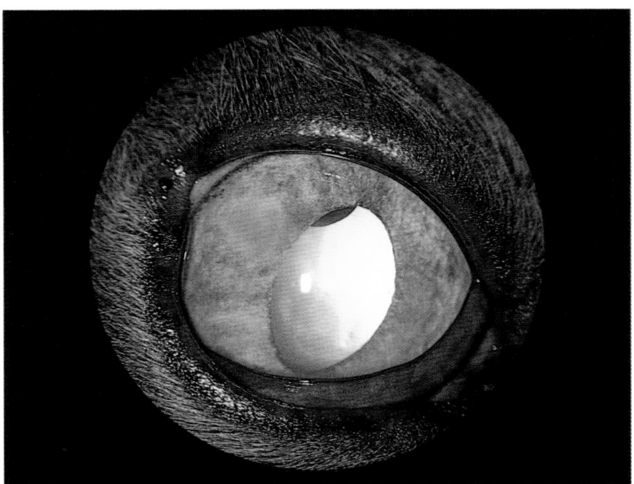

Fig. 12.17 *A 14-year-old Burmese. Edge of uveal cyst apparent at dorsolateral pupillary margin. There was a penetrating injury to the cornea some years earlier and the site of the corneal scar (nebula) lies just ventrolateral to the cyst.*

Cysts may be distinguished from primary tumours of the iris because of their location and smooth round to elliptical shape. There is no reaction to their presence, no apparent effect on vision and they can be transilluminated with a bright light even when they are heavily pigmented.

Synechiae

These are adhesions which form as a result of iris inflammation and they should be differentiated from persistent pupillary membrane. There are a great number of possible causes.

Anterior synechiae, adherence of the iris to the cornea, is a common complication of corneal penetrating injuries (see Chapter 3). Posterior synechiae, adherence of the iris to the anterior lens capsule, is a common sequel to iritis and the commonest reason for a fixed, irregular pupil (Figs. 12.18–12.20). Peripheral anterior synechiae affect the peripheral iris and thus may impede aqueous outflow; they are usually a complication of severe inflammation.

Inflammatory disease of the uveal tract

Anterior uveitis may primarily involve the iris (iritis) or both the iris and the anterior part of the ciliary body (iridocyclitis). Intermediate uveitis predominantly involves the posterior part of the ciliary body (pars planitis). Posterior uveitis primarily involves the choroid (choroiditis), but close association of the retina means that inflammation of both choroid and retina is the usual situation. Panuveitis is inflammation of the entire uveal tract – iris, ciliary body and choroid (Crispin, 1993).

Exogenous causes of uveitis include ocular insults such as trauma and corneal ulcers (see also Chapters 3 and 9).

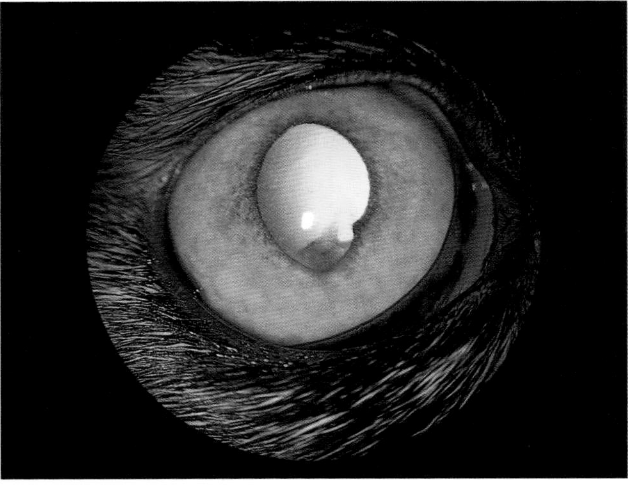

Fig. 12.18 *A 2-year-old Domestic shorthair with acute bilateral panuveitis of unknown cause. The right eye is shown. Note the mild corneal opacity, aqueous flare, sparse keratic precipitates, loss of iris detail, irregular pupil with posterior synechiae in the '5 o'clock' position and an inflammatory deposit behind the iris and in front of the lens. Examination of the posterior segment indicated vitritis and active chorioretinitis.*

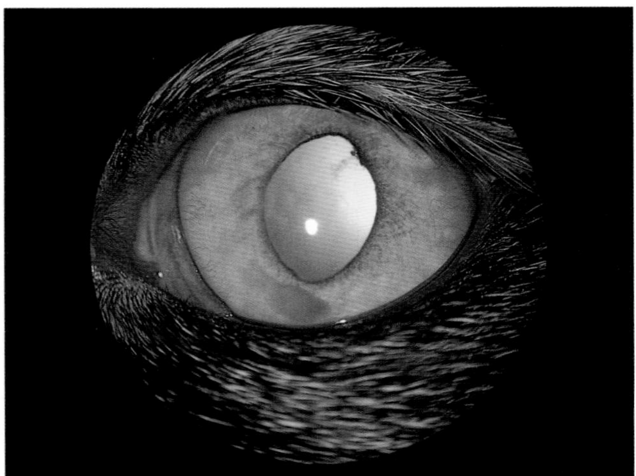

Fig. 12.19 *The left eye of the cat shown in Fig. 12.18. The changes are similar to those of the right eye, but have been present for slightly longer. Fine neovascularization of the cornea is present and the inflammatory deposit in this eye is in the anterior chamber.*

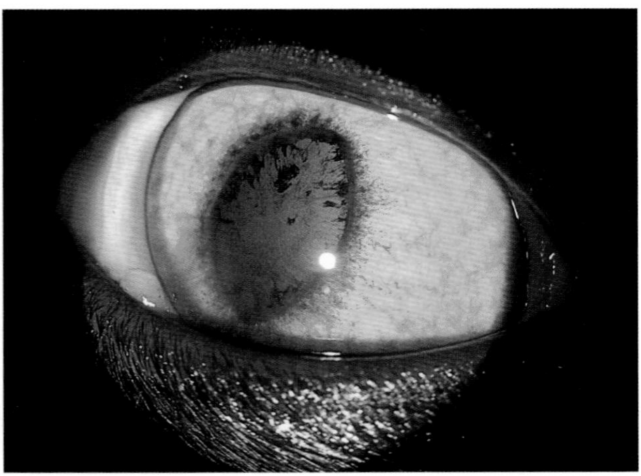

Fig. 12.20 *Domestic shorthair with chronic unilateral uveitis of unknown cause (idiopathic). Keratic precipitates are apparent on the posterior cornea, new blood vessels have formed on the surface of the iris; posterior synechiae have formed around almost the entire periphery of the pupil. Extensive deposits of pigment on the anterior lens capsule (iris rests) are a legacy of previous adhesions between the posterior iris and anterior lens capsule and there is also fine vascularization on the anterior lens capsule.*

Endogenous uveitis is commonly associated with a range of infectious agents, less commonly with neoplasia and certain types of lens pathology. In those cases of endogenous uveitis where the cause is unknown the uveitis is termed idiopathic and lymphocytic–plasmacytic anterior uveitis is a frequent histopathological finding (Davidson *et al.*, 1991).

Inflammatory diseases of the uveal tract must be distinguished from other problems such as triglyceride-rich lipid within the anterior chamber (see Chapter 10), hypertension associated with hyphaema (see Chapters 3, 10 and 14) and neoplasia with a range of appearances (see below). Effective management depends upon establishing the cause.

The standard ophthalmic examination can be supplemented in a number of simple ways to help in assessment of the uveal tract.

(1) The pupil and drainage angle are examined as a matter of routine.
(2) A beam of light is shone directly across the anterior chamber from a number of different directions, but particularly lateral to medial, so as to gain an estimate of the depth of the anterior chamber, which may be notably shallower than usual if the iris is very swollen, or deeper than usual if the lens has ruptured or its contents have resorbed.
(3) A narrow beam of light, rather than diffuse illumination, should be used when checking for possible aqueous flare.
(4) Transillumination can be helpful to distinguish solid from fluid-filled masses.
(5) More specialist techniques such as tonometry and gonioscopy will also be required on occasion.
(6) A complete physical examination should always be performed in addition to ophthalmic examination.
(7) If the cause of any uveal tract problem is not obvious, routine haematology, blood biochemistry and specific diagnostic tests should be performed.
(8) Serodiagnosis may be useful, but not necessarily diagnostic, for feline leukaemia virus, feline immunodeficiency virus and feline infectious peritonitis, mycotic infections (not available in the UK) and toxoplasmosis.
(9) Diagnostic imaging techniques such as ultrasonography and magnetic resonance imaging (MRI) are particularly valuable when ocular changes make comprehensive examination of the eye impossible.
(10) Radiogaphy may be indicated on occasion; for example, if neoplasia with metastases is likely, or if there is a possibility that the animal has been shot.
(11) Aqueous and vitreous paracentesis are rarely used as diagnostic tools, they may be helpful for the diagnosis of mycotic disease.

Clinical Signs of Uveitis

The clinical signs are usually not diagnostic of the cause of endogenous uveitis, whereas the cause of exogenous types is often apparent on clinical examination (Chavkin *et al.*, 1992).

Acute uveitis is unusual in cats except for that associated with trauma. There is rarely the intense pain seen in dogs and horses and many cats are first presented when the ocular manifestations have become subacute. Clinical signs include pain, photophobia, blepharospasm, lacrimation, inflammation hyperaemia of visible vessels, aqueous flare, hyphaema, miosis, low intraocular pressure and a swollen iris with loss of iris detail. There may also be posterior segment involvement, including optic neuritis and intraocular haemorrhage. Vision can also be affected.

Chronic uveitis is the commonest presentation of feline uveal tract inflammation and the extensive range of appearances are rarely diagnostic for any specific cause (Table 12.1). Owners often cite alteration of appearance, especially a change of iris colour (Fig. 12.21), as a reason for seeking professional advice.

Viral Causes of Uveitis

Feline infectious peritonitis virus (FIPV) Feline infectious peritonitis (FIP) is one of the most common causes of uveitis in cats. FIP is found more frequently in younger cats than older cats and is more common in pedigree cats kept in multicat households. Nonophthalmic signs of this immune-mediated disease are very variable but usually include non-specific signs of illness such as lethargy, pyrexia, inappetence and weight loss. Neurological signs are common (Kline *et al.*, 1994) and progressive, although they may be initially subtle (see Chapter 15). FIP is invariably fatal.

The ocular lesions of FIP usually involve the anterior uveal tract and may also affect the posterior uvea (Figs. 12.22–12.28). Both eyes are often involved, although the

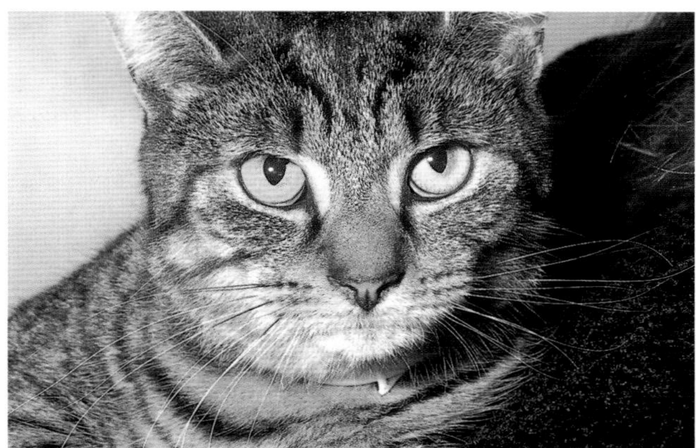

Fig. 12.21 *A 6-year-old Domestic shorthair neutered male. The darker iris in the right eye is associated with a previous iritis.*

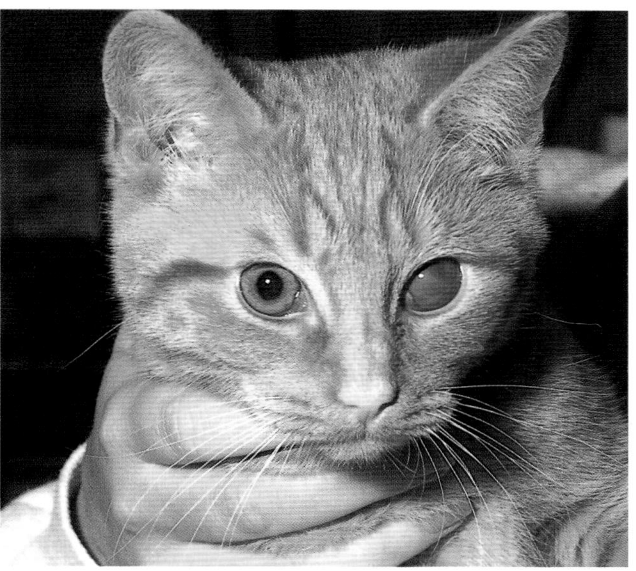

Fig. 12.22 *An 8-month-old Domestic shorthair male with bilateral anterior uveitis associated with feline infectious peritonitis. The changes in the right eye are limited to aqueous flare, slight loss of iris detail and vasculitis. In the left eye haemorrhage (hyphaema) and fibrin obscure the underlying changes in the iris which are more severe and have been present for longer than those of the right eye. The kitten also had neurological deficits.*

Table 12.1 Common Clinical Features of Feline Uveitis

General	Usually mildly uncomfortable or painless
	Effects on vision variable, from no effect to incapacitating
Anterior	Eye may or may not be inflamed (variable/absent redness)
	Aqueous flare less common than keratic precipitates/mutton fat precipitates/hypopyon
	Swollen iris/vasculitis/iris nodules/synechiae/changes of iris colour
	Fibrin and/or frank haemorrhage may be present
	Pupil may be normal or irregular with a normal or slightly sluggish reaction to bright light
	Inflammatory debris (opacities) may be present on the anterior lens capsule
Intermediate	Inflammatory cells on posterior lens capsule, pars plana and in anterior vitreous (snowball opacities)
Posterior	Vitritis
	Vitreous opacities
	Chorioretinitis
	Retinal haemorrhage/retinal detachment
	Optic neuritis

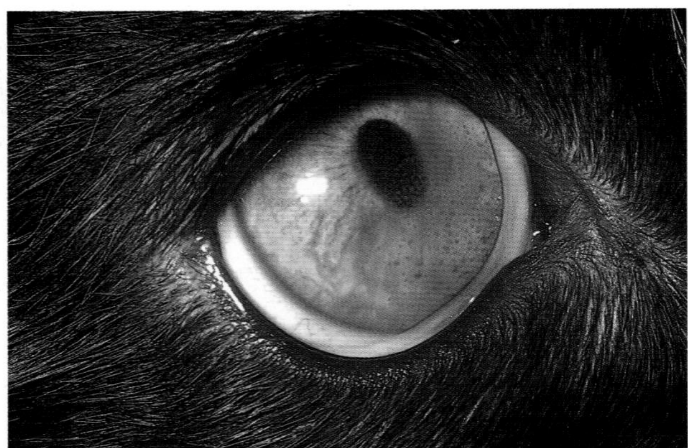

Fig. 12.23 *A 16-month-old Domestic shorthair neutered male with bilateral anterior uveitis associated with feline infectious peritonitis; the right eye is shown. A single corneal blood vessel is present at '6 o'clock' and inflamed blood vessels and new blood vessels are visible on the iris. There are also numerous keratic precipitates, some of which are so large that the designation mutton fat deposits is appropriate.*

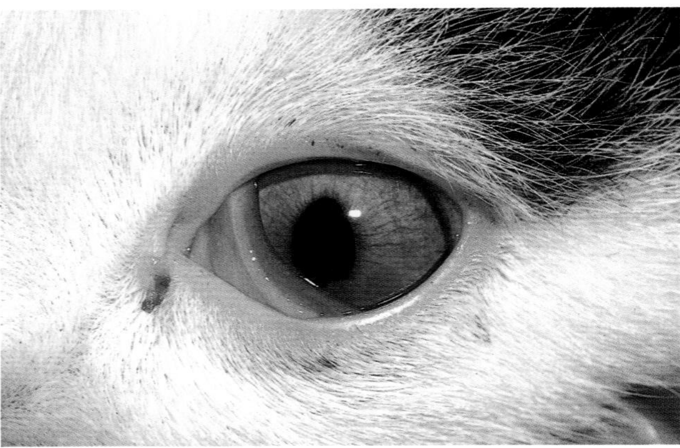

Fig. 12.24 *An 8-month-old Domestic shorthair neutered male with bilateral anterior uveitis associated with feline infectious peritonitis; the left eye is shown. In addition to sparse keratic precipitates there is hypopyon. Note also the intense vasculitis of iris blood vessels. A littermate was similarly affected.*

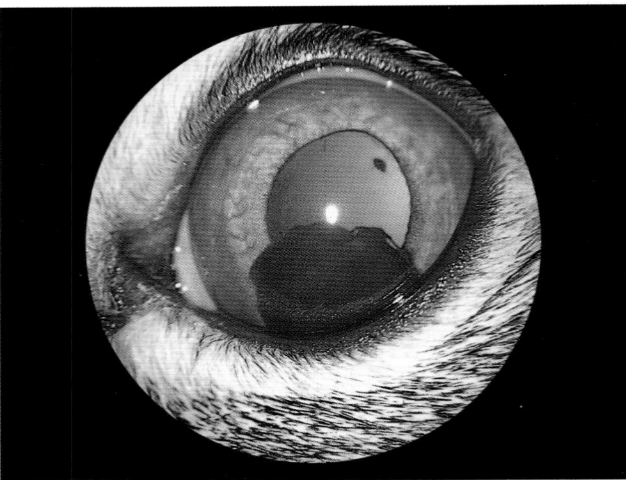

Fig. 12.25 *A 7-month-old Domestic shorthair neutered male with bilateral anterior uveitis associated with feline infectious peritonitis; the hyphaema present in the left eye is shown; but hyphaema of the right eye was more extensive. Optic neuritis was also present in the right eye; the posterior segment of the left eye could not be visualized. The hyphaema is a direct consequence of whole blood leaking from the inflamed iris blood vessels.*

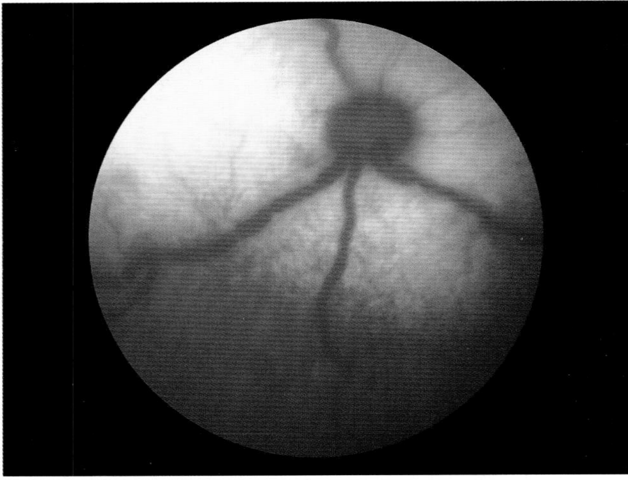

Fig. 12.26 *A 12-month-old Siamese neutered male with posterior segment changes associated with feline infectious peritonitis. Hyperviscosity (best observed in the primary retinal venules) associated with hyperproteinaemia (gammaglobulins >70 g/l, plasma proteins >120 g/l).*

lesions are not bilaterally symmetrical. The pathogenesis is associated with perivascular pyogranulomatous inflammation and subsequent breakdown of the blood aqueous barrier. Inflammatory cells and plasma proteins such as fibrin leak into the aqueous or vitreous, giving rise to aqueous flare, keratic precipitates and hypopyon in the anterior chamber or vitritis when the vitreous is involved. Inflammation of the iris vessels is usually obvious and there may be microhaemorrhages from the inflamed vessels, and sometimes frank hyphaema. If it is possible to examine the fundus a range of abnormalities may be observed (see also Chapter 14). Serum hyperproteinaemia is associated with characteristic hyperviscosity if total protein levels are high enough (see Chapter 14). Intense vasculitis and perivascular exudates; focal or diffuse areas of chorioretinitis, choroidal exudation, retinal oedema and/or haemorrhage may be observed. Retinal detachments (usually focal) can occur in some cases. Optic neuritis may be present.

FIP is almost impossible to confirm in the live animal (Sparkes *et al.*, 1994). Interpretation of serology is confusing for several reasons. Cats may be infected by a number of

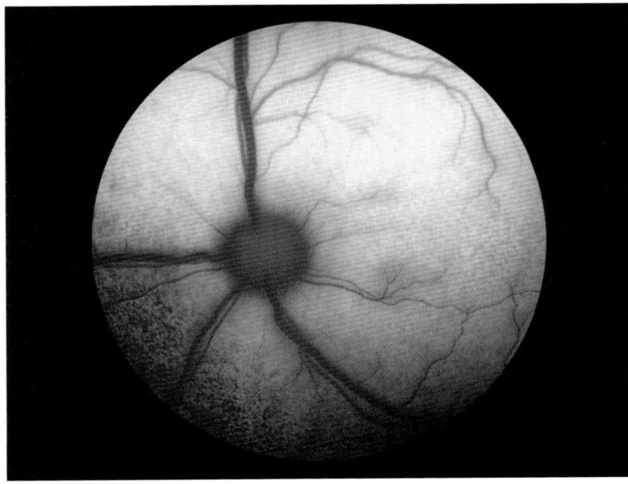

Fig. 12.27 *An 8-month-old Domestic shorthair female with bilateral posterior uveitis. Intense vasculitis associated with feline infectious peritonitis.*

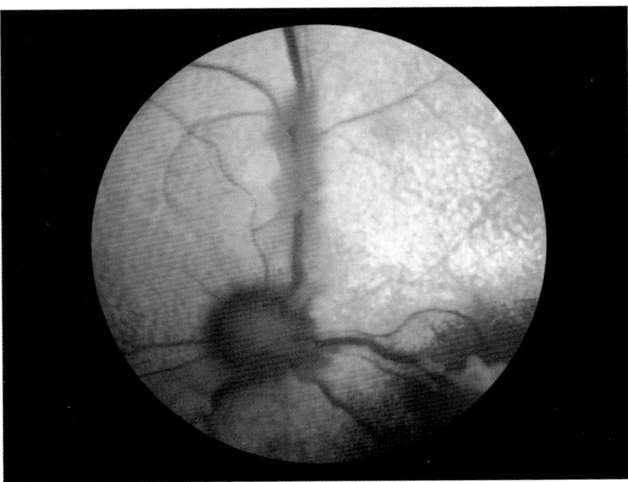

Fig. 12.28 *A 14-month-old Chinchilla female with bilateral posterior uveitis associated with feline infectious peritonitis; the right eye is shown. Note the obvious perivascular exudates (white material). There are also rather less obvious acquired retinal folds, indicative of subretinal effusion and early detachment.*

coronaviruses, few of which may lead to clinical disease and antibodies cannot determine whether a cat has been exposed to a pathogenic strain of coronavirus. Although cats with confirmed FIP often have high coronavirus titres, low and even zero titres may occur and, in addition, many healthy cats have high titres. Titres may also vary according to which diagnostic technique (and laboratory) is used; in general, immunofluorescence (IFA) is more reliable than the commercial enzyme-linked immunosorbent assay (ELISA) kits. Most importantly, the experimental evidence that frequent and rapid mutations of feline enteric coronaviruses can produce pathogenic feline infectious peritonitis phenotypes (Poland *et al.*, 1996) is of crucial importance in understanding the complexities of this disease.

Provisional diagnosis of FIP in the live animal is based on an appropriate history, exclusion of other diseases and a diversity of clinical signs in addition to uveitis. Protein analysis of effusions is a helpful diagnostic aid, but effusions are not usually a feature of cats with ocular involvement. Clinicopathological changes which include raised total proteins, hypergammaglobulinaemia, lymphopenia and a coronavirus titre of ≥160, taken in conjunction with other clinical findings, are strongly suggestive of FIP (Sparkes *et al.*, 1994). However, it is important to emphasize that, at present, FIP can only be confirmed by histological examination of biopsy or post mortem material.

Feline leukaemia–lymphosarcoma complex (FeLLC) Cats of all ages may be infected by feline leukaemia virus (FeLV), although infection is much more common in young cats and rare in cats over 10 years old. Feline leukaemia virus *per se* is possibly not a cause of primary ocular disease and the range of uveal tract manifestations is postulated to be a consequence of two processes: lymphosarcomatous invasion and severe anaemia (Brightman *et al.*, 1991). Ocular lymphosarcoma most commonly affects the uveal tract (Corcoran *et al.*, 1995), but other parts of the eye, adnexa and body may also be infiltrated by neoplastic cells and thorough clinical examination and imaging techniques are necessary to establish the extent of the lesions.

Chronic uveitis can occur as a result of generalized uveal infiltration by neoplastic cells. Immune-mediated inflammation in response to immune complex deposition may also be involved in the pathogenesis. Aqueous flare, keratic precipitates, hypopyon, hyphaema, neovascularization of the iris, change of iris colour, iris nodules, anterior and posterior synechiae, with thickening and pigmentary changes of the iris are the most frequently observed signs (Figs 12.29–12.31). Secondary glaucoma may arise because neoplastic cells obstruct the drainage angle (Fig. 12.32). Posterior segment changes occur less frequently and in addition may be difficult or impossible to observe because of anterior uveal lesions. Vitreous opacities sometimes develop and a variety of fundic lesions including chorioretinal infiltrates, pigment proliferation, retinal haemorrhage, retinal degeneration, partial or complete retinal detachment and optic neuritis may be present (see Chapter 14). Anterior and posterior segment haemorrhage is likely to be secondary to the marked anaemia and thrombocytopenia which is present in many clinical cases.

Immunofluorescent and ELISA-based techniques are generally reliable for confirmation of FeLV infection in cats with uveitis. The definitive laboratory test, however, involves virus recovery.

Treatment of lymphosarcoma can be attempted using various regimes of corticosteroids, cytotoxic drugs and interferon, but treatment is unlikely to reverse the viraemia.

Feline immunodeficiency virus (FIV) A significant proportion of cats with uveitis are infected with FIV, usually in the absence of infection with any other agent commonly

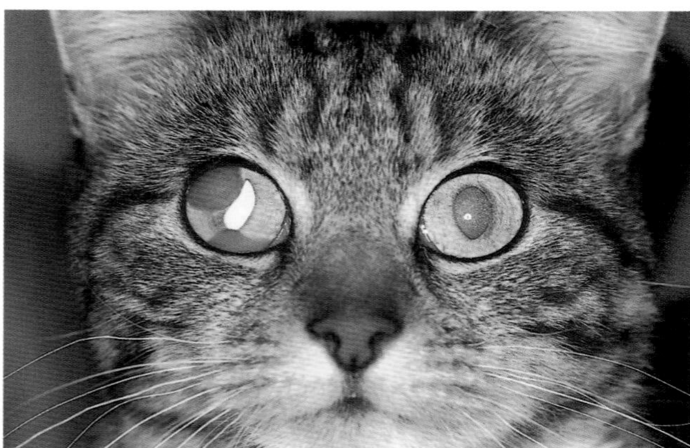

Fig. 12.29 *Adult Domestic shorthair, approximately 2 years, with bilateral anterior uveitis associated with the feline leukaemia–lymphosarcoma complex. In the right eye there is a solid mass dorsally and hypopyon (neoplastic cells) ventrally, the pupil is markedly distorted by the solid mass. In the left eye there is aqueous flare and a loss of lens transparency because of deposits on the anterior lens capsule.*

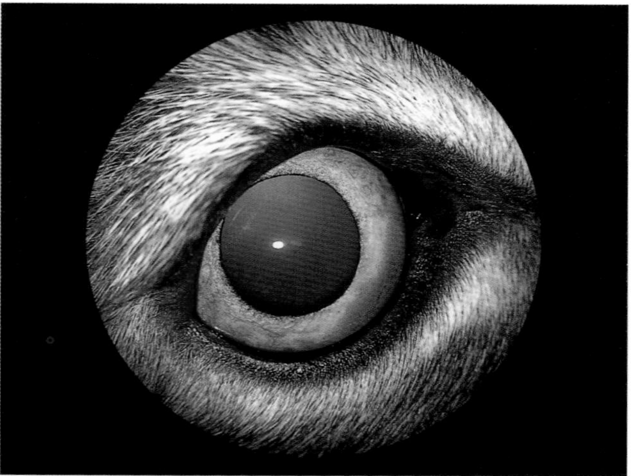

Fig. 12.30 *A 4-year-old Domestic shorthair neutered male with bilateral anterior uveitis associated with the feline leukaemia–lymphosarcoma complex, the right eye is shown. Note the accumulation of keratic precipitates on the posterior surface of the ventromedial cornea and the thickened, inflamed, peripheral iris.*

associated with uveitis. The pathogenesis of uveal lesions is unclear but may be related to immune-mediated mechanisms (e.g. through the deposition of immune complexes, or because of the localization of FIV in uveal lymphoid tissue). The virus is associated with neuropathogenicity and encephalitis has been described in association with naturally occurring disease (Gunn-Moore *et al.*, 1996). Cats in the later stages of FIV infection may develop uveitis as a result of secondary infection with a variety of organisms, including *Toxoplasma gondii*.

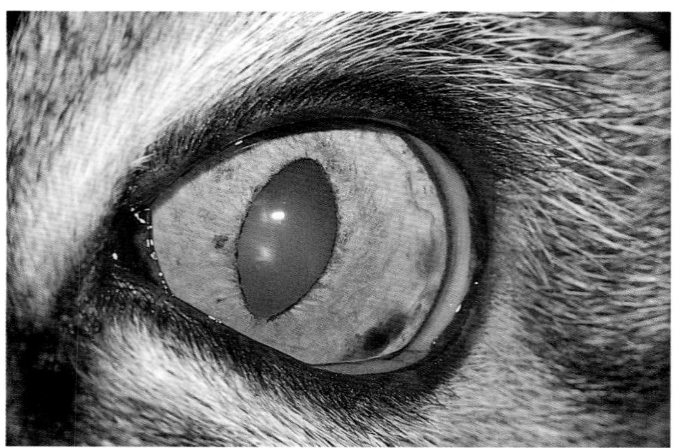

Fig. 12.31 *A 6-year-old Domestic shorthair neutered female with bilateral anterior hyphaema associated with the feline leukaemia–lymphosarcoma complex; the left eye is shown, the right eye had more extensive hyphaema. Note the source of anterior chamber haemorrhage; whole blood can be seen escaping from the major arterial circle of the iris. The cat was anaemic.*

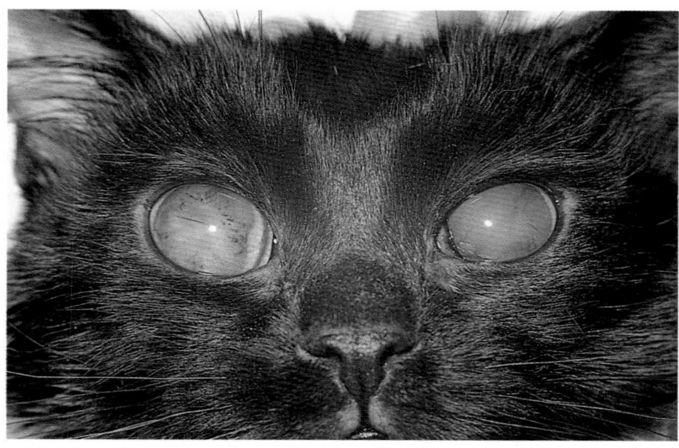

Fig. 12.32 *A Domestic shorthair, neutered female, approximately 3-years-old with bilateral anterior uveitis and secondary glaucoma associated with the feline leukaemia–lymphosarcoma complex. Both eyes are enlarged (hydrophthalmos).*

FIV occurs most often in adult, free-roaming, non-pedigree cats and is more common in males than females (Hopper *et al.*, 1989). Clinical problems associated with FIV infection rarely occur in isolation and other signs, together with haematological changes, are often found. Cats may present with acute uveitis but chronic or recurrent uveitis is more usual. It may be difficult clinically to distinguish lesions associated with FIP or FeLV infection from those of FIV, except that the time course is usually slower and the lesions are less florid with the latter (Figs 12.33–12.39). Corneal oedema, aqueous flare, keratic precipitates, hypopyon, irregularity of pupil size, iris thickening, iris nodules, iris neovascularization, synechiae formation and hyphaema may all be present.

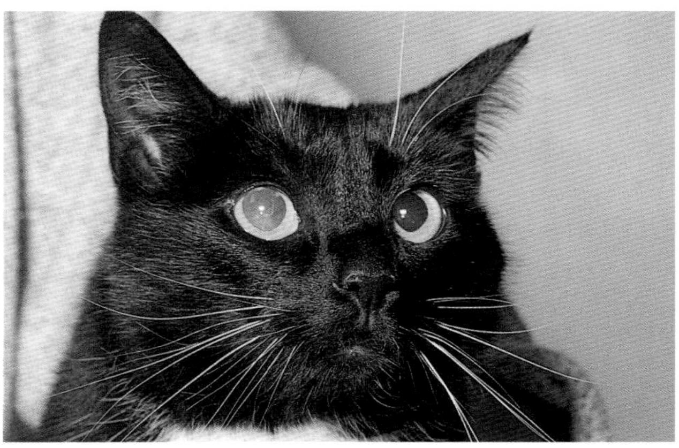

Fig. 12.33 *A 12-year-old Domestic shorthair neutered male with bilateral intermediate uveitis (pars planitis) associated with FIV. Note the anisocoria (the intraocular pressure was normal: 14 mmHg in the right eye and 13 mmHg in the left). In the right eye (in which the pupil is more dilated) white material is apparent in the ventral pupil (leukocoria) and this is the typical appearance of 'snowbanking', produced by inflammatory cells on the posterior lens capsule and within the anterior vitreous.*

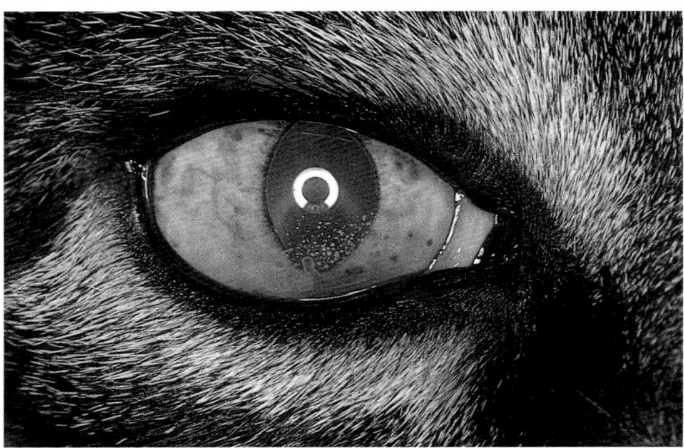

Fig. 12.35 *A 4-year-old Domestic shorthair neutered male with unilateral anterior uveitis associated with FIV. The fine detail of the iris has been lost as a consequence of the inflammation, but the keratic precipitates (KPs) on the posterior surface of the ventral cornea form the most obvious feature. Note that some of the KPs are darker than others (almost black), which is a feature of ageing. The appearance of the KPs can thus be used to indicate whether early active inflammation is present (pale KPs only), whether chronic inflammation is present (pale and dark KPs) and whether the eye is quiet (dark KPs only).*

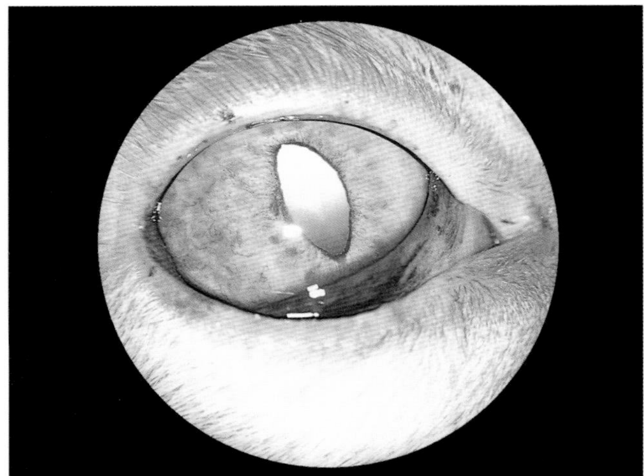

Fig. 12.34 *A 4-year-old Domestic shorthair neutered male with bilateral anterior uveitis associated with FIV; the right eye is shown. Note the faint opacity in the pupil which is a consequence of inflammatory debris adherent to the anterior lens capsule; posterior synechiae are also present, but the pupil shape is fairly regular. In addition to the very obvious iris blood vessels there are numerous iris nodules; smaller ones surround the pupil and larger ones are located on the surface of the iris away from the pupil. In humans, iris nodules are typical of granulomatous anterior uveitis, those situated at the pupillary border are termed Koeppe nodules, the larger ones are termed Busacca nodules.*

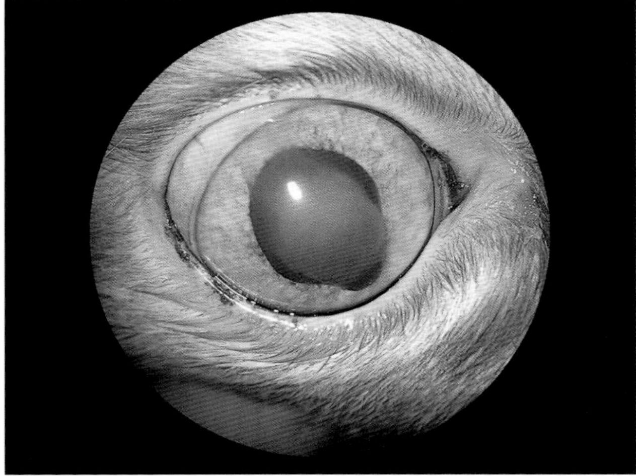

Fig. 12.36 *An 11-year-old Domestic shorthair neutered male with bilateral anterior uveitis associated with FIV; the right eye is shown. The reaction in this eye is more florid than usual, with a fibrinous mass and dependent haemorrhage filling the pupillary aperture. The left eye was also affected, but the predominant finding in this eye was infiltration of the iris by a solid mass which appeared to be neoplastic.*

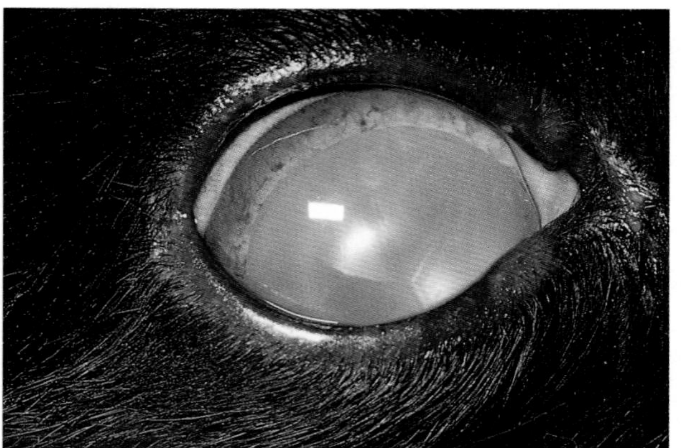

Fig. 12.37 *A 9-year-old Domestic shorthair neutered male with bilateral anterior uveitis associated with FIV; the right eye is shown. In this eye, but not the left eye, there was an anterior lens luxation and the luxated lens has become secondarily cataractous. Note that the eye is neither painful nor glaucomatous (intraocular pressure 13 mmHg).*

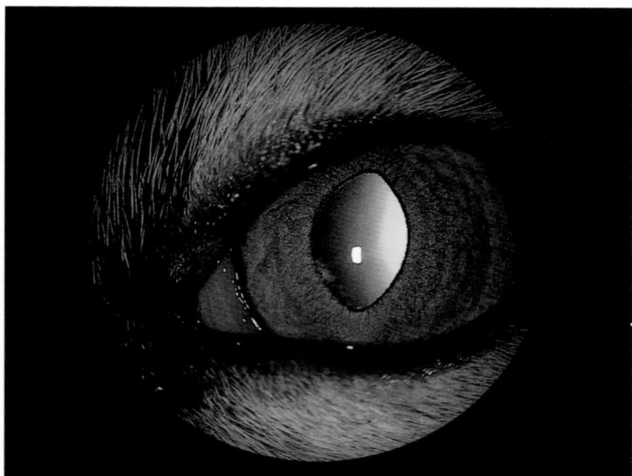

Fig. 12.38 *A 4-year-old Domestic shorthair neutered male with bilateral intermediate uveitis associated with FIV; the left eye is shown. If the pupil is dilated the extent of the pars planitis will become obvious. In this figure, prior to mydriasis, snowball opacities (in the anterior vitreous and on the posterior lens capsule) are evident in the ventromedial pupil.*

Intermediate uveitis (pars planitis) seems to occur more frequently with FIV than with other viral causes of feline uveitis; the changes are typical and the result of inflammatory cells (snowball opacities) accumulating in the anterior vitreous and adhering to the posterior lens capsule (snowbanking). Fundic lesions are unusual but can include vasculitis, focal chorioretinitis, retinal haemorrhage and retinal detachment. Invasion by opportunistic organisms, notably *T. gondii*, may occur in some cases.

Routine testing involves the detection of antibody to FIV and a positive result is conclusive. However, a significant proportion of FIV infected cats have no detectable antibody and therefore a negative antibody result does not preclude FIV infection.

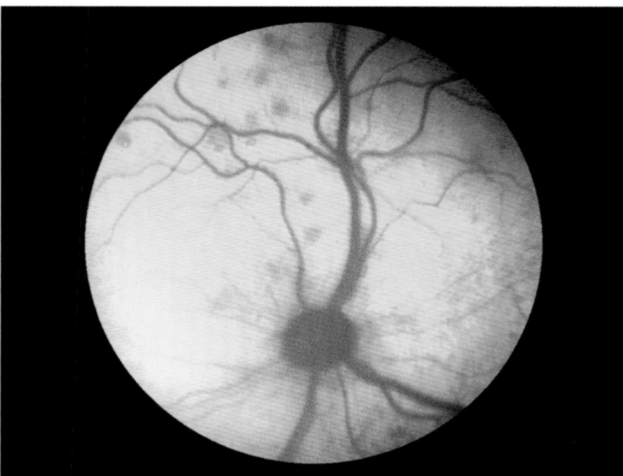

Fig. 12.39 *A 10-year-old Domestic shorthair neutered male. Originally presented because of a tumour in the left eye (see Fig. 12.60) demonstrated on histopathology to be a ciliary body adenocarcinoma. At the time of presentation the cat was also found to be FIV positive and a variety of FIV-related problems (e.g. gingivitis, capricious appetite) were managed successfully for 3 years before the cat deteriorated rapidly and was humanely destroyed. This was the appearance of the right fundus at the time of the deterioration in health and it was assumed that intercurrent infection (e.g. toxoplasmosis) was possible; post mortem examination was not performed.*

Treatment of cats with FIV tends to be symptomatic (see below) and supportive; they can be given good quality of life for some years after the diagnosis has been made through the judicious use of systemic corticosteroids and attention to any accompanying problems such as gingivitis.

Parasitic Causes of Uveitis

Toxoplasmosis *Toxoplasma gondii* is an intracellular coccidian parasite found throughout the world. The domestic cat and other felidae are the only definitive hosts, whereas any mammal may act as the intermediate host. The life cycle is very complex.

Clinical signs of toxoplasma infection are uncommon in the cat, particularly during the primary phase of infection, which occurs soon after the ingestion of infective cysts found in the tissues of intermediate hosts (e.g. mice and birds). It is much more usual for cats to present with chronic secondary toxoplasmosis following the recrudescence of encysted organisms, although this occurs only in a minority of infected cats. A wide range of clinical signs may develop, including pyrexia, weight loss, diarrhoea, vomiting, uveitis, neurological and respiratory signs. Any form of stress or debilitation, including concurrent infection with viruses or other parasites, is likely to predispose to the development of secondary disease. Neonatal infections in cats congenitally infected with *T. gondii* are rarely recognized but have been reported following experimental oral inoculation of pregnant queens with *T. gondii* tissue cysts.

Ocular lesions are rare in primary disease but frequently occur in secondary toxoplasmosis. Anterior uveitis, posterior uveitis and panuveitis have all been observed but the main ocular lesion of early cases is retinitis; lesions may be unilateral or bilateral (Figs 12.40–12.48).

Anterior uveitis is typically chronic in nature and may be a consequence of granulomatous infiltration or a hypersensitivity reaction of the iris. The appearance is clinically indistinguishable from other forms of infectious uveitis. Posterior segment changes may be restricted initially to the retina: affected animals have focal retinitis lesions and the choroid becomes involved secondarily. In more advanced cases both focal and diffuse inflammatory changes are seen and older, inactive focal chorioretinopathies may coexist with more recent active lesions. There may be associated exudative (bullous) retinal detachments. Panuveitis is usually accompanied by vitritis and the classical snowball opacities of pars planitis, in addition to the features already described. Secondary glaucoma is a likely complication of the uveitis associated with *T. gondii* seropositive cats and the reasons for this are unclear (Chavkin *et al.*, 1992). *T. gondii* infection has also been suggested as an important risk factor for the development of lens luxation (Chavkin *et al.*, 1992).

Serological confirmation of the diagnosis is ideally based on the use of ELISA for detection of *T. gondii*-specific immunoglobulin M (IgM), G (IgG) and circulating antigens (Lappin *et al.*, 1989). The clinical signs, serological evidence of infection (IgM titres > 1:256, increasing IgG titres or circulating antigen without antibodies) and response to treatment are helpful, but not definitive, in determining antemortem aetiology. Histopathology is an additional means of confirming diagnosis but, practically, restricted to post mortem material (Dubey and Carpenter, 1993).

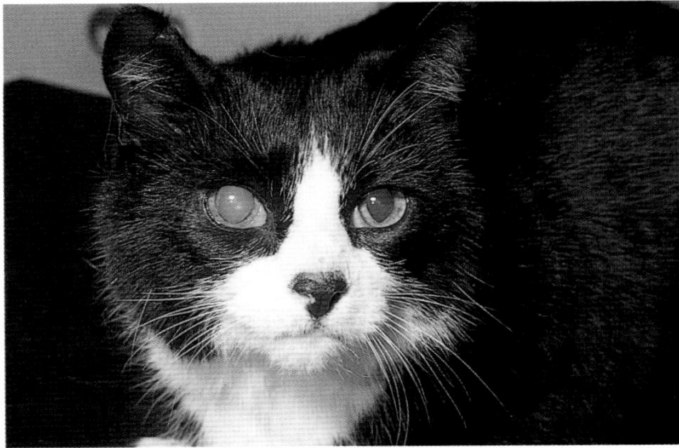

Fig. 12.40 *A 4-year-old Domestic shorthair neutered male with bilateral anterior uveitis associated with toxoplasmosis. Note the ansiocoria, in this case arising as a complication of glaucoma secondary to uveitis in the right eye (intraocular pressure of right eye 46 mmHg and left eye 17 mmHg).*

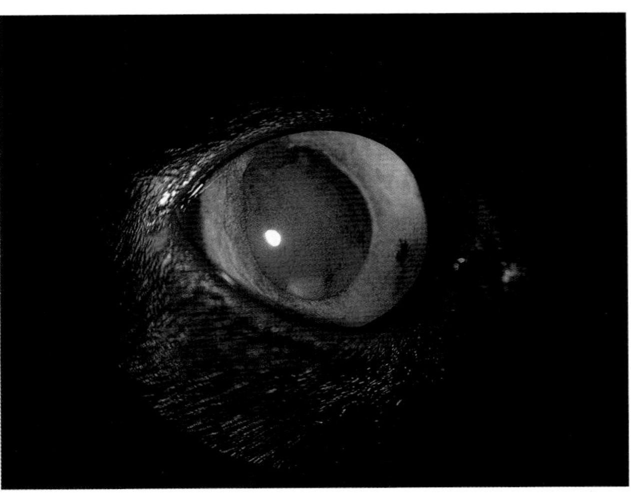

Fig. 12.41 *A 10-month-old Domestic shorthair neutered female with bilateral anterior uveitis associated with toxoplasmosis; the right eye is shown. This cat was the smallest of the litter and had not grown normally. At initial presentation there was an active, but chronic, uveitis with bilateral total cataracts; that of the left eye was denser than that of the right. In both eyes aqueous flare was present, together with keratic precipitates and inflammatory material on the anterior lens capsule. It was not possible to examine the posterior segment. In this eye it is apparent that lens rupture is likely to occur at the most dorsal aspect of the lens visible in the pupil. The cat was given a course of systemic clindamycin and topical corticosteroids; this photograph was taken approximately 1 week after treatment had started.*

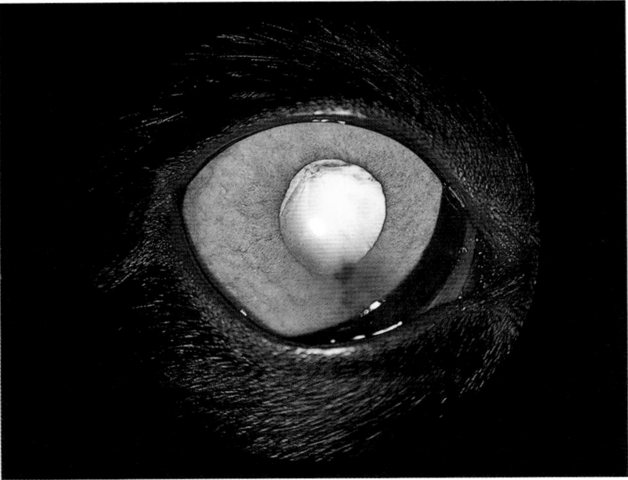

Fig. 12.42 *The same eye as shown in Fig. 12.41 2 months later. The lens has ruptured and the cataract has resorbed. It was now possible to examine the posterior segment which was normal and the cat could now see out of this eye. Subsequently, the cataract of the left eye underwent a degree of natural resorption, a Morgagnian cataract resulted, and there was useful vision in this eye also.*

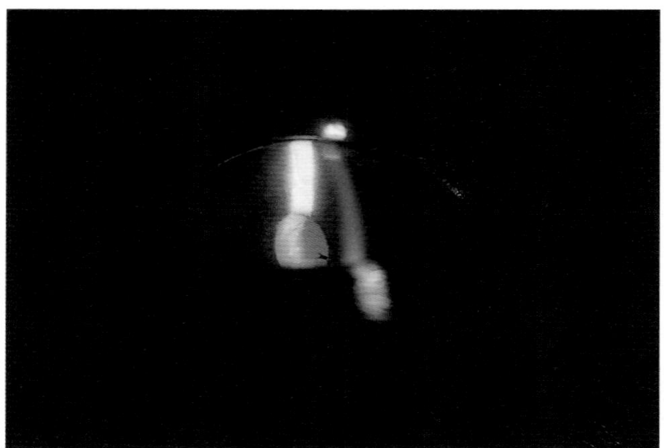

Fig. 12.43 *Slit lamp photograph of the same eye as shown in Figs 12.41 and 12.42 taken at the same time as Fig. 12.42 to demonstrate deepening of the anterior chamber associated with lens resorption.*

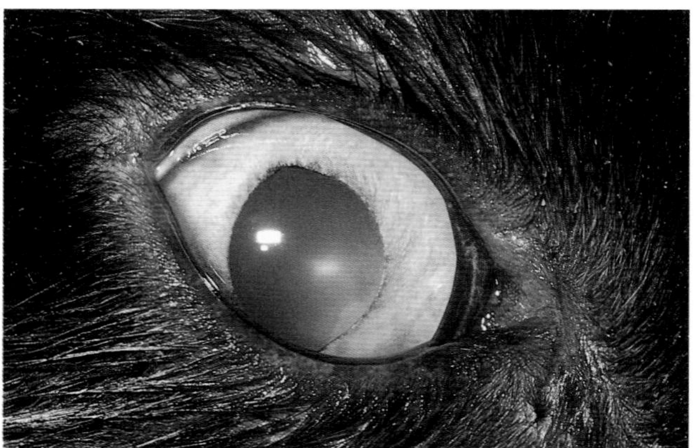

Fig. 12.44 *An 11-year-old Domestic shorthair neutered male with bilateral anterior uveitis and pars planitis associated with toxoplasmosis; the right eye is shown. Note the keratic precipitates (grey) on the posterior surface of the ventral cornea and the snowbanking (posterior lens capsule and anterior vitreous) in the ventromedial aspect of the pupil. This eye subsequently developed secondary glaucoma.*

Attempts to determine specific aetiology are further complicated, because serological evidence of *T. gondii* co-infection may be demonstrated in a proportion of cats with uveitis seropositive for FIP (coronavirus antibody titres of ≥ 1:1,600), FeLV and FIV (Chavkin *et al.*, 1992; Lappin *et al.*, 1992).

Treatment of toxoplasmosis involves either topical and/or systemic corticosteroids (see below) according to the site of uveal tract involvement, combined with a course of oral clindamycin hydrochloride (25 mg/kg daily in two divided doses for a minimum of 3 weeks); clindamycin appears more effective and without the side-effects of the sulphonamides and pyrimethamine used previously (Lappin *et al.*, 1992). The disease may recur.

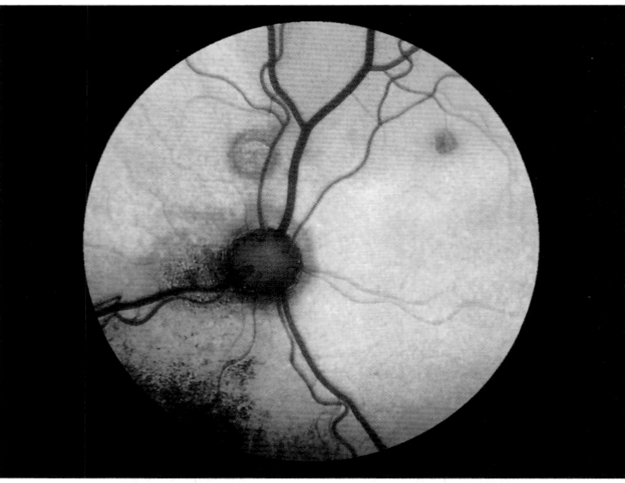

Fig. 12.45 *Domestic shorthair, age and sex unknown, with bilateral posterior uveitis associated with toxoplasmosis; the left eye is shown. Multiple focal active and inactive retinochoroiditis lesions.*

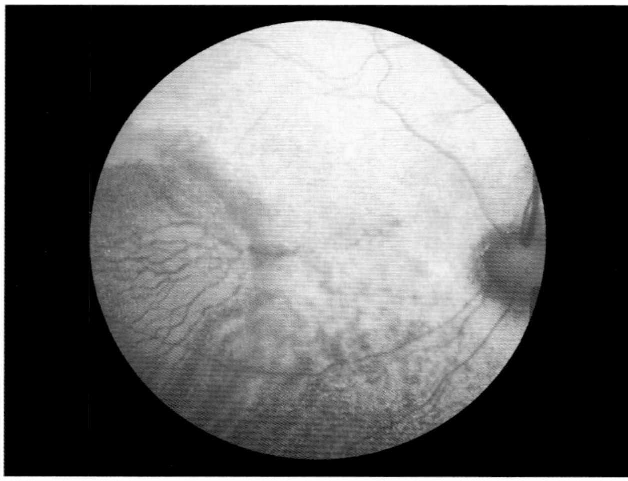

Fig. 12.46 *A 9-year-old Siamese neutered male with unilateral posterior uveitis associated with toxoplasmosis; the right eye is shown. A large focal area of chorioretinitis is apparent almost lateral to the optic disc.*

Others Other rare causes of parasitic uveitis are limited to single case reports (Bussanich and Rootman, 1983; Johnson *et al.*, 1988) and include aberrant nematodes (e.g. *Dirofilaria immitis*) and dipteran larvae (e.g. *Cuterebra* spp. larvae).

Mycotic Uveitis

Uveitis as a consequence of cryptococcosis, histoplasmosis, blastomycosis, coccidiomycosis and candidiasis have all been reported in cats. However, reports of these infections are rare and tend to be limited to countries where mycoses are endemic. They are very unlikely to occur in the United Kingdom unless the cat has been imported from such a country. Nevertheless, when investigating uveitis of possible infectious origin, it is sensible to enquire if the cat has been abroad at any time in the past.

All these species of fungi have yeast forms capable of growth in animal tissues. In general, ocular lesions occur only when the infection, acquired by inhalation or possible ingestion, becomes systemic. The principal lesion involves the retina and the anterior uvea may not be involved at all, or only in the later stages of the disease. The lesions are almost always bilateral, but are rarely symmetrical. It is not possible to distinguish between these infections by ocular examination, but vitreocentesis and identification of the organism is diagnostic in those cases with posterior segment involvement. Serological diagnosis of mycotic infections is not available in the UK, moreover the results of serology are inconclusive and interpretation of titres can be difficult.

Cryptococcosis *Cryptococcus neoformans* infection is the most common of the systemic mycoses in the cat (Figs 12.49, 12.50 and 5.22). The organism is widespread in the United States but may also occur in most other parts of the world, including Europe. Cats of all ages may be infected and there are no breed or sex predispositions. Intraocular involvement has been described by a number of authors, following the original report by Fischer (1971). In most cases the organism rapidly becomes disseminated and the site most commonly affected is the upper respiratory tract,

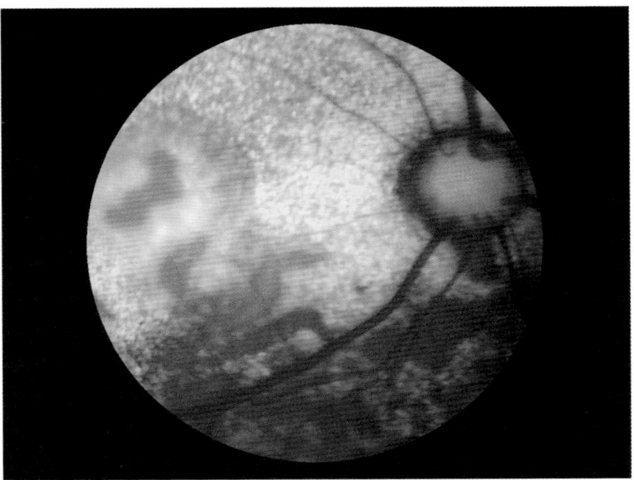

Fig. 12.47 *A 7-year-old Domestic shorthair neutered male. This cat was presented because of widely dilated pupils and acute onset blindness. On admission the toxoplasma antibody titre was 1:8192 and bizarre vermiform lesions and bullous detachments were present.*

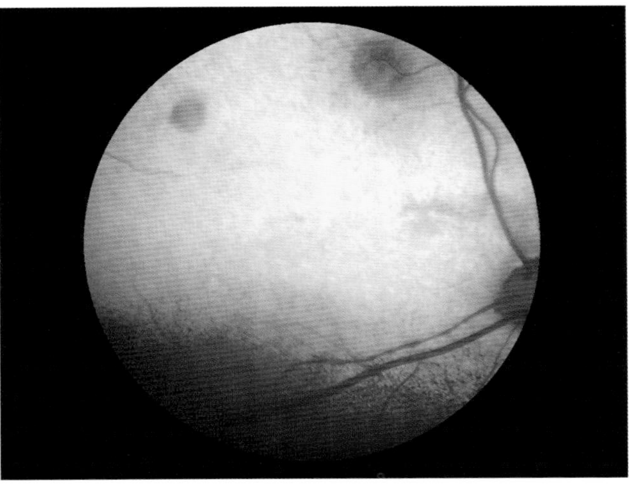

Fig. 12.49 *A 12-year-old Siamese neutered female with bilateral posterior uveitis associated with cryptococcosis. The cat had come to England via Venezuela and New York. Note the active, focal granulomatous chorioretinitis lesions.*

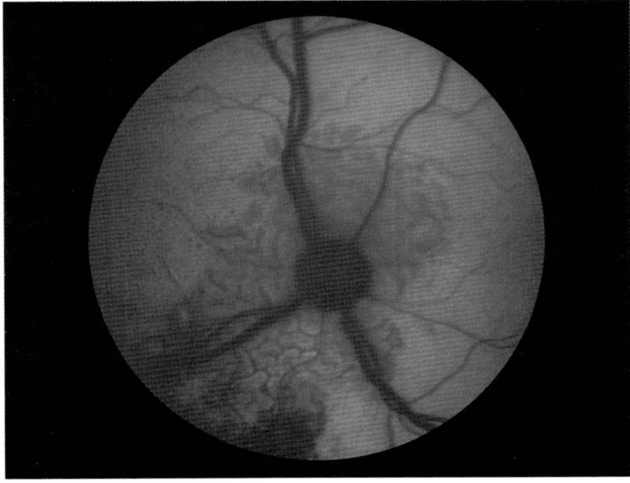

Fig. 12.48 *A 2-year-old Tonkinese neutered male with bilateral posterior uveitis associated with toxoplasmosis. Peripapillary serous retinal detachment has occurred.*

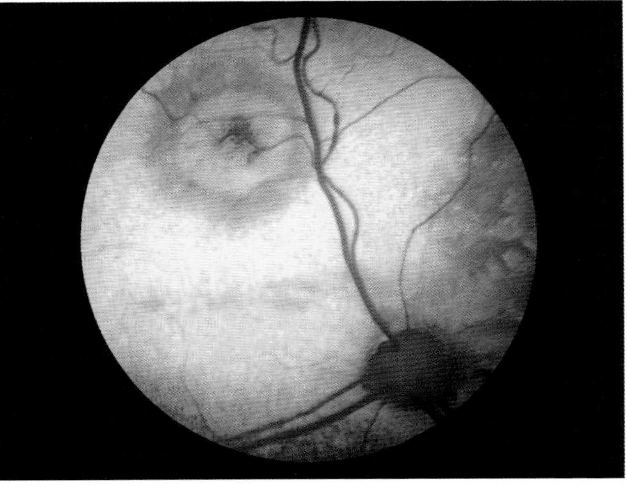

Fig. 12.50 *The same cat as shown in Fig. 12.49 after treatment with ketaconazole and 5-fluorocytosine. Note the change of appearance of the focal granulomatous lesions as active inflammation is no longer present.*

followed by the skin, eyes and central nervous system (CNS). However, the course of the disease is usually fairly slow, unless the CNS is involved. Affected animals may present with pneumonia, sinusitis or meningitis in addition to any ocular manifestations.

Ocular involvement may arise from haematogenous spread or by direct invasion from the paranasal sinuses, the nasal cavity or the optic meninges. Posterior uveitis usually occurs, with dark, raised focal granulomatous lesions or a more obvious exudative chorioretinitis. In the latter, there may be intraocular haemorrhage and retinal detachment leading to blindness. Anterior uveitis occurs in relatively few cases.

Treatment has variable success rates. A combination of 5-fluorocytosine, ketaconazole (Mikicuik *et al.*, 1990) and/or itraconazole may be effective in some cases, but long term results can be disappointing.

Histoplasmosis *Histoplasma capsulatum* is endemic in the major river valleys of the temperate and tropical regions of the world and it is not uncommon for cats living in, or travelling through, these areas to be infected with the organism. Infection is more common in younger cats, under 4 years old. A small proportion of infected cats develop disseminated histoplasmosis and associated clinical illness (Peiffer and Belkin, 1979; Wolf and Belden, 1984), usually in the form of acute weight loss, anorexia, depression, pyrexia and anaemia. Specific signs depend on organ involvement but respiratory signs are common because cats are initially infected by inhalation. Gross ocular lesions are apparent in only about 10% of cases but considerably more have fundic changes which are obvious on examination. Focal granulomatous chorioretinitis is usually observed, with occasional retinal detachment. Anterior uveitis is rare.

Disseminated histoplasmosis is usually confirmed by bone marrow aspiration and demonstration of the causative organism. The prognosis is poor, despite treatment with a variety of antifungal agents (e.g. amphotericin B and ketaconazole).

Blastomycosis Infection with *Blastomyces dermatitidis* is rare in cats. The organism is found principally in North America, but has also been reported in Africa and Central America. Cats usually become infected by inhalation of spores and the primary lesions tend to be in the lungs, although CNS signs may also develop (Nasisse *et al.*, 1985).

Clinical signs, usually seen only in the last 1–3 weeks of infection, include nonspecific signs such as weight loss, depression and pyrexia. Specific signs relate to the distribution of lesions. The ocular lesions consist of greyish-white choroidal granulomas, sometimes with retinal detachments and, in some cases, chronic granulomatous anterior uveitis.

Others Coccidiomycosis is caused by *Coccidioides immitis*, a soil fungus found in the south western United States and parts of Central and South America. This may be an occasional cause of feline mycotic uveitis (Angell *et al.*, 1985). Candidiasis, caused by *Candida albicans*, has been reported as a rare cause of feline uveitis (Miller and Albert, 1988; Gerding *et al.*, 1994).

Miscellaneous Forms of Infectious Uveitis

Disseminated bacterial causes of uveitis are virtually non-existent in the cat. Isolated cases of uveitis associated with tuberculosis (Hancock and Coates, 1911; Formston, 1994) are the exception (Figs 12.51 and 12.52) and tubercular choroiditis with retinal detachment is the commonest ocular manifestation.

Local injury, usually as a result of a fight, may result in direct intraocular inoculation of bacteria (e.g. *Pasteurella multocida*) and this is a relatively common cause of uveitis which is amenable to symptomatic treatment for the uveitis, together with topical administration of antibiotic solutions such as chloramphenicol or newer generation penicillins (see Chapter 3).

Traumatic Uveitis

See Chapter 3.

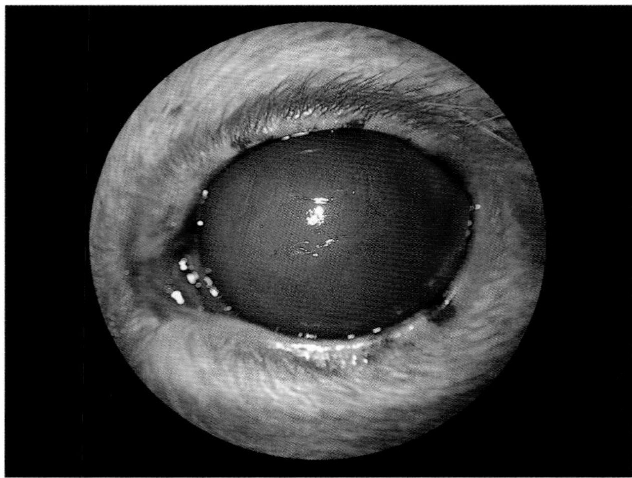

Fig. 12.51 *A 20-year-old Domestic shorthair neutered male with mycobacterial uveitis (see also Fig. 9.54).*

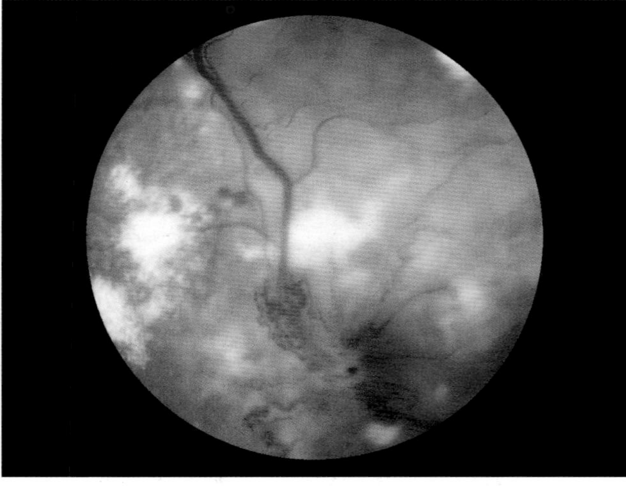

Fig. 12.52 *A 4-year-old Domestic shorthair neutered male with mycobacterial choroiditis.*

Lens-induced uveitis Lens-induced uveitis is most likely to be encountered in conjunction with lens trauma, especially rupture of the lens capsule (see Chapters 3 and 11).

Idiopathic and Other Forms of Uveitis

In a proportion of cases it is not possible to establish a precise aetiology and there may be other causes of feline uveitis which await discovery. For example, *Bartonella henselae*, the cause of cat scratch fever in humans, has been isolated from cats with uveitis, but its exact role is unknown.

Idiopathic lymphocytic–plasmacytic uveitis (Peiffer and Wilcock, 1991) is believed to be an example of immune-mediated disease (Wilcock *et al.*, 1990). In this condition (Figs 12.53 and 12.54), which may be unilateral or bilateral, affected animals are not systemically ill and older cats (mean age approximately 9 years) are affected (Davidson *et al.*, 1991; Gemensky *et al.*, 1996). Because a lymphocytic–plasmacytic response is not unusual in cats with chronic disease, it is possible that this type of uveitis may reflect the poor sensitivity of diagnostic tests, including those for FIV and toxoplasmosis, rather than representing a specific disease. The long-term prognosis for affected eyes is poor as the condition is only partly controlled by anti-inflammatory and immunosuppressive therapy. Complications include visual loss, cataract, glaucoma and lens luxation.

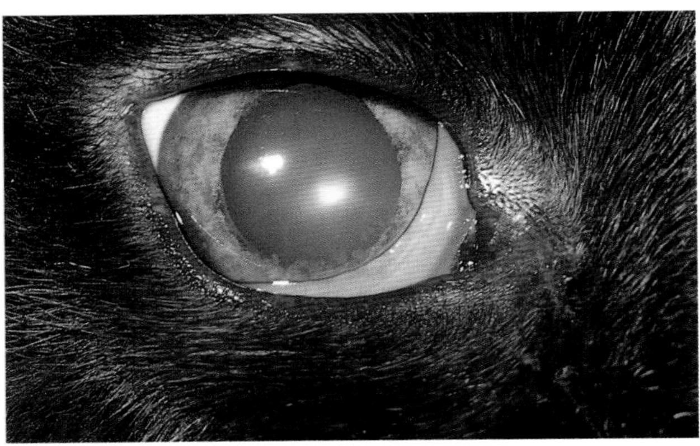

Fig. 12.53 *A 12-year-old Domestic longhair neutered male with idiopathic unilateral anterior uveitis. Note the darkened, rather dull, iris and the very dark keratic precipitates on the posterior surface of the ventral cornea. Examination of the posterior segment indicated some retinal degeneration and cupping of the optic disc. The clinical course was marked by fluctuations of intraocular pressure and poor response to treatment.*

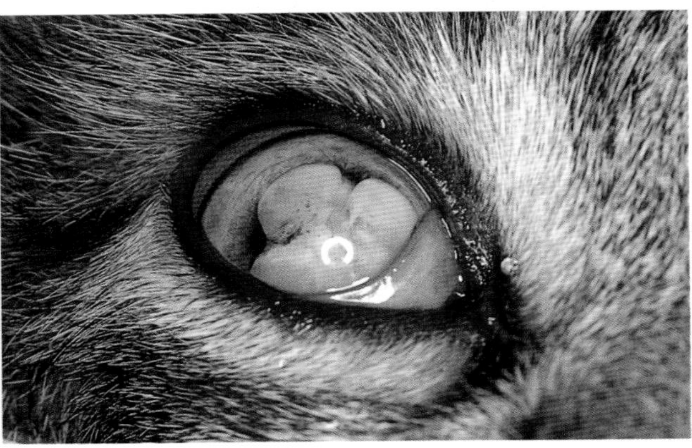

Fig. 12.54 *A 9-year-old Domestic shorthair neutered female with lens luxation secondary to idiopathic anterior uveitis. Note the dorsal posterior synechiae. The cataract is hypermature and the lens is shrunken.*

Periarteritis nodosa, a possible hypersensitivity response to collagen, has been described as a cause of lymphocytic-plasmacytic infiltration of the feline uveal tract (Campbell *et al.*, 1972).

Symptomatic Treatment of Uveitis

Successful management of uveitis depends upon establishing the cause and giving specific treatment whenever possible. In addition to specific treatment of the underlying cause, the clinical signs of uveitis will require symptomatic treatment which usually consists of anti-inflammatory agents and mydriatic cycloplegics.

Corticosteroids Corticosteroids topically and/or systemically are the commonest type of anti-inflammatory agent used in the treatment of uveitis. Prednisolone acetate 1%, dexamethasone 0.1% and betamethasone sodium phosphate 0.1% are potent topical preparations for the treatment of anterior uveitis; prednisolone acetate is probably the most effective topical agent.

Oral prednisolone is indicated for the treatment of intermediate and posterior uveitis. Both topical and oral corticosteroids will be required for the treatment of panuveitis and for those situations in which immune-mediated mechanisms are suspected. A dose rate of 1 mg/kg of prednisolone every 12 h is used initially and the treatment should be tapered off after 5–14 days. Treatment with these corticosteroids should not be stopped abruptly.

Corticosteroids should not be used, or used with caution, if the cause of the uveitis is not apparent, or there is corneal ulceration. Systemic corticosteroids should be avoided in the treatment of uveitis resulting from viral or mycotic infection. Reactivation of latent feline herpesvirus infection is a potential complication of corticosteroid usage.

Nonsteroidal anti-inflammatory agents Flurbiprofen sodium can be used topically in situations where topical corticosteroids would be absolutely contraindicated as, for example, with ulceration. However, these agents will modify wound healing, so patients should be monitored carefully. Topical nonsteroidal anti-inflammatory agents are most often used as an adjunct to intraocular surgery.

Nonsteroidal anti-inflammatory agents can be used orally as an alternative to systemic corticosteroids. Their side-effects include gastrointestinal haemorrhage and inhibition of platelet function. The risk of gastro-intestinal haemorrhage is considerably increased when they are used in conjunction with corticosteroids and they should therefore not be used in combination.

Oral acetylsalicylic acid may be used with caution at a total dose of 80 mg every 48–72 h.

Mydriatic cycloplegics Atropine 1% ointment is the drug of choice. Phenylephrine 10% is not particularly effective in cats (possibly because the dilator muscle of the cat's iris has both an adrenergic and cholinergic nerve supply) and is not used therapeutically.

The patient's progress should be monitored closely and the aim is to eliminate pain (by relaxing ciliary spasm) and to reduce the risk of synechiae formation. This can be achieved with moderate pupillary dilation and mydriatic cycloplegics should then be applied only as often as is necessary to maintain this state.

Treatment should be started as soon as possible after the onset of uveitis and continued for up to 10 days after the clinical signs have resolved.

Complications of Uveitis

Some types of infectious uveitis respond poorly to symptomatic treatment and if the underlying cause cannot be identified and eliminated then such animals can only be managed according to their quality of life.

Glaucoma as a complication of uveitis is less common in cats than dogs (see Chapters 3 and 10), but when it does occur, particularly in those cats which are seropositive for *T. gondii*, it can be very difficult to treat, especially if additional problems arise in the form of corneal decompensation with epithelial erosion, visual loss, or globe enlargement. For active uveitis and secondary glaucoma more intensive use of anti-inflammatories, possibly combined with a short-acting mydriatic (tropicamide 1%) and carbonic anhydrase inhibitor may be required, but such cases often respond poorly. When active uveitis is accompanied by both secondary glaucoma and corneal erosion, effective management becomes impossible and, if the underlying uveitis cannot be controlled, it is better to remove the affected eye. Cats manage loss of vision extraordinarily well and their quality of life will be affected more by the presence of a blind painful eye than by its absence.

Lens luxation is not an uncommon complication of chronic uveitis (Fig. 12.54), but in cats, unlike dogs, it is not an emergency and secondary glaucoma is less likely as a consequence of the initial luxation. Effective management is centred around establishing and treating the cause of the underlying uveitis (as described earlier). Once the uveitis has been brought under control, lens removal can be considered.

UVEAL NEOPLASIA

PRIMARY NEOPLASIA

Although the cat is subject to a range of uveal tract tumours, the commonest primary intraocular tumour is a melanoma and it is usually uniocular (Figs 12.55–12.58); other types of tumour (Figs 12.59 and 12.60) are much less common (Bellhorn and Henkind, 1970; Williams *et al.*, 1981; Dubielzig, 1990). The iris and ciliary body are more frequently affected than the choroid (which tends to be involved because of extension from the anterior uvea) and uveal melanomas may be benign or malignant. There is no single morphological feature that enables the behaviour of these tumours to be predicted; however, the prognosis is good in cats in which neoplastic cells are limited to the anterior face of the iris and becomes poorer if transformed cells infiltrate the iris stroma, or extend beyond the iris (Duncan and Peiffer, 1991). Malignancy is associated with potential for distant metastases to sites such as the lungs and liver and more than 50% of melanomas will metastasize (Patnaik and Mooney, 1988; Duncan and Peiffer, 1991).

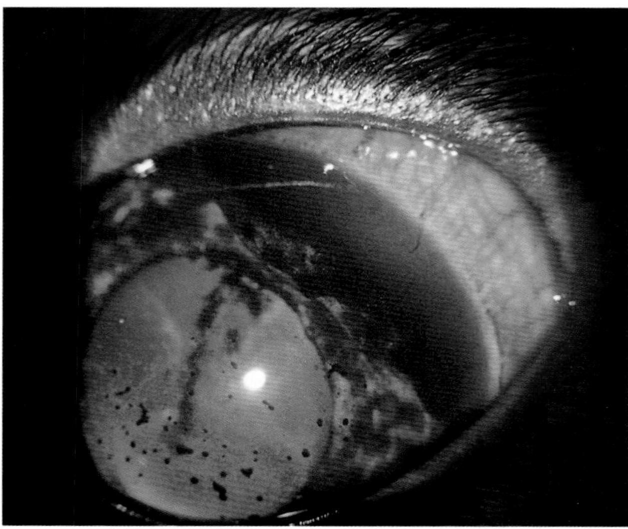

Fig. 12.55 *A 13-year-old Domestic shorthair with diffuse iris melanoma. The eye is reddened and there is marked pigment shedding, secondary glaucoma is developing.*

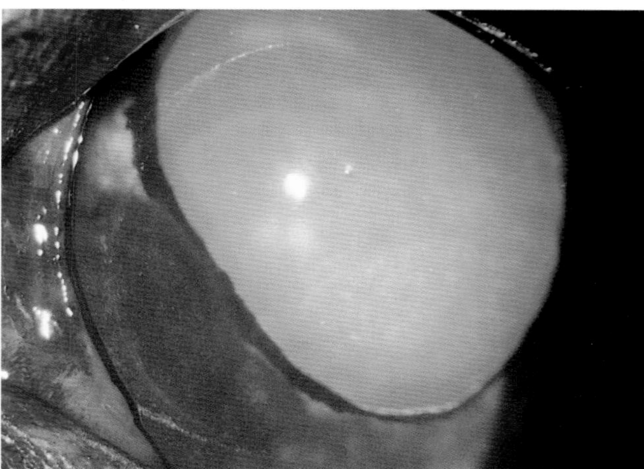

Fig. 12.56 *Adult domestic shorthair with iris melanoma. Note that the tumour has infiltrated most of the iris, but a small sector of normal colour is apparent. The pupil is slightly distorted and ectropion uveae is apparent. There is no pigment shedding.*

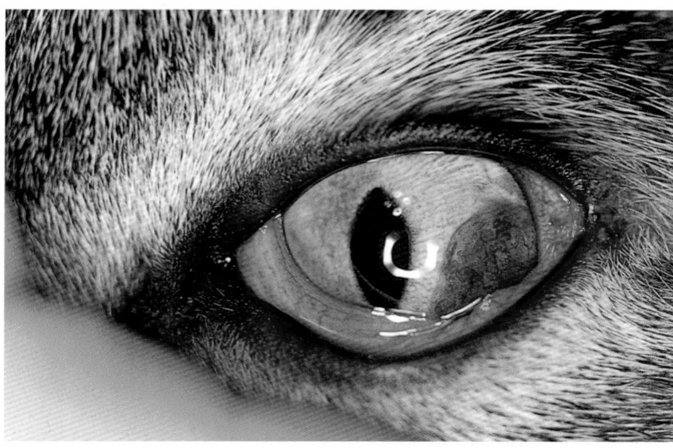

Fig. 12.57 Adult domestic shorthair with iris melanoma. The eye is reddened and the tumour is associated with a marked vascular response. (Courtesy of J. P. Oleshko.)

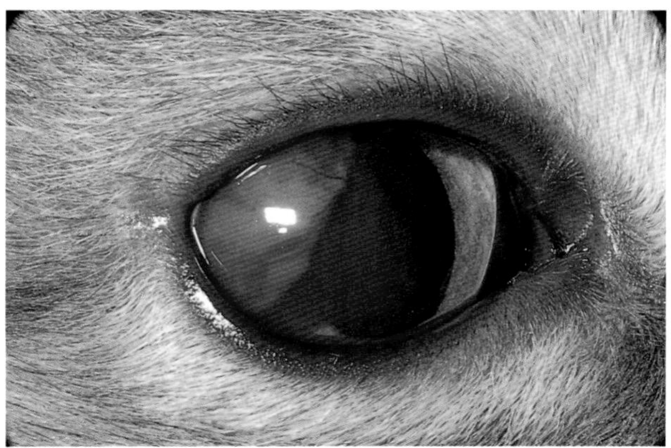

Fig. 12.58 A 5-year-old Domestic shorthair. Iris melanoma, with more extensive iris involvement and hyphaema.

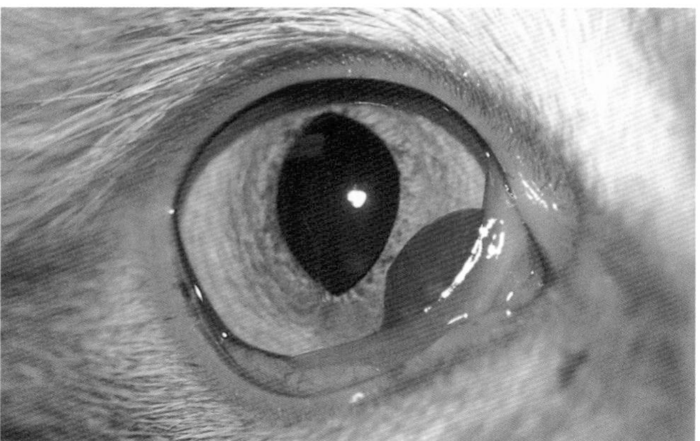

Fig. 12.59 Domestic shorthair with ciliary body adenoma (courtesy of J. Wolfer).

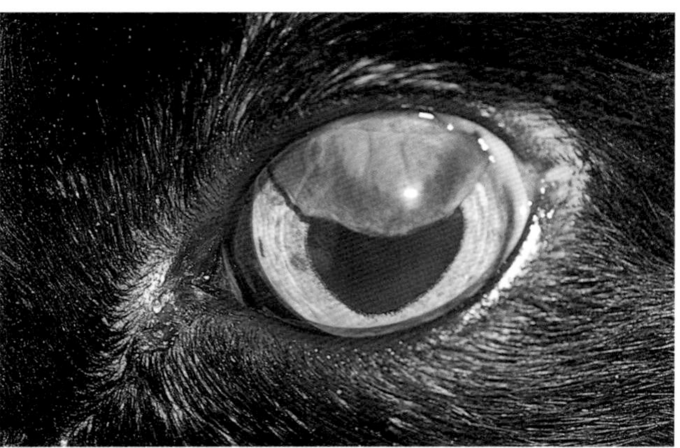

Fig. 12.60 A 7-year-old Domestic shorthair neutered male with ciliary body adenocarcinoma affecting the left eye. The right eye is shown in Fig. 12.39. The cat was FIV positive.

Iridal neoplasia provides a range of clinical presentations, whether or not a visible mass is present; they include a change of iris appearance, or position, increased prominence of intraocular and occasionally extraocular vessels, changes in the depth of the anterior chamber, pigment dispersal, uveitis and glaucoma. Both pigmented and nonpigmented lesions occur. Diagnosis is aided by careful examination of the appearance of the iris, the pupil and the depth of the anterior chamber, together with transillumination, gonioscopy, tonometry and ultrasonography or MRI. Biopsy is not usually indicated. Sequential observation may be necessary to confirm that a mass is getting larger.

Primary tumours of the ciliary body are not detected on clinical examination as readily as those of the iris, but when they enlarge they tend to displace the iris and may also displace the lens.

Primary feline ciliary body tumours include melanomas and also those of epithelium (e.g. adenoma and adenocarcinoma) and possibly smooth muscle (e.g. leiomyoma).

Early enucleation is usually the treatment of choice for anything other than small, well-circumscribed discrete primary uveal tumours, or those which involve a change of pigmentation of the anterior iris surface as the only abnormality. Careful physical examination and chest radiographs should be taken if the benign nature of the tumour is in doubt prior to performing the surgery. In all cases the globe should be submitted for histopathology.

Secondary Neoplasia

Lymphosarcoma associated with FeLV is the commonest secondary neoplasm affecting the feline eye and orbit and the uveal tract is most commonly involved (Figs 12.61–12.64) as discussed above. There is a spectrum of clinical appearances involving both anterior and, less commonly, posterior uvea and it is not always possible to differentiate the ocular manifestations of the feline leukaemia–lymphosarcoma complex from other problems affecting the uveal tract.

Plasma cell myeloma (multiple myeloma) usually produces clinical problems because of infiltration of organs by neoplastic plasma cells and the damaging effects of the plasma cell M component (paraprotein). Plasma cell myeloma is a rare cause of secondary neoplasia in cats.

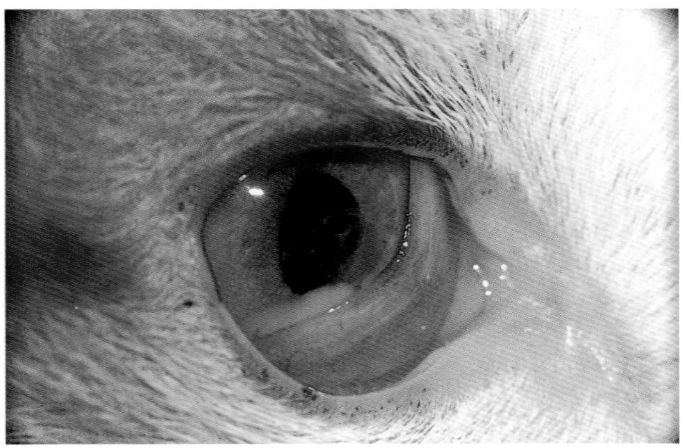

Fig. 12.61 A 2-year-old Domestic shorthair with generalized lymphosarcoma. Note the presence of fibrin and neoplastic cells in the anterior chamber and mild infiltration of the peripheral iris.

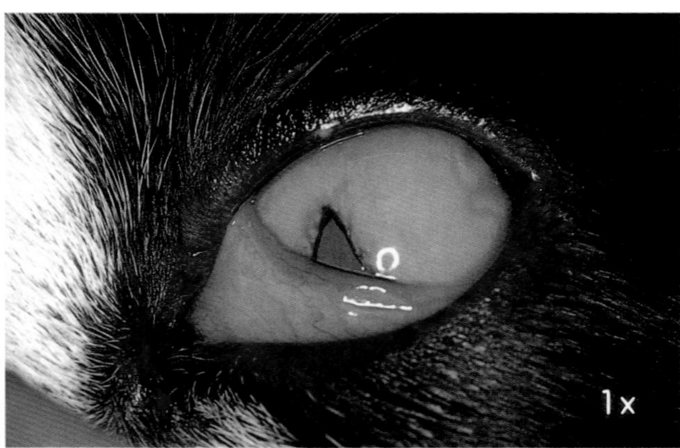

Fig. 12.62 Domestic shorthair with lymphosarcoma infiltrating the iris. The anterior chamber is shallow because of the extent of iris infiltration.

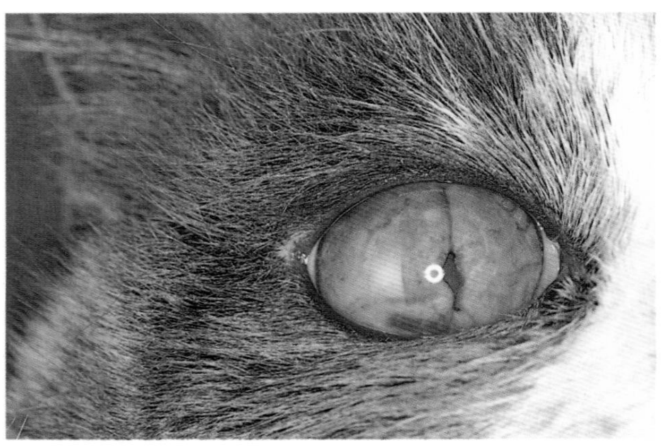

Fig. 12.63 A 7-year-old Domestic shorthair neutered female. Lymphosarcoma infiltrating the iris. In addition to the shallow anterior chamber note the iris vessels and the pupil distortion.

Metastatic carcinomas (e.g. adenocarcinoma, squamous cell carcinoma) and sarcomas (e.g. haemangiosarcoma, fibrosarcoma) should also be considered as a cause of secondary uveal neoplasia; they arise from a number of primary sites such as uterus, mammary gland, lung and kidney and may metastasize to the choroid and anterior uvea (Fig. 12.65). The prognosis is grave.

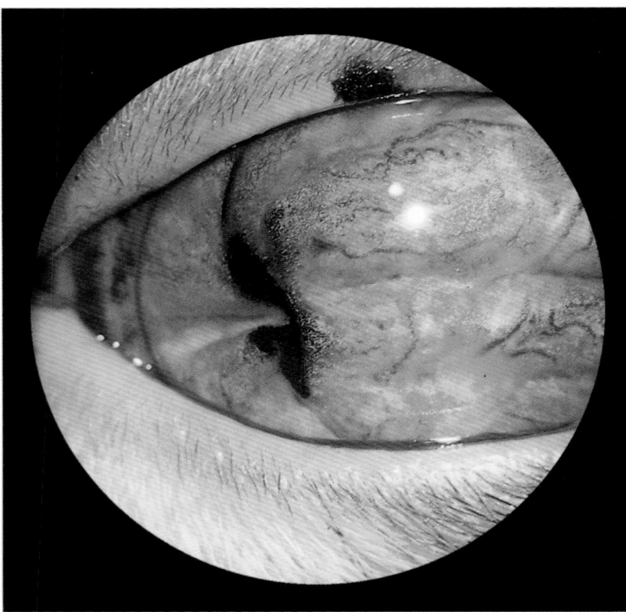

Fig. 12.64 A 15-year-old Domestic shorthair with lymphosarcoma infiltrating the iris. As in Fig. 12.62 there is a shallow anterior chamber, vascular response and pupil distortion.

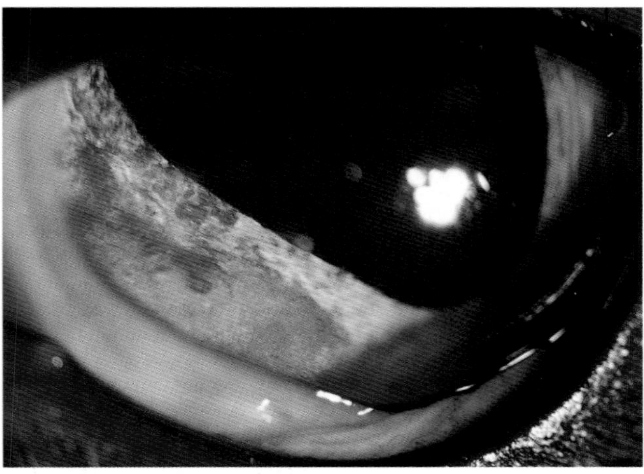

Fig. 12.65 Domestic shorthair with metastases from mammary gland adenocarcinoma (involving the eye and many other sites). Mammary gland surgery had been performed only weeks before.

References

Acland GM, McLean IW, Aguirre GD, Trucksa R (1980) Diffuse iris melanoma in cats. *Journal of the American Veterinary Medical Association* **176**: 52–56.

Angell JA, Shively JN, Merideth RE, Reed RE, Jamison KC (1985) Ocular coccidiomycosis in a cat. *Journal of the American Veterinary Medical Association* **187**: 167–169.

Bellhorn RW, Henkind P (1970) Intraocular malignant melanoma in domestic cats. *Journal of Small Animal Practice* **10**: 631–637.

Bergsma DR, Brown KS (1971) White fur, blue eyes and deafness in the domestic cat. *Journal of Heredity* **62**: 171–185.

Bill A (1966) Formation and drainage of aqueous humour in the cat. *Experimental Eye Research* **5**: 185–190.

Brightman AH, Ogilvie GK, Tompkins M (1991) Ocular disease in FeLV-positive cats: 11 cases (1981–1986). *Journal of the American Animal Hospital Association* **198**: 1049–1051.

Bussanich MN, Rootman J (1983) Intraocular nematode in a cat. *Feline Practice* **13**: 24–26.

Campbell LH, Fox JG, Drake DF (1972) Ocular and other manifestations of periarteritis nodosa in a cat. *Journal of the American Veterinary Medical Association* **161**: 1122–1126.

Chavkin MJ, Lappin MR, Powell CC, Roberts SM, Parshall CJ, Reif JS (1992) Seroepidemiologic and clinical observations of 93 cases of uveitis in cats. *Progress in Veterinary and Comparative Ophthalmology* **2**: 29–36.

Crispin SM (1993) The uveal tract. In Petersen-Jones SM, Crispin SM (eds), *Manual of Small Animal Ophthalmology*, pp. 173–190. BSAVA Publications, Cheltenham.

Corcoran KA, Peiffer RL, Koch SA (1995) Histopathologic features of feline ocular lymphosarcoma: 49 cases (1978–1992). *Veterinary and Comparative Ophthalmology* **5**: 35–41.

Davidson MG, Nasisse MP, English RV, Wilcock BP, Jamieson V (1991) Feline anterior uveitis: a study of 53 cases. *Journal of the American Animal Hospital Association* **27**: 77–83.

Dubey JP, Carpenter JL (1993) Histologically confirmed clinical toxoplasmosis in cats – 100 cases (1952–1990). *Journal of the American Veterinary Medical Association* **203**: 1556–1566.

Dubielzig RR (1990) Ocular neoplasia in small animals. *Veterinary Clinics of North America: Small Animal Practice* **20**: 837–848.

Duncan DE, Peiffer RL (1991) Morphology and prognostic indicators of anterior melanomas in cats. *Progress in Veterinary and Comparative Ophthalmology* **1**: 25–32.

Fischer CA (1971) Intraocular cryptococcosis in two cats. *Journal of the American Veterinary Medical Association* **158**: 191–199.

Formston C (1994) Retinal detachment and bovine tuberculosis in cats. *Journal of Small Animal Practice* **35**: 5–8.

Gemensky A, Lorimer D, Blanchard G (1996) Feline uveitis: A retrospective study of 45 cases. *Proceedings of the American College of Veterinary Ophthalmologists* **27**: 19.

Gerding PA, Morton LD, Dye JA (1994) Ocular and disseminated candidiasis in an immunosuppressed cat. *Journal of the American Veterinary Medical Association* **204**: 10, 1635–1638.

Gunn-Moore DA, Pearson GR, Harbour DA, Whiting CV (1996) Encephalitis associated with giant cells in a cat with naturally occurring feline immunodeficiency virus infection demonstrated by *in situ* hybridisation. *Veterinary Pathology* **33**: 699–703.

Hancock and Coates (1911) Tubercle of the choroid in the cat. *Veterinary Record* **23**: 433–436.

Hopper CD, Sparkes AH, Gruffydd-Jones TJ, Crispin SM, Muir P, Harbour DA, Stokes CR (1989) Clinical and laboratory findings in cats infected with feline immunodeficiency virus. *Veterinary Record* **125**: 341–346.

Johnson BW, Helper LC, Szajerski ME (1988) Intraocular *Cuterebra* larva in a cat. *Journal of the American Veterinary Medical Association* **193**: 829–830.

Kline KL, Joseph RJ, Averill DR (1994) Feline infectious peritonitis with neurologic involvement: Clinical and pathological findings in 24 cats. *Journal of the American Animal Hospital Association* **30**: 111–118.

Lappin MR, Greene CE, Winston S, Toll SL, Epstein ME (1989) Clinical feline toxoplasmosis. *Journal of Veterinary Internal Medicine* **3**: 139–143.

Lappin MR, Marks A, Greene GE, Collins J, Carman J, Reif JS, Powell CC (1992) Serologic prevalence of selected infectious diseases in cats with uveitis. *Journal of the American Veterinary Medical Association* **201**: 1005–1009.

Mikicuik MG, Fales WH, Schmidt DA (1990) Successful treatment of feline cryptococcosis with ketoconazole and flucytosine. *Journal of the American Animal Hospital Association* **26**: 199–201.

Miller WM, Albert RA (1988) Ocular and systemic candidiasis in a cat. *Journal of the American Animal Hospital Association* **24**: 521–524.

Nasisse MP, van Ee RT, Wright B (1985) Ocular changes in a cat with disseminated blastomycosis. *Journal of the American Veterinary Medical Association* **187**: 629–631.

Patnaik AK, Mooney S (1988) Feline melanoma: A comparative study of ocular, oral and dermal neoplasms. *Veterinary Pathology* **25**: 105–112.

Peiffer RL, Belkin PV (1979) Ocular manifestations of disseminated histoplasmosis in a cat. *Feline Practice* **9**: 24–29.

Peiffer RL, Wilcock BP (1991) Histopathological study of uveitis in cats: 139 cases (1978–1988). *Journal of the American Veterinary Medical Association* **198**: 135–138.

Poland AM, Vennema H, Foley JE, Pedersen NC (1996) Two related strains of feline infectious peritonitis virus isolated from immunocompromised cats infected with a feline enteric coronavirus. *Journal of Clinical Microbiology* **34**: 3180–3184.

Sparkes AH, Gruffydd-Jones TJ, Harbour DA (1994) An appraisal of the value of laboratory tests in the diagnosis of feline infectious peritonitis. *Journal of the American Animal Hospital Association* **30**: 345–350.

Wilcock BP, Peiffer RL, Davidson MG (1990) The causes of glaucoma in cats. *Veterinary Pathology* **27**: 35–40.

Williams DL (1993) A comparative approach to anterior segment dysgenesis. *Eye* **7**: 607–616.

Williams LW, Gelatt KN, Gwin R (1981) Ophthalmic neoplasms in the cat. *Journal of the American Animal Hospital Association* **17**: 999–1008.

Wolf AM, Belden MN (1984) Feline histoplasmosis: A literature review and retrospective study of 20 new cases. *Journal of the American Animal Hospital Association* **20**: 995–998.

13 Vitreous

Introduction

The vitreous, vitreous body or vitreous humour, occupies the posterior segment of the eye and constitutes two-thirds in volume of the globe. The vitreous is a transparent jelly-like substance consisting of approximately 99% water with collagen and hyaluronic acid and very few cells. Embryologically, vitreous is derived from ectoderm and is divided into primary (hyaloid artery system), secondary (adult vitreous), which forms around the primary, and tertiary (lens zonular fibres).

The vitreous base is the attachment of vitreous in the region of the ora ciliaris retinae. The vitreous cortex occupies the peripheral part next to the retina. In the cat the cortex is more fluid than the denser centre portion. The patellar fossa is the concave anterior face of the vitreous which holds the lens and in the cat there is a prominent pseudo-membrane attached to the posterior surface of the lens. Cloquet's canal contains initially the hyaloid artery and travels from the optic disc to the posterior pole of the lens; the hyaloid artery is present at birth in the kitten but disappears by 8–9 weeks. Mittendorf's dot is a small opacity on the posterior lens capsule marking the hyaloid artery attachment.

The functions of the vitreous are to support the retina, to transmit light and to maintain the shape of the eyeball.

With age, holes and liquefaction (syneresis) occur within the vitreous.

Congenital anomalies

The congenital condition of persistent hyperplastic primary vitreous (PHPV), which occurs in the dog as isolated cases and also as a form of congenital hereditary eye disease in such breeds as the Dobermann and Staffordshire Bull Terrier, has not been described in the cat.

Persistent hyaloid artery would appear to be rare in the cat. Ketring and Glaze (1994) record a case with anterior lens luxation and Fig. 13.1 shows another, uniocular and in a young cat.

Diseases of the vitreous

Vitreous infiltrates do occur in the cat in cases of posterior uveitis and severe anterior uveitis (iridocyclitis), with or without aqueous flare. Figures 13.2 and 13.3 both show inflammatory cells in the anterior vitreous in cases of pars planitis.

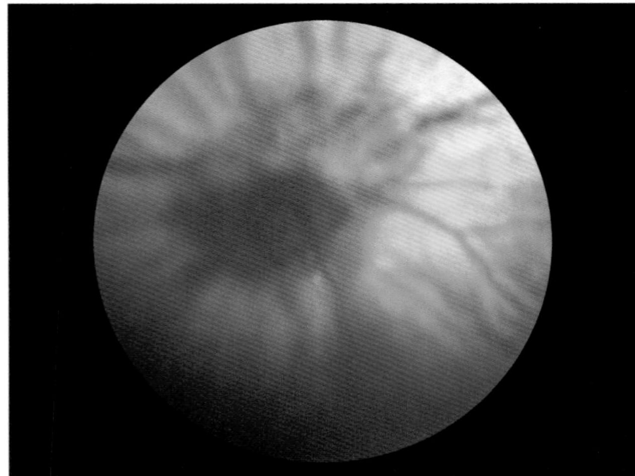

Fig. 13.1 *A 7-month-old Ragdoll male. Uniocular persistent hyaloid and small vitreal haemorrhage.*

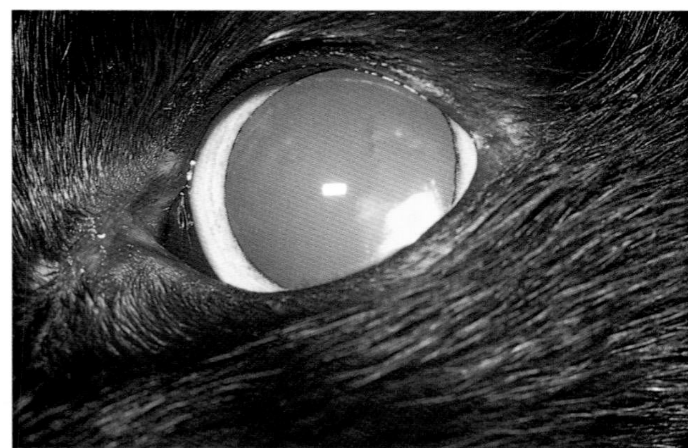

Fig. 13.2 *An 11-year-old Domestic shorthair neutered female. Pars planitis: inflammatory cells in anterior vitreous and on posterior lens capsule. Possible toxoplasmosis case.*

Haemorrhage into the vitreous is the most likely condition to be encountered clinically and may result from inflammation, trauma, neoplasia, clotting disorders and, in particular, hypertension. In such cases vitreal haemorrhages may be accompanied by retinal haemorrhages and examples of the former are shown in Figures 13.4–13.6 (see also Chapter 14). Haemorrhage into the vitreous may also occur in severe anaemia.

Folds of detached retina may also be seen in the vitreous, particularly in cases of hypertension from various causes (see Chapter 14).

A case of ophthalmomyiasis interna, with a larva in the vitreous body, has been recorded by Brooks *et al.* (1984). A single bilateral case of asteroid hyalosis, a degenerative condition of the vitreous, is recorded in a white Persian by Walde *et al.* (1990).

References

Brooks DE, Wolf ED and Merideth R (1984) Ophthalmomyiasis interna in two cats. *Journal of the American Animal Hospital Association* **20**: 157–160.

Ketring KL and Glaze MB (1994) *Atlas of Feline Ophthalmology*, p. 95. Veterinary Learning Systems, New Jersey.

Walde I, Schaffer EH and Kostlin RG (1990) *Atlas of Ophthalmology in Dogs and Cats*, p. 295. B.C. Decker Inc., Toronto.

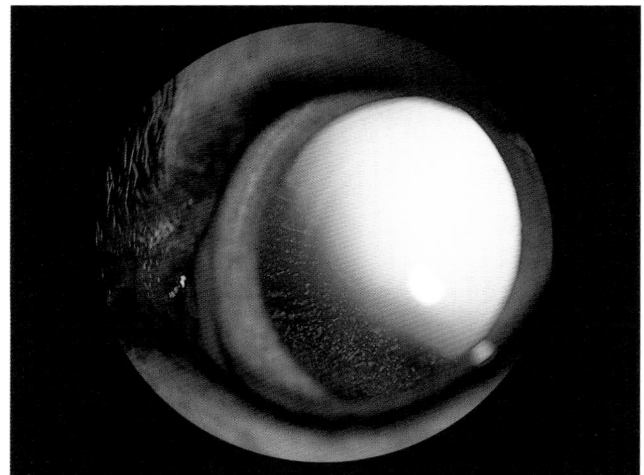

Fig. 13.3 *A 4-year-old Domestic shorthaired neutered male. Pars planitis, FIV positive.*

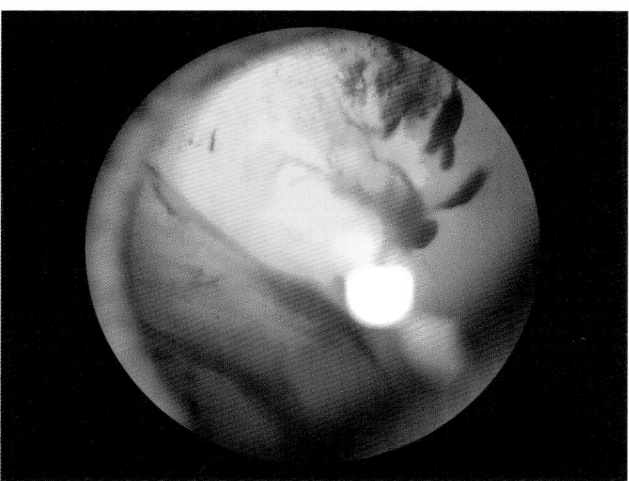

Fig. 13.5 *A 10-year-old Domestic shorthaired neutered male with anterior vitreal haemorrhage and retinal detachment; hypertension secondary to diabetes mellitus following long-term treatment with megestrol acetate.*

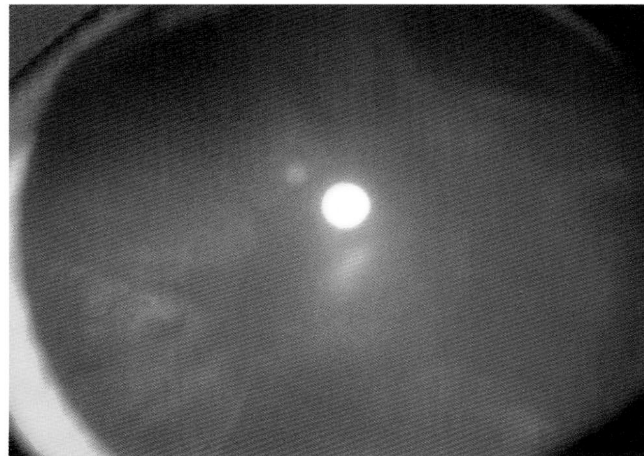

Fig. 13.4 *An 8-year-old Domestic shorthaired neutered female with diffuse vitreal haemorrhage and bilateral retinal detachment; hypertension secondary to renal failure.*

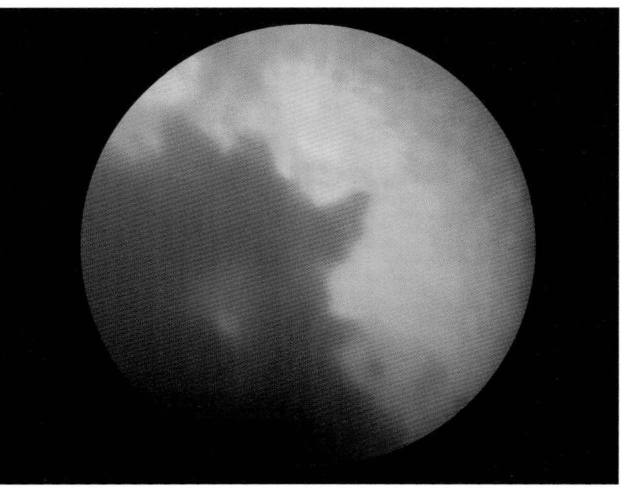

Fig. 13.6 *A 14-year-old Domestic shorthaired male. Massive vitreal haemorrhage; primary hypertension.*

14 Fundus

Introduction

The fundus of the eye is the posterior part of the globe viewed ophthalmoscopically and includes the appearance of the retina, superimposed over the underlying choroid and sclera and divided into tapetal and nontapetal portions, the optic disc (optic nerve head or papilla) and the retinal blood vessels. The gross appearance of the fundus is illustrated in Fig. 14.1, which shows the relative sizes and positions of both tapetal and nontapetal portions and also the usual position of the optic disc. The histological appearance of tapetal and nontapetal fundus is shown in Figs 14.2 and 14.3. The feline fundus is more regular and shows less variation than any of the other domestic animals and certainly less than that of the dog.

The retina is usually considered to have ten layers. The outermost layer, the retinal pigment epithelium, which lies next to the choroid, is derived from the outer layer of the optic cup (ectoderm) whereas the remaining nine layers, the neuro-sensory retina, develop from the inner layer of the optic cup (also ectoderm). The pigment epithelium is pigmented except over the tapetum, as is the case in all animals with a tapetal fundus.

The vascular pattern of the feline retina is classified as holangiotic, as is the case in the dog, with a direct blood supply to most of the retina. There are three major pairs of cilioretinal arterioles and slightly larger, and usually less tortuous, veins which leave at or near the edge of the optic disc and extend towards the periphery, leaving the central portion of the disc, unlike the dog, free from blood vessels. A central retinal artery is not usually present in this species but has been reported (Szymanski, 1987).

Figures 14.4 and 14.5 are fluoroscein angiograms showing arteriolar and arteriolar and venous filling, respectively.

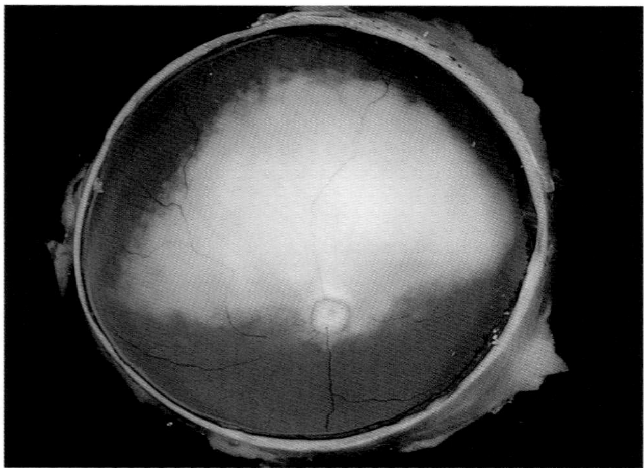

Fig. 14.1 The normal feline fundus in a young adult Domestic shorthaired cat. Posterior segment showing the shape and size of the tapetal fundus and position of the optic disc.

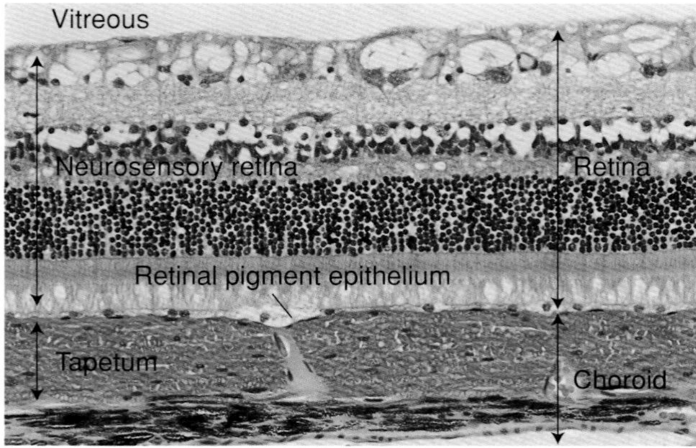

Fig. 14.2 Histological section (haematoxylin and eosin) of feline tapetal fundus. Note cellular tapetum below retina, absence of pigment in retinal pigment epithelium, and small vessel arising from choroid perforating tapetum.

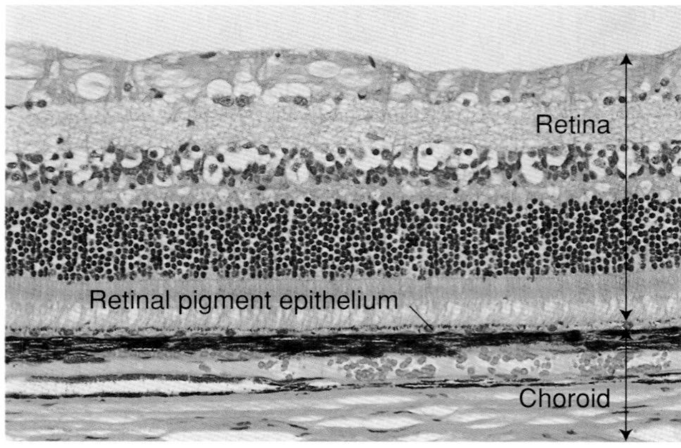

Fig. 14.3 Histological section (haematoxylin and eosin) of feline nontapetal fundus. Note melanin in retinal pigment epithelium and absence of tapetum.

Note the obvious but normal cupping of the optic disc with dipping of blood vessels at its edge.

The classification of feline retinal diseases differs between authors and is complicated by the fact that many cases may have an unknown aetiology, even after detailed investigation. Feline retinal disease is often asociated with systemic disease and a full eye examination, in particular examination of the fundus, should always be included as part of the clinical examination of the sick cat and in a significant number of cases may be of considerable aid in diagnosis. Ophthalmoscopic findings, although not necessarily pathognomonic of a specific disease, may well indicate systemic disease. In this chapter, following *The Normal Fundus, Congenital and Early Onset Abnormalities* are described including retinal dysplasia, colobomatous defects and lysosomal storage diseases. *Acquired Diseases of the Ocular Fundus* follow and include Vascular Anomalies and Abnormalities (anaemia, hyperviscosity, lipaemia retinalis and haemorrhage); Retinal Detachment; and Hypertension. There then follow three specific degenerative retinal diseases of known aetiology, *Taurine Deficiency Retinopathy* and two separate forms of *Hereditary Progressive Retinal Atrophy* in the Abyssinian cat. *Inflammatory Retinopathies* (viral, bacterial, parasitic and mycotic) complete this section on the retina. *The Optic Nerve* is divided into Congenital Problems (aplasia or hypoplasia and colobomatous defects) and Acquired Problems (papilloedema, optic neuritis, glaucomatous cupping and optic atrophy). Finally, *Neoplasia of the Ocular Fundus* describes tumours of the retina and choroid, optic nerve and meninges.

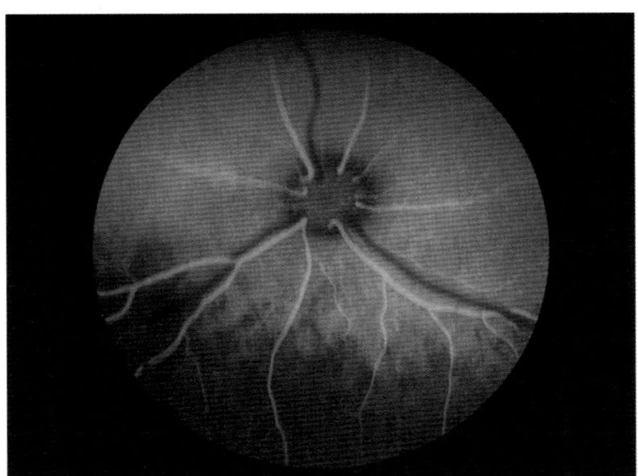

Fig. 14.4 *Fluoroscein angiogram of adult Domestic shorthaired cat at 5 s showing arteriolar filling (courtesy of A. Leon).*

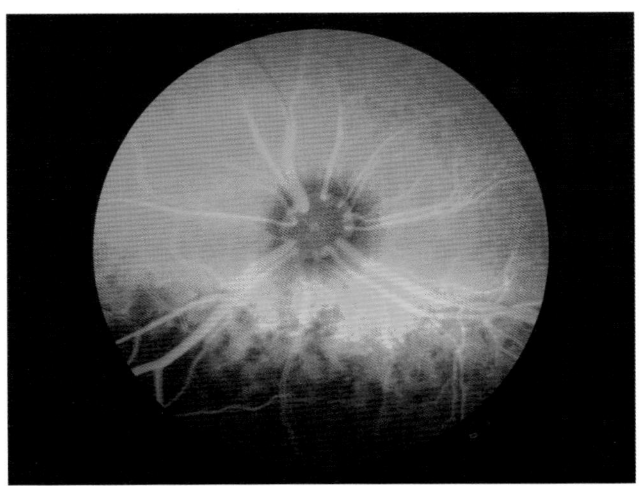

Fig. 14.5 *Fluoroscein angiogram of same cat at 22 s showing arteriolar and venous filling (courtesy of A. Leon).*

THE NORMAL FUNDUS

The cat has a very well developed, highly reflective, cellular tapetum. The shape is triangular, the appearance granular and the colour usually yellow to green, sometimes blue (Figs. 14.6 to 14.9). Incomplete tapetal development with many

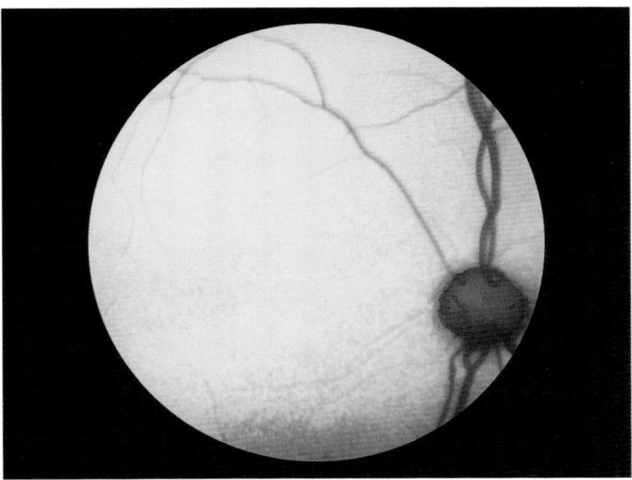

Fig. 14.6 *Yellow tapetal fundus.*

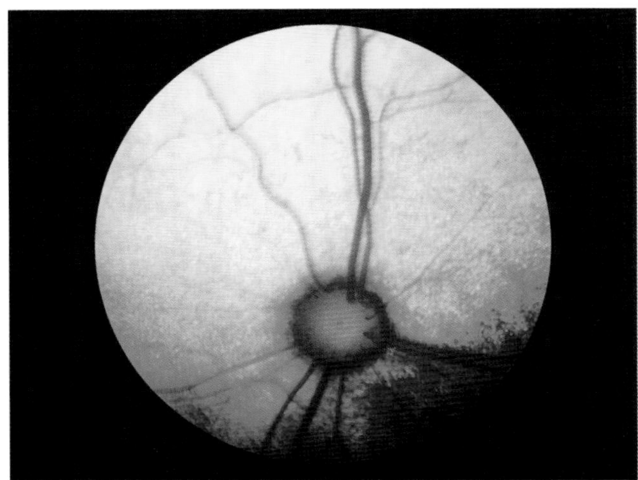

Fig. 14.7 *Yellow-green tapetal fundus.*

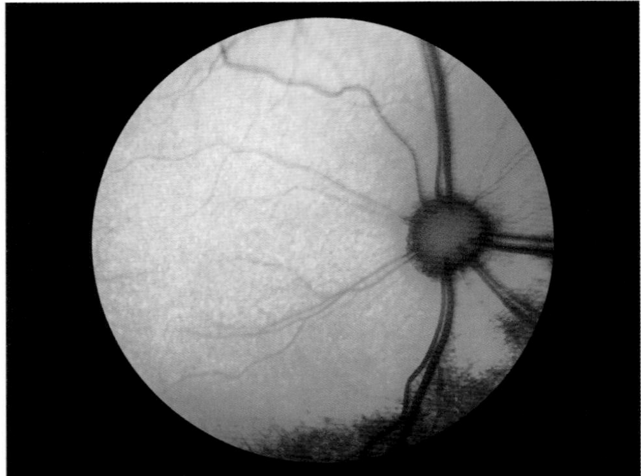

Fig. 14.8 Green tapetal fundus.

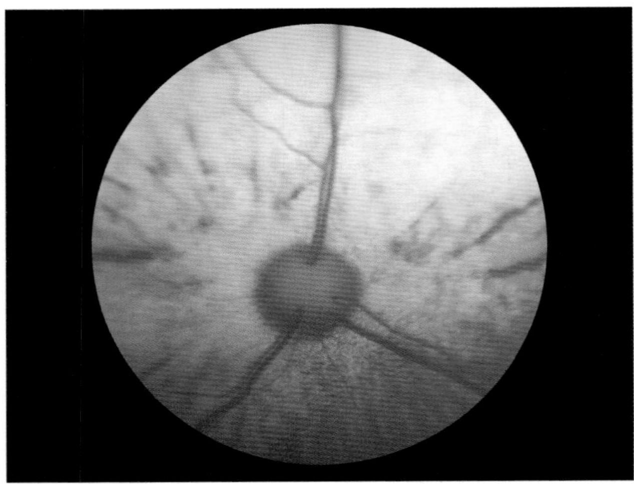

Fig. 14.10 Pale and thin tapetal fundus with some visible choroidal vessels in a white Domestic shorthaired cat.

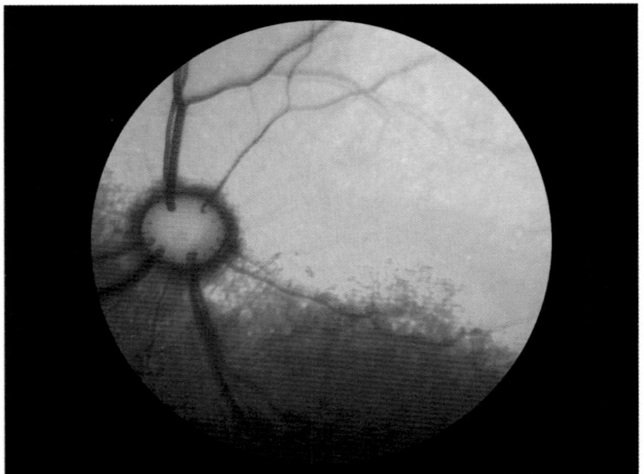

Fig. 14.9 Green-blue tapetal fundus.

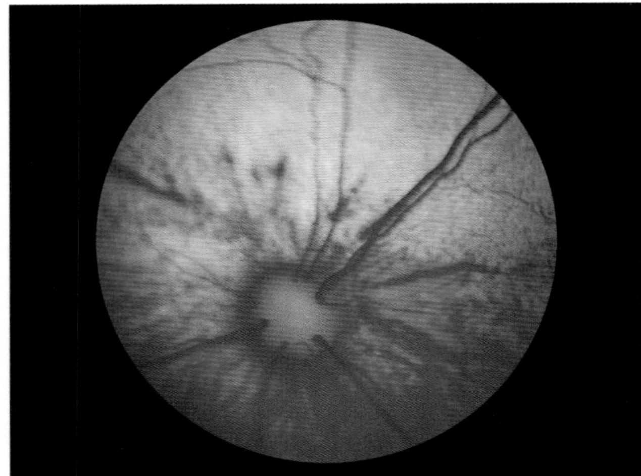

Fig. 14.11 Similar pale and thin tapetal fundus in a blue-eyed white young adult Domestic shorthaired cat.

islets of colour on a pigmented background is rare in the cat, but has been recorded (Rubin, 1974). Absence of the tapetum occurs in some blue-eyed, white, colour-dilute cats, in others the tapetum is thin with visible choroidal vessels similar to that in blue merle dogs (Figs 14.10–14.12). The area centralis, an area of maximum cone density similar to the fovea, is situated approximately 3 mm lateral to the optic disc (Fig. 14.13). This region is devoid of blood vessels and is sometimes a darker green in colour (Fig. 14.14). This part of the tapetal fundus is of particular importance in taurine deficiency retinopathy or feline central retinal degeneration (see later section). Peripapillary rings of pigment or hyper-reflectivity (conus) are often present (Figs 14.15 and 14.17) or may be absent (Fig. 14.16).

The nontapetal fundus is usually heavily pigmented and dark grey-brown in colour (Fig. 14.18). In breeds such as the Siamese and Himalayan, which lack ocular pigment, the nontapetal fundus may be described as tigroid with

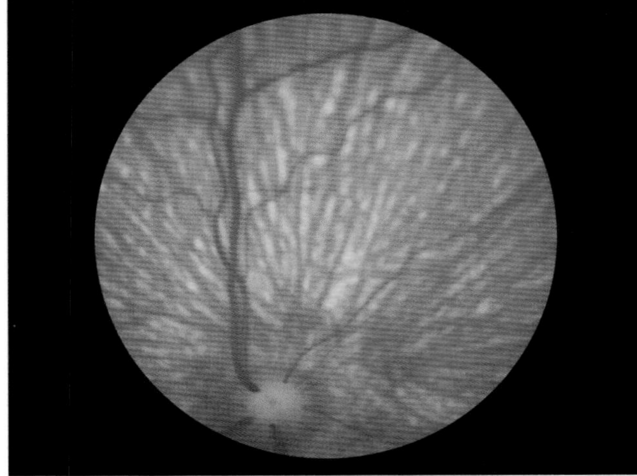

Fig. 14.12 Absence of tapetum and subalbinism of the whole fundus in a blue-eyed white cat.

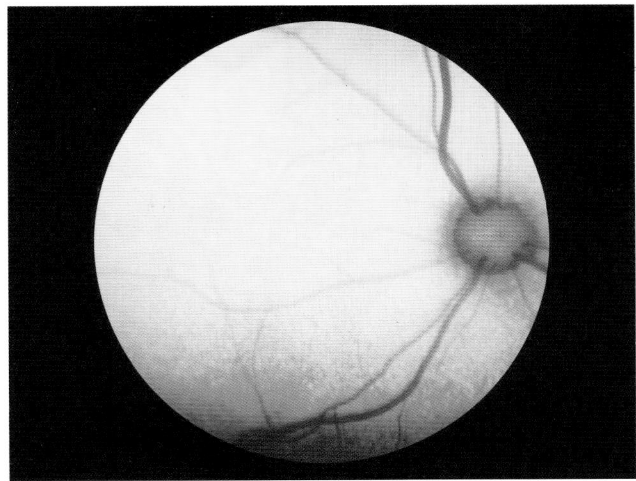

Fig. 14.13 *Area centralis lateral to the optic disc (right eye). Note absence of blood vessels in this region.*

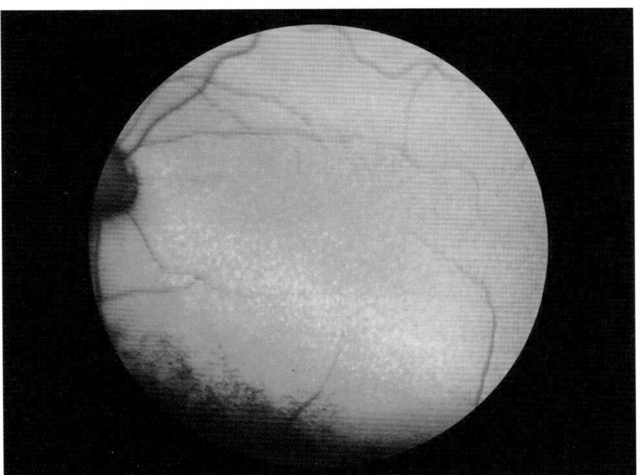

Fig. 14.14 *Area centralis lateral to disc (left eye). Note darker green colour in this region.*

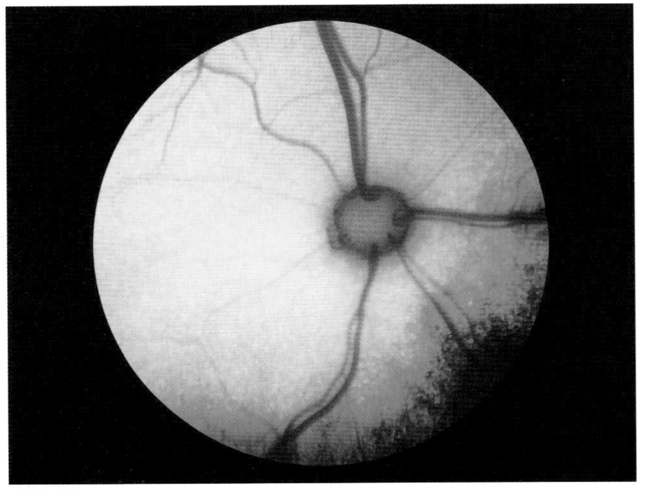

Fig. 14.15 *Pigmented and coloured peripapillary ring.*

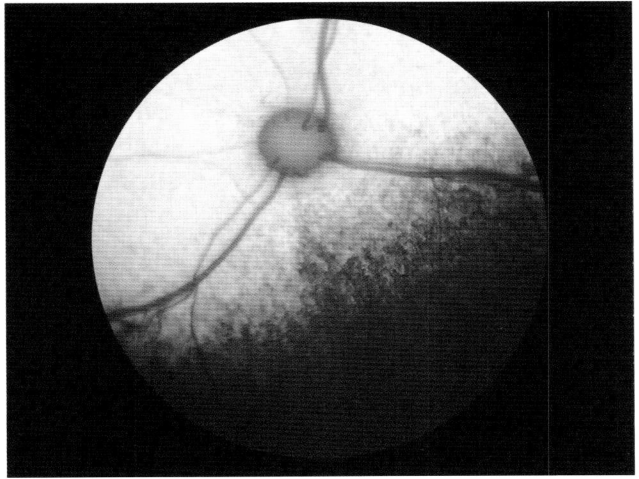

Fig. 14.16 *Absence of peripapillary rings.*

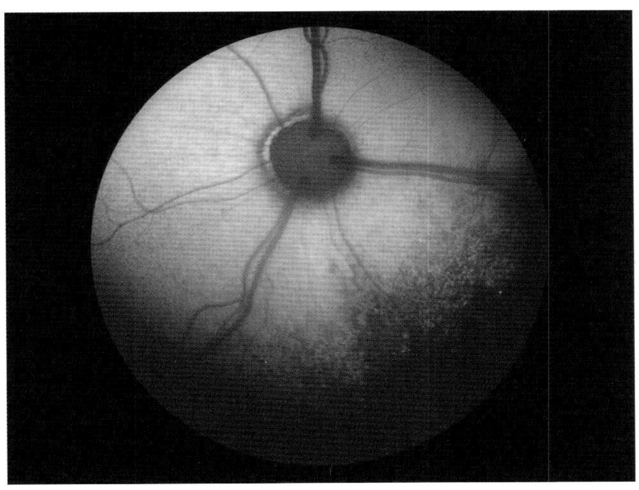

Fig. 14.17 *Hyper-reflective peripapillary ring or physiological conus.*

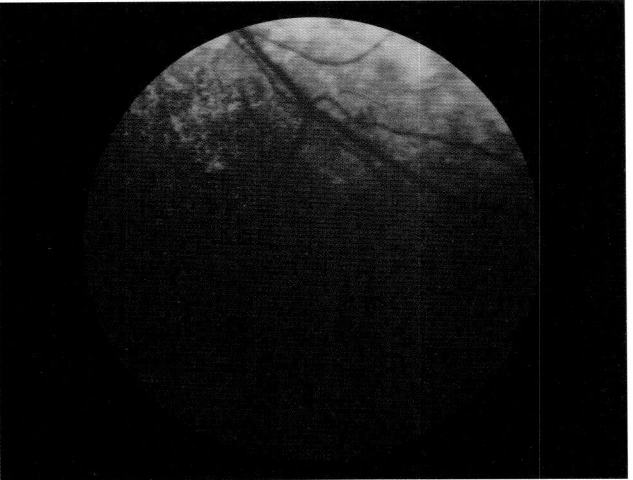

Fig. 14.18 *Nontapetal fundus in an adult tabby Domestic shorthaired.*

visible choroidal vessels due to lack of pigment in the retinal pigment epithelium (Fig. 14.19); choroidal pigment may also be lacking in some blue-eyed, white individuals (Fig. 14.20) and a few cats have patches of subalbinism in the nontapetal area (Figs 14.21 and 14.23). The tapetal junction with the nontapetal area is usually clearly defined but occasionally tapetal islets may be present (Fig. 14.21).

The feline optic disc is small, roughly circular, cupped and with a well-defined edge. In those animals with a tapetum the disc appears completely within the tapetum and is in a position slightly lateral and ventral to the posterior pole of the eye. Occasionally, the tapetum may not extend to include the disc (Fig. 14.24). The optic disc is grey and not myelinated (unlike the dog), and the lamina cribrosa is visible ophthalmoscopically (Fig. 14.25). Myelination usually begins posterior to the lamina cribrosa, although myelinated or opaque nerve fibres are occasionally visible ophthalmoscopically from part of

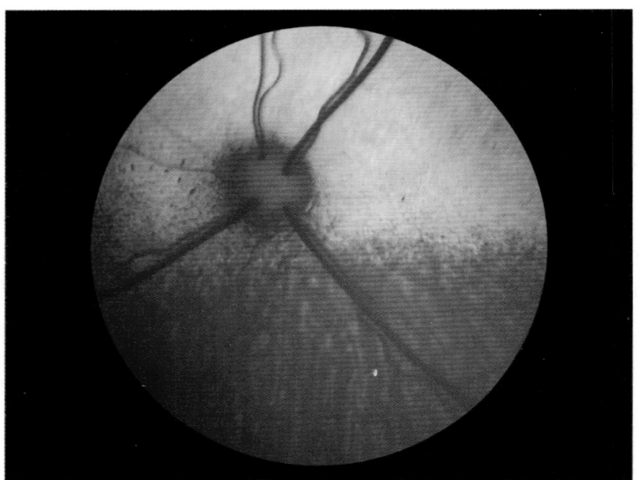

Fig. 14.19 *Tigroid nontapetal fundus (seal-point Siamese).*

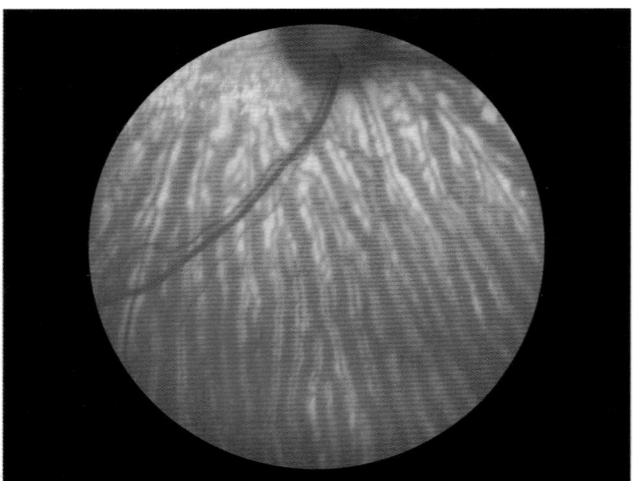

Fig. 14.20 *Subalbinism of nontapetal fundus in a blue-eyed white Domestic shorthaired. Note visible choroidal vessel and little choroidal pigmentation.*

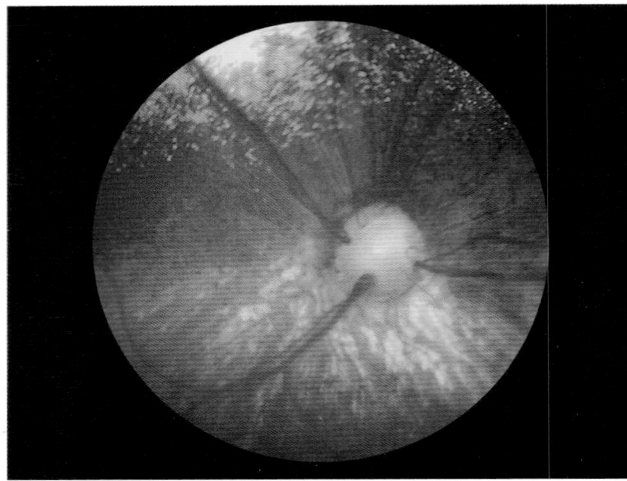

Fig. 14.21 *Partial subalbinism of nontapetal fundus in a white Persian cat.*

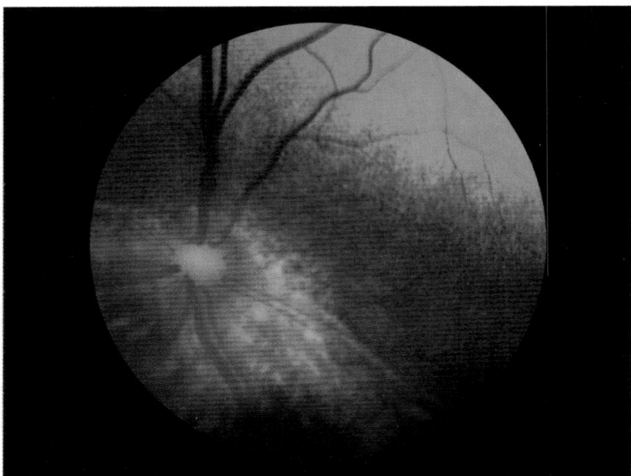

Fig. 14.22 *Patch of subalbinism in an otherwise heavily pigmented nontapetal fundus.*

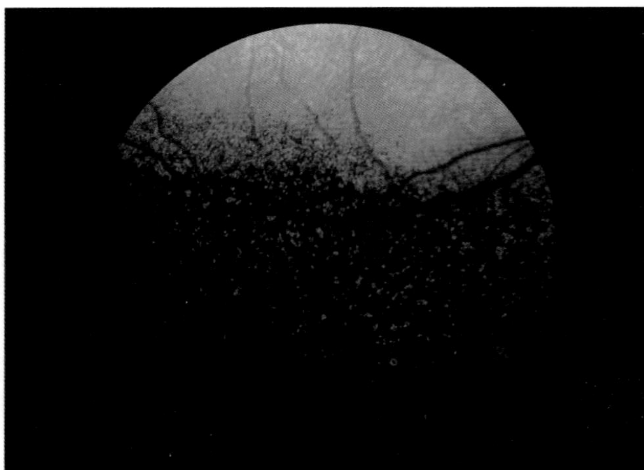

Fig. 14.23 *Islets of tapetum at junction with nontapetal fundus.*

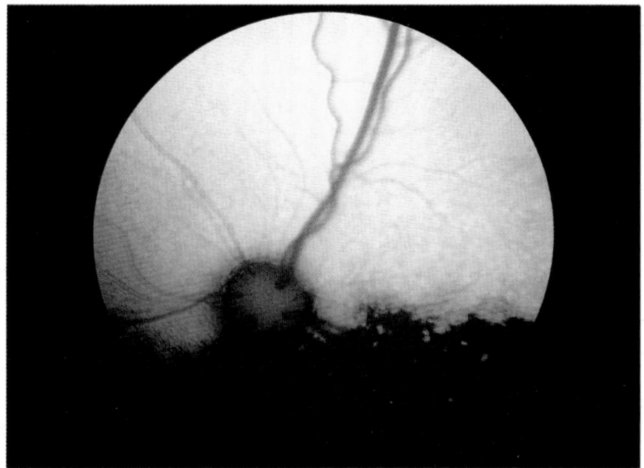

Fig. 14.24 Unusual position of optic disc adjacent to junction between tapetal and nontapetal regions (the disc in the cat is commonly well inside the tapetal fundus).

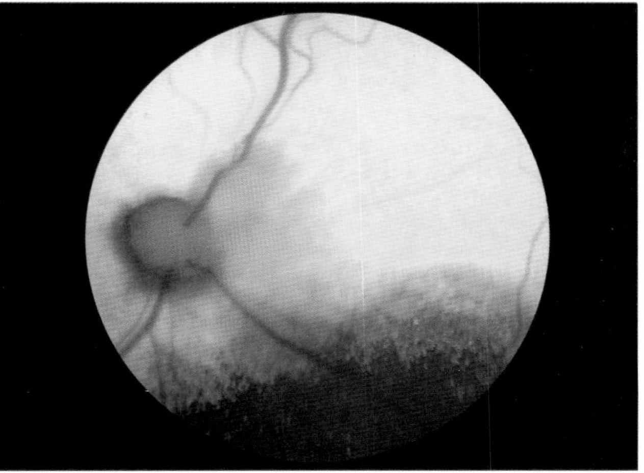

Fig. 14.26 Medullated nerve fibres visible ophthalmoscopically from '1 o'clock' to '5 o'clock'.

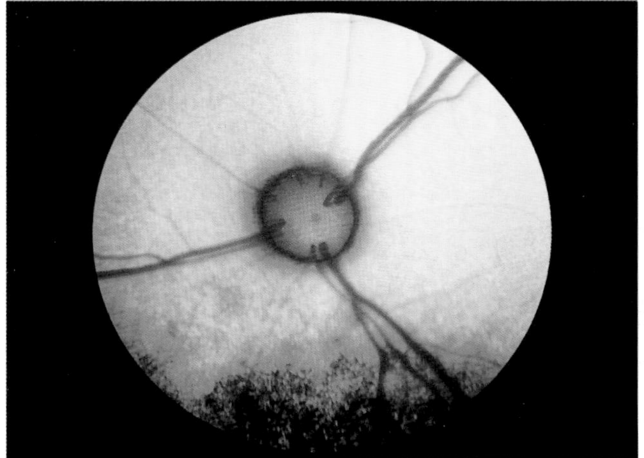

Fig. 14.25 Nonmyelinated grey disc showing lamina cribrosa.

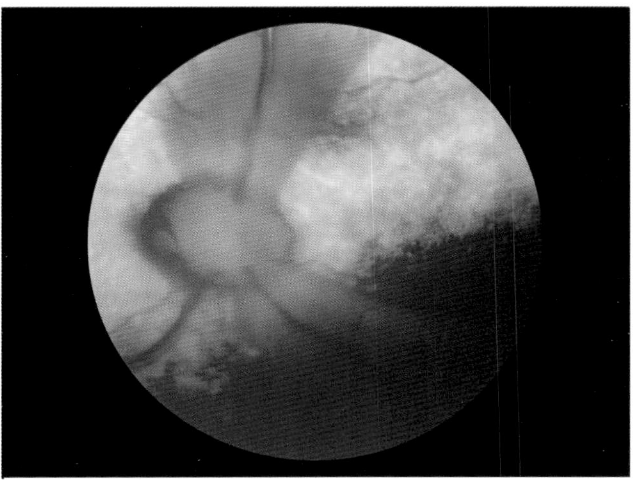

Fig. 14.27 Medullated nerve fibres visible dorsally and ventrally (the optic disc also shows an abnormality).

the disc (Figs 14.26 and 14.27). This is a normal variation and may be present in one or both eyes.

The feline optic disc is normally cupped with blood vessels hooking over its edge (Figs 14.28, 14.4 and 14.5). Figure 14.29 depicts an unusual vascular pattern on the disc. Excessive tortuosity of arterioles in the feline fundus is uncommon (Fig. 14.30). Variation in size of disc between cats is not great but minor degrees do occur (Figs 14.31 and 14.32).

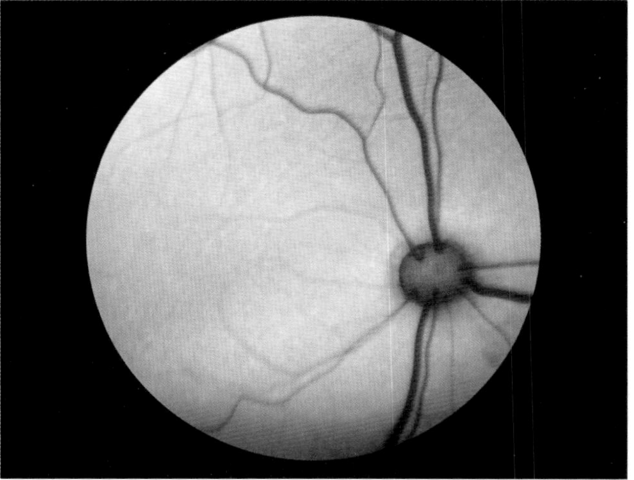

Fig. 14.28 Normal cupped optic disc showing hooking of blood vessels over its edge.

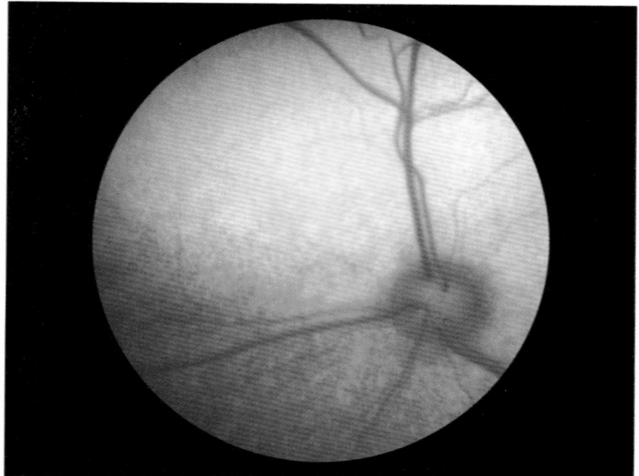

Fig. 14.29 *Unusual vascular pattern on the optic disc.*

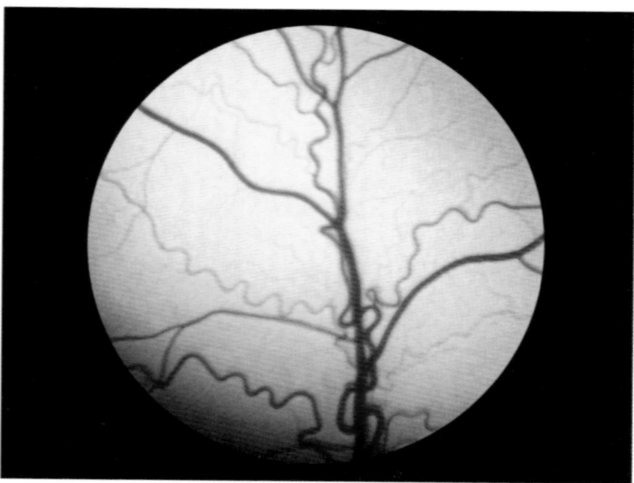

Fig. 14.30 *Unusual and excessive tortuosity of retinal arterioles in an otherwise apparently healthy cat.*

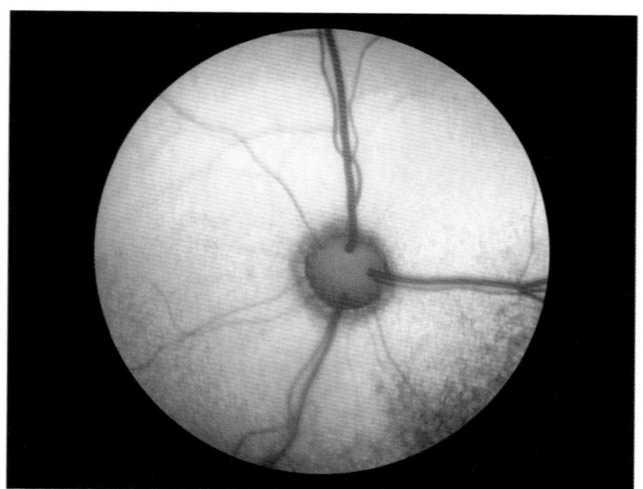

Fig. 14.31 *Moderately large optic disc.*

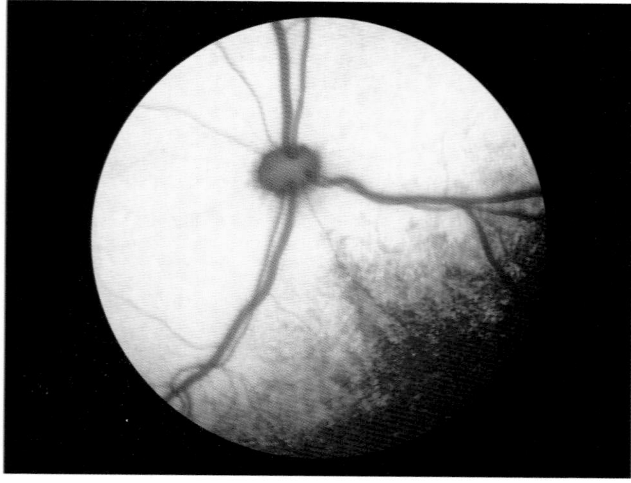

Fig. 14.32 *Small optic disc (micropapilla).*

Congenital and early onset abnormalities

Retinal dysplasia

There are sporadic reports of retinal dysplasia in the cat, usually secondary to viral infections such as panleukopenia and feline leukaemia (Albert *et al.*, 1977), but also associated with physical and chemical insults. Retinal dysplasia may occur as an isolated finding, or in conjunction with other ocular defects such as cataracts and microphthalmos. Sometimes the cause is not obvious (Fig. 14.33).

The teratogenic effects of feline panleukopenia virus are well documented (Percy *et al.*, 1975). In addition to causing cerebellar hypoplasia, the virus may damage the developing retina, resulting in large focal or multifocal areas of retinal degeneration. There is no treatment.

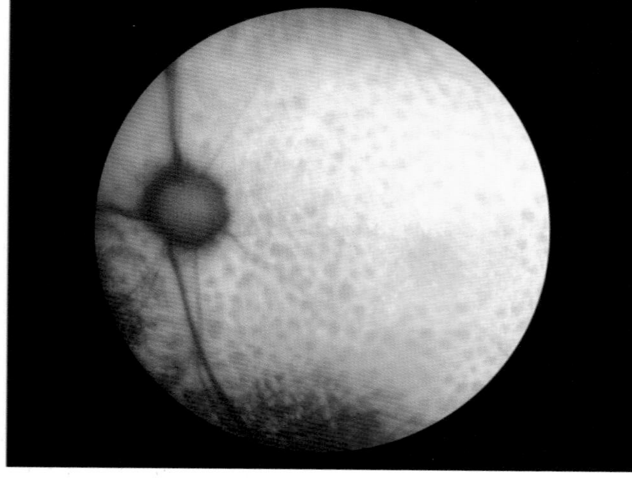

Fig. 14.33 *Domestic shorthair kitten with retinal dysplasia of unknown cause.*

Colobomatous defects

Colobomatous defects (Figs 14.34 and 14.35) involving some or all of the optic disc, peripapillary area, choroid and sclera are rare in cats (Bellhorn *et al.*, 1971). Visual problems are unlikely and the defects may be discovered incidentally during ophthalmic examination. Occasionally, other congenital defects may be present.

Lysosomal storage diseases

Retinal changes, in the form of multiple small spots, which represent the accumulation of glycolipid within the ganglion cells, have been reported in cats with GM_1-gangliosidosis (Murray *et al.*, 1977). A dull, grey, granularity of the area centralis has been described in α-mannosidosis (Blakemore, 1986). In a proportion of cats with mucopolysaccharidosis type VI (Haskins *et al.*, 1979) and the single case of mucolipidosis type II reported by Hubler *et al.* (1996) the appearance was described as diffuse generalized retinal degeneration. All affected animals show neurological signs in the first few months of life (see Chapter 15).

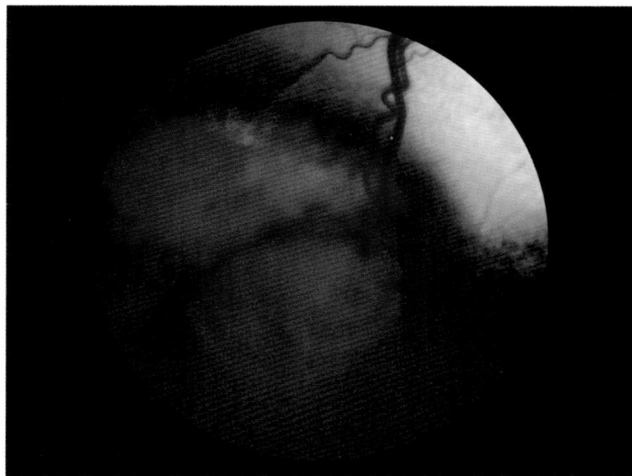

Fig. 14.34 A 1-year-old Domestic shorthair with coloboma of the optic disc and adjacent retina and choroid.

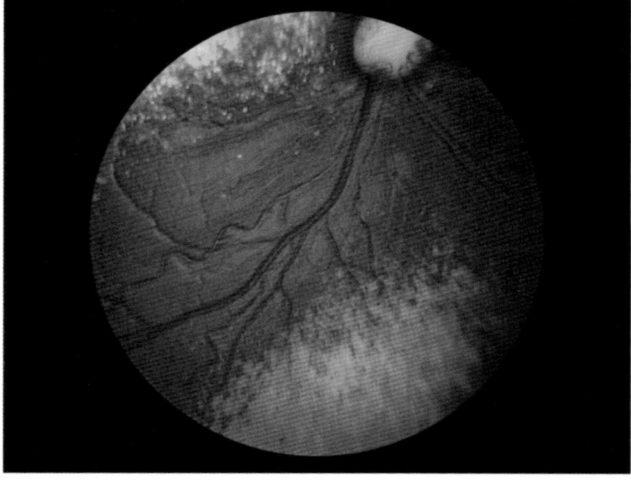

Fig. 14.35 A 10-month-old Domestic shorthair with a colobomatous defect as a 'tigroid' area ventral to the optic disc in the right eye. In the left eye, fundus examination was incomplete as there was a large corneal opacity associated with persistence of the pupillary membrane, but a similar defect appeared to be present ventral to the disc.

Acquired diseases of the ocular fundus

Vascular anomalies and abnormalities

Anaemia

Anaemia will produce a loss of colour in the visible vessels of the fundus and the optic disc may also appear paler than normal. The distinction between arteries and veins, which is never obvious in the smaller vessels, will become even more difficult because of loss of colour contrast and slight widening of the vessels. Retinal haemorrhage is also a likely finding (Fig. 14.36) when the haematocrit is less than 10% and haemoglobin levels are below 5g/dl. The pathophysiology of haemorrhage probably rests with increased vessel fragility, itself a consequence of altered vascular dynamics in response to anaemia-induced hypoxia. Concurrent thrombocytopenia will also make haemorrhage more likely.

The causes of anaemia may be obvious, as for example, the acute and chronic effects of blood loss after major trauma. In many cases, however, detailed investigation is necessary to establish the precise aetiology, which includes aplastic anaemia, autoimmune haemolytic anaemia, thrombocytopenia (which has a variety of causes), neoplasia (e.g. lymphosarcoma), panleukopenia, haemobartonellosis and various toxaemias.

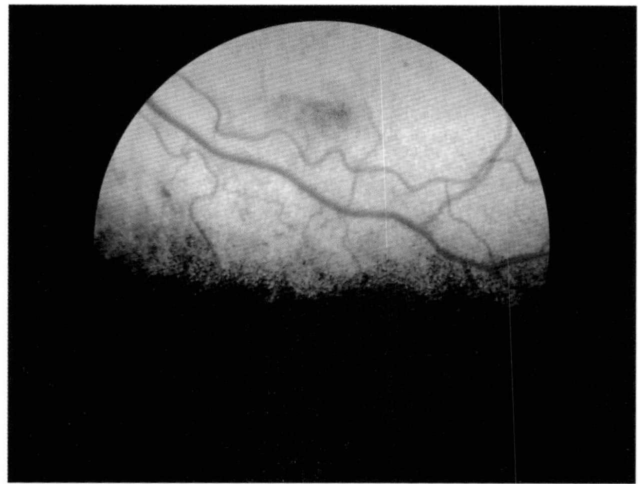

Fig. 14.36 A 3-year-old Domestic shorthair neutered male. Anaemic retinopathy with slight pallor of the retinal vessels and retinal haemorrhage at the level of the retinal nerve fibre layer. The cat had thrombocytopenia and anaemia of unknown cause.

Hyperviscosity

Hyperviscosity may be a consequence of too many circulating red cells (polycythaemia) or raised plasma protein levels (hyperproteinaemia). Polycythaemia may be primary or secondary (Figs 14.37 and 14.38). Secondary poycythaemia may be a consequence of heart disease or various types of pulmonary insufficiency. Congenital heart diseases such as the tetralogy of Fallot (ventricular septal defect, pulmonary stenosis, dextraposed aorta and right ventricular hypertrophy) are associated with secondary polycythaemia because of arterial hypoxaemia and affected animals will also be cyanotic because of right to left shunting.

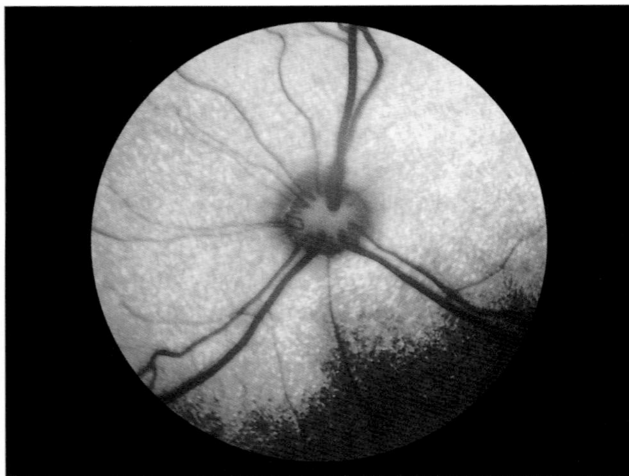

Fig. 14.37 *An 8-year-old Domestic shorthair neutered male with primary polycythaemia. The vascular changes are more obvious in the venules, retinal vessels appear darker and wider than usual.*

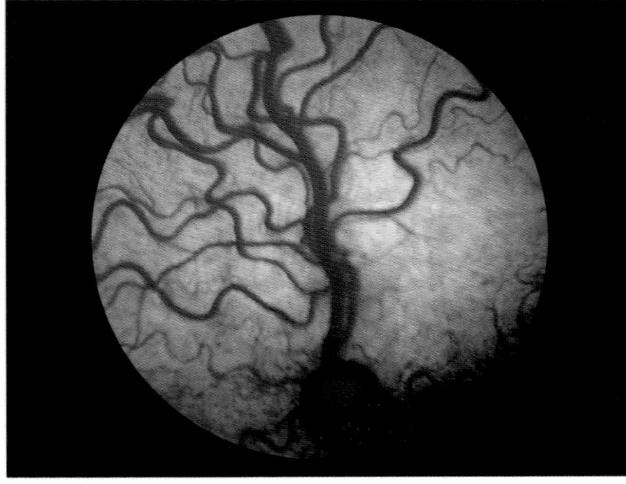

Fig. 14.38 *A 10-month-old Domestic shorthair with secondary polycythaemia (tetralogy of Fallot). The conjunctiva of this cat is illustrated in Fig. 8.33. Note the dark, congested and tortuous retinal vessels (packed cell volume 62%).*

There are many possible reasons for hyperproteinaemia (see also Chapter 12), they include monoclonal gammopathies such as plasma cell myeloma and plasmacytoma and polyclonal gammopathies associated with immune-mediated disorders (e.g. systemic lupus erythematosus) and chronic antigenically stimulating diseases (e.g. feline infectious peritonitis).

The ocular features are striking and characteristically affect the retinal veins which appear engorged (sometimes like a string of sausages) and tortuous (Fig. 12.26). A few retinal haemorrhages may also be present and the optic disc may be oedematous. Effective management of hyperviscosity syndromes depends upon establishing and treating the underlying cause.

Lipaemia Retinalis

Lipaemia retinalis is an ocular manifestation of chylomicronaemia (excessive quantities of large triglyceride-rich lipoproteins) and it may be seen in association with both primary and secondary hyperlipoproteinaemia, or more specifically hypertriglyceridaemia (Crispin, 1993).

A primary inherited type has been demonstrated to be caused by defective lipoprotein lipase activity as a consequence of mutation in the lipoprotein lipase gene (Ginzinger *et al.*, 1996); all affected kittens have fasting lipaemia and a high proportion have peripheral neuropathies which are progressive unless a low-fat dietary regime is instituted.

A transient hyperlipoproteinaemia associated with anaemia (a packed cell volume of less than 11%) has been reported by Gunn-Moore *et al.* (1997) and in these 4–5-week-old kittens the chylomicronaemia occurred at about the time of weaning. While there may be an hereditary element in this type, other factors (fleas, *Haemobartonella felis* and high fat intake) are involved and provided that the condition is recognized and treated (oxygen-enriched atmosphere and whole-blood transfusion for the acute anaemia, doxycycline for *H. felis* infection, reduction of flea burden by daily combing and weaning onto a low-fat diet) the condition resolves completely.

In older animals secondary hyperlipoproteinaemia associated with raised triglycerides is seen most commonly in association with diabetes mellitus and megestrol acetate administration.

Lipaemia retinalis is most readily observed against the dark background of the nontapetal fundus and lipaemia is easier to observe if the patient has a low haematocrit as there are fewer red cells to obscure the creamy plasma. The colour of the blood column within the retinal vessels varies from salmon-pink to creamy white, the vessels are wider than normal and it may be more difficult than usual to distinguish arteries and veins when lipaemia retinalis is marked (Figs 14.39 and 14.40).

Haemorrhage

Retinal haemorrhage is not unusual in the cat and may have a variety of causes. Blunt and penetrating injuries (Figs 3.5

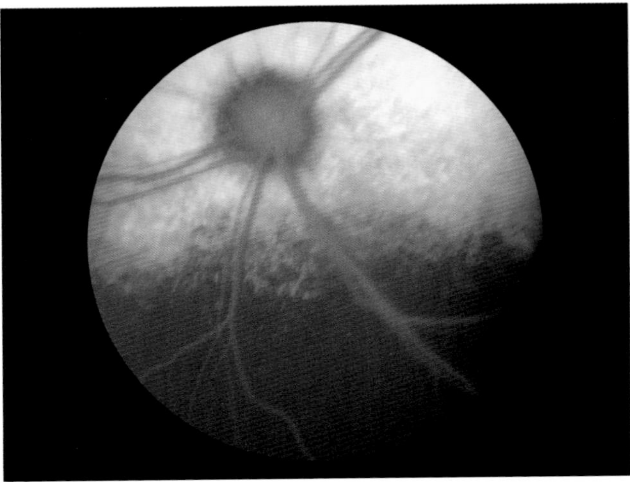

Fig. 14.39 *A 4-year-old Domestic shorthair neutered female with lipaemia retinalis. Lipid keratopathy developed precipitously at the site of a cat scratch in the right eye (Fig. 9.60). Ophthalmoscopy indicated lipaemia retinalis. Raised serum cholesterol and triglyceride (9.89 and 79.8 mmol/l, respectively), chylomicronaemia and an abnormal lipoprotein profile were found on laboratory examination.*

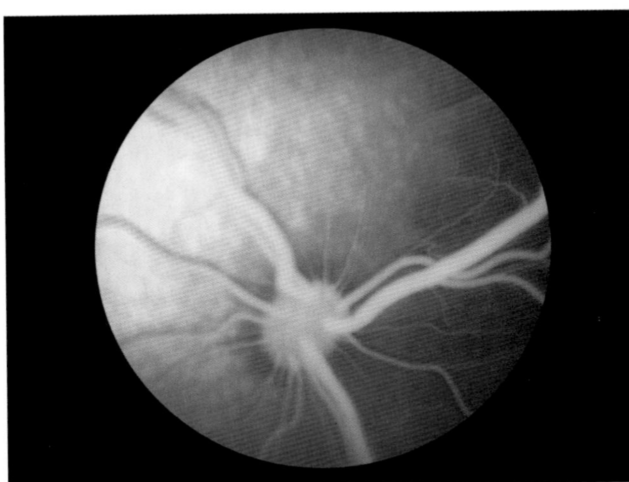

Fig. 14.40 *A 4-week-old Domestic shorthair kitten with lipaemia retinalis and anaemia (serum cholesterol 6.97 mmol/l, serum triglyceride 41.6 mmol/l, abnormal lipoprotein profile, chylomicronaemia, packed cell volume 8%). This kitten was one of an affected litter, all of which became normal after treatment.*

and 3.6) are common causes of retinal and choroidal haemorrhage. Anaemic retinopathy has been discussed earlier (Fig. 14.36). Thiamine deficiency, as a consequence of thiaminase-rich diets or low thiamine content has a variety of effects which include dilated retinal vessels, retinal haemorrhages, neovascularization and peripapillary oedema (Fig. 14.41) as well as neurological signs (see Chapter 15), and culminates in coma and death in unrecognized cases. Inflammatory retinopathies may be associated with haemorrhage

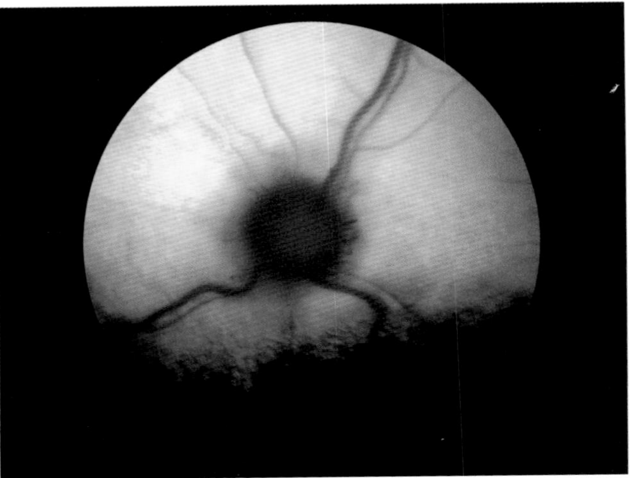

Fig. 14.41 *Domestic shorthair with thiamine deficiency. the pupils were dilated and responded poorly to light. Neurological signs included spinal hypersensitivity and ventriflexion of the head and neck. Note the dilated retinal vessels, retinal haemorrhages, neovascularization and peripapillary oedema.*

(e.g. feline infectious peritonitis) and migrating parasites can produce haemorrhage. Haemorrhage may also be a consequence of primary and secondary neoplasia. Hypertension (see below) is one of the commonest causes of retinal and choroidal haemorrhage. Haemostatic disorders are not regularly associated with intraocular haemorrhage.

Retinal detachment

Retinal detachment results when the neurosensory retina separates from the underlying retinal pigment epithelium. The causes of retinal detachment include hypertension (see below), inflammation (see Chapter 12), trauma (Figs 3.6 and 14.42), neoplasia (see below), hyperviscosity syndromes and ethylene glycol poisoning (Barclay and Riis, 1979). The pathogenesis of retinal detachment depends upon the cause; hypertensive changes, inflammatory choroidal and/or retinal exudates can result in bullous and exudative detachment; trauma-induced and post-surgical holes and tears can produce rhegmatogenous detachments; neoplasia can infiltrate the choroid and/or retina to produce a solid detachment. Traction detachments as a result of the formation of post-inflammatory vitreal traction bands are not usually recognized in cats.

Management of retinal detachment depends upon establishing the cause. Unfortunately, degeneration of the feline retina begins within 1 h of detachment and the changes are progressive and usually irreversible, so prompt treatment to initiate retinal reattachment is critical for retinal regeneration (Dziezyc and Millichamp, 1993).

Hypertension

Sudden onset blindness associated with retinal detachment and/or intraocular haemorrhage is the most perceptible

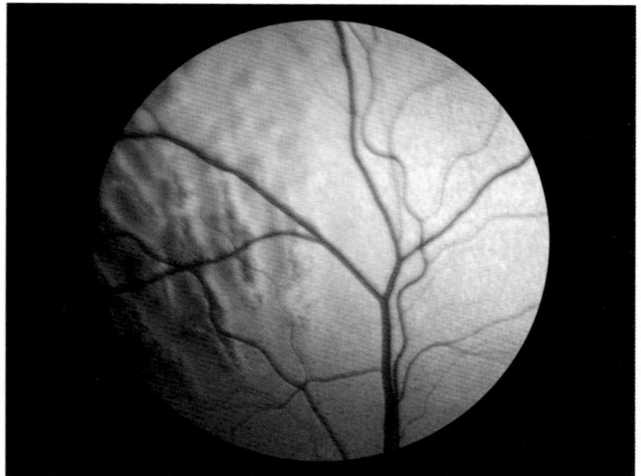

Fig. 14.42 A 3-year-old Domestic shorthair neutered male. This cat was injured in a road traffic accident and suffered facial injuries, a fracture of the left zygomatic arch, facial nerve damage and proptosis of the left eye. The right eye is shown and the folds apparent dorsolaterally are indicative of retinal reattachment. The retinal detachment in the right eye was apparent at the time of initial examination and this case demonstrates the importance of assessing both eyes, so that the full extent of injuries can be established and treated (see also Fig. 15.10).

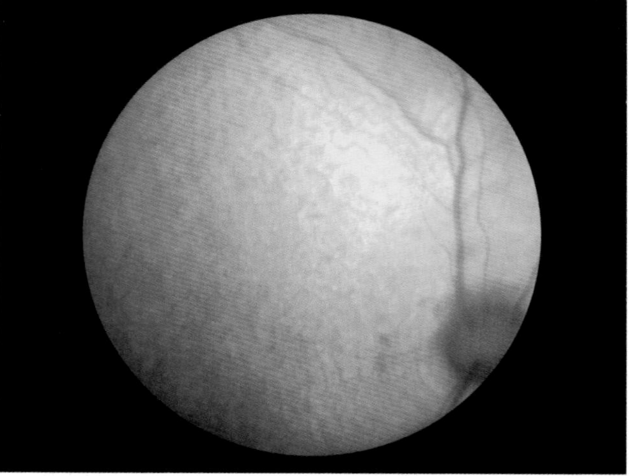

Fig. 14.43 A 12-year-old Domestic shorthair with primary hypertension (systolic blood pressure 245 mmHg). Note the subtle fuzzy areas in the peripapillary region where exudation is occurring. Multiple linear folds are also present, indicating retinal detachment and reattachment.

indicator of the presence of systemic hypertension (Boldy, 1983; Morgan, 1986; Christmas and Guthrie, 1989; Kobayashi *et al.*, 1990; Turner *et al.*, 1990; Labato and Ross, 1991; Littman, 1994; Sansom *et al.*, 1994; Stiles *et al.*, 1994). Unfortunately, advanced, irreversible pathology underlies these ocular manifestations and it must be stated unequivocally that the successful management of hypertension in cats depends upon early recognition, accurate diagnosis and effective, well-monitored treatment. The problem is most commonly recognized in older cats (on average 14–15 years), although regular health checks of older cats indicate that early hypertensive changes may be detected at a younger age (on average 11–12 years). It is, however, important to emphasize that hypertension can be a clinical problem in younger animals.

Hypertension is a common feline problem; it may be primary or secondary. Secondary causes of feline hypertension include renal disease, thyroid disease (hyperthyroidism), chronic anaemia, diabetes mellitus, megestrol acetate administration, chronic corticosteroid usage (iatrogenic hyperadrenocorticism) and primary aldosteronism. Detailed laboratory investigation is therefore essential and the situation is futher complicated because established hypertension will cause other organs to dysfunction (e.g. glomerulosclerosis, left-ventricular hypertrophy, hypertensive encephalopathy). Further information on the pathophysiology can be obtained from a comprehensive review of hypertension by Dukes (1992).

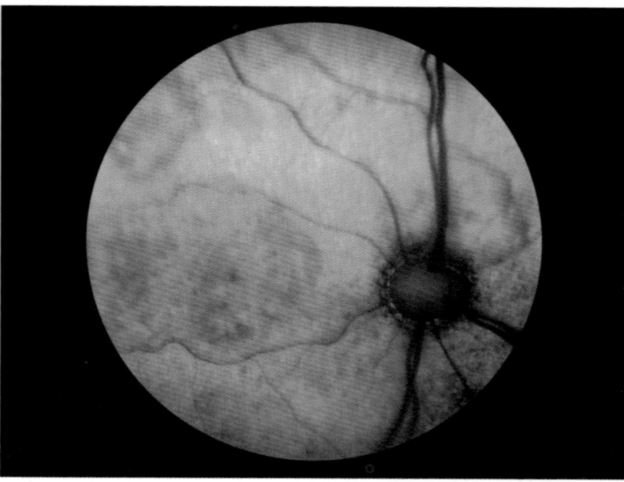

Fig. 14.44 A 13-year-old Domestic shorthair with hypertension. Multiple bullous detachments because of exudation.

The eye appears to be particularly susceptible to the effects of hypertension (Mould, 1993) and it is fortunate that it is so accessible to detailed examination. A range of ophthalmoscopic appearances may be encountered and they largely reflect the underlying pathogenesis (Figs 14.43–14.52). The earliest changes of hypertension which are likely to be observed on fundoscopy probably originate from choroidal vessels and consist of focal, slightly hazy, opacities overlying the choriocapillaris which are easiest to observe against a tapetal background; these might reflect incompetence of the choriocapillaris with leakage of plasma and fibrinogen. It may be that choroidal vessels are affected earlier and more severely than retinal vessels because of their anatomical

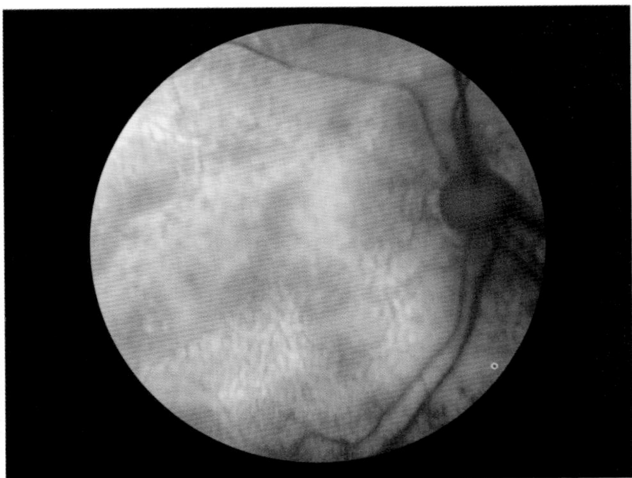

Fig. 14.45 *A 14-year-old Domestic shorthair with primary hypertension (systolic blood pressure 280 mmHg). Bullous detachments and areas of retinal reattachment. A single focal haemorrhage is also present at '10 o'clock'.*

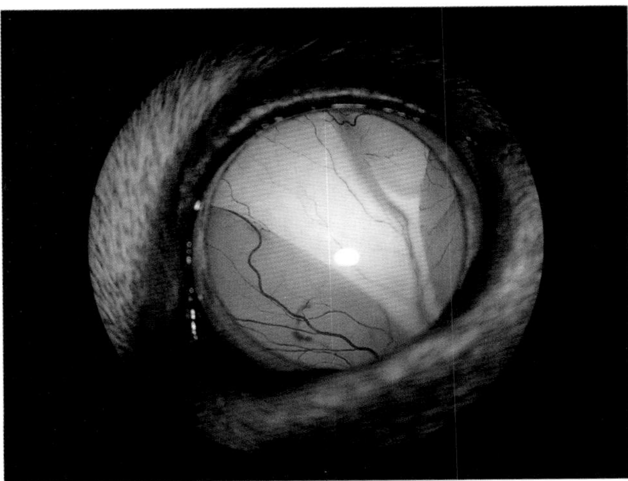

Fig. 14.47 *A 13-year-old Domestic shorthair with hypertension (systolic blood pressure 270 mmHg). Total exudative detachment of the retina. The cat was also in renal failure.*

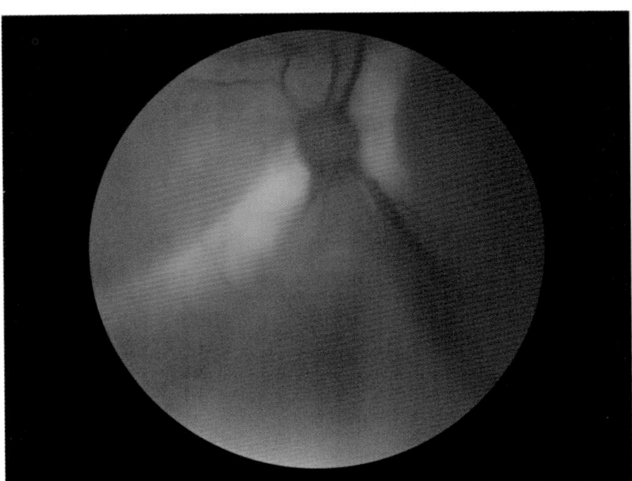

Fig. 14.46 *An 11-year-old Domestic shorthair with hypertension. Total exudative detachment, the hypertension was secondary to hyperthyroidism.*

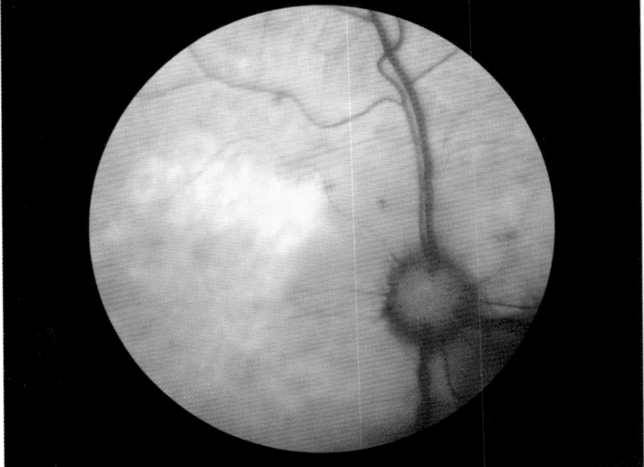

Fig. 14.48 *A 7-year-old Domestic shorthair with primary hypertension (systolic blood pressure 290 mmHg). Presented because of episodic collapse. Hyphaema was present in the other eye.*

arrangement and because they lack the autoregulatory control of blood flow found in the retinal vessels. If hypertension persists there will be further damage to the choroidal vessels and small, focal intra-retinal haemorrhages may be observed.

Retinal detachment is a likely consequence of ischaemic damage to the retinal pigment epithelium and sub-retinal exudation. Diurnal fluctuations of blood pressure probably account for the variations of appearance (flat detachments, reattachments with retinal folds) which may be seen in many early cases on sequential examination. Flat detachments typically accompany the early changes detectable ophthalmoscopically, but more extensive bullous retinal detachment (usually multiple bullae), perhaps even total detachment, will follow if blood pressure remains high.

Early changes in the retinal vessels are difficult to recognize and consist of subtle narrowing and straightening of the arterioles as the vessels vasoconstrict in an attempt to maintain tissue perfusion. As the retinal vessels become more damaged, the changes are easier to observe and consist of variations of calibre (vasodilation, vascular sheathing, sclerosis and luminal occlusion), aneurysmal dilations, increased tortuosity and even frank haemorrhage. Haemorrhage will become more extensive if the hypertension remains unrecognized and hyphaema, because of haemorrhage from iris vessels, is also likely (see Chapter 10).

Haemorrhagic serous retinal detachment probably carries a less favourable prognosis than serous retinal detachment

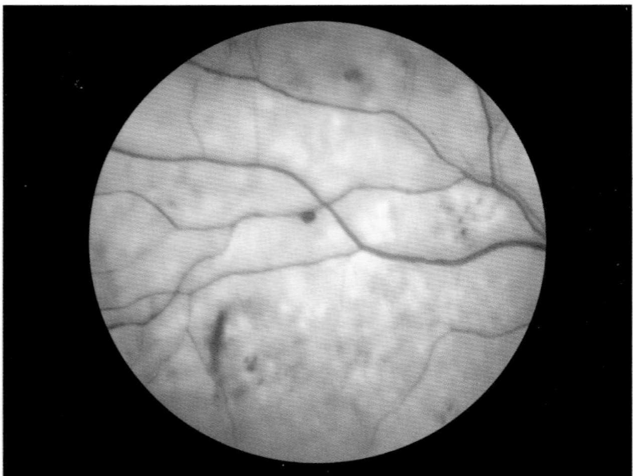

Fig. 14.49 A 12-year-old Domestic shorthair with hypertension (systolic blood pressure 210 mmHg). Note the multiple small focal haemorrhages and retinal detachment and also the obvious changes in retinal vessels. Changes in the retinal vessels include aneurysmal dilation in the centre of the photograph and marked variation of calibre producing a beaded appearance in places.

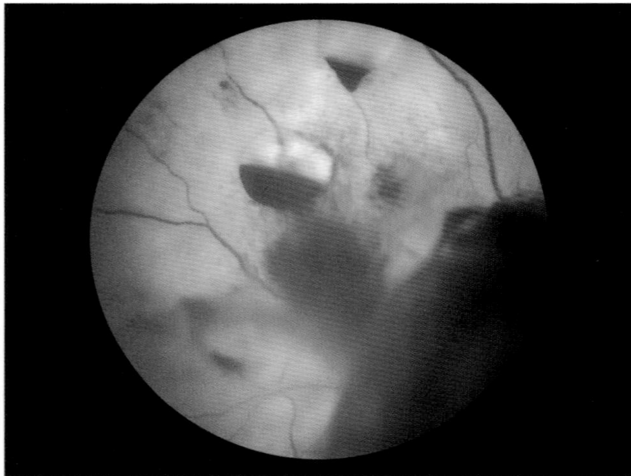

Fig. 14.50 A 13-year-old Domestic shorthair; right eye. Primary hypertension (systolic blood pressure 360 mmHg). Presented as a case of 'sudden blindness' there is advanced and irreversible fundus pathology. Both retinas had detached, in this eye there was a large detachment ventrally (4 o'clock to 8 o'clock) and extensive intraocular haemorrhage. Note that some of the haemorrhage dorsally originates from ruptured aneurysms (blood-filled bullae). The cat was depressed, lethargic and anorexic on presentation.

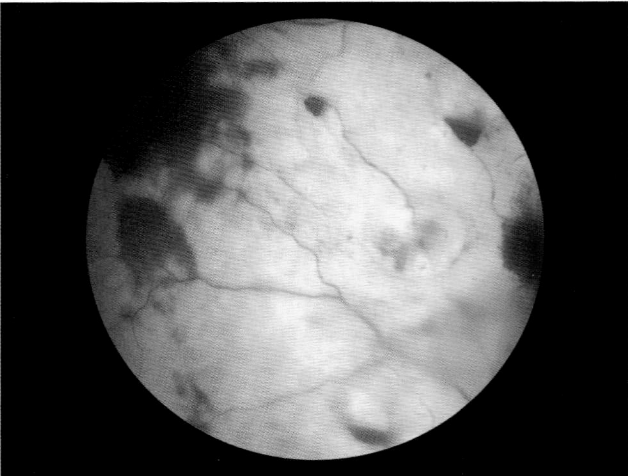

Fig. 14.51 The same eye as illustrated in Fig. 14.50. Two weeks after treatment had started, the haemorrhage has diminished; systolic blood pressure was 220 mmHg.

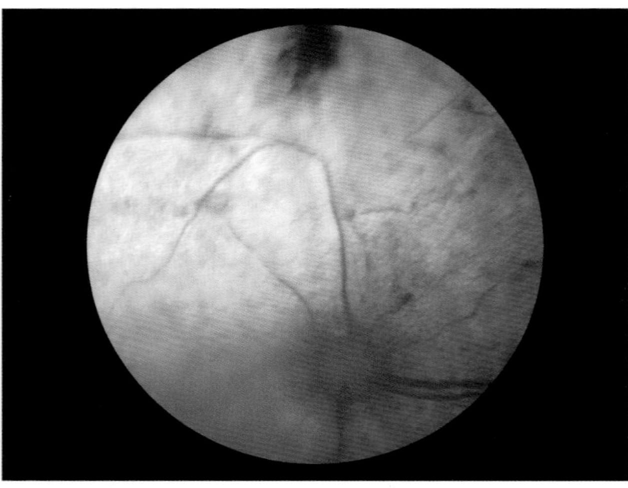

Fig. 14.52 The same eye as illustrated in Figs 14.50 and 14.51, 4 months after treatment had started. Systolic blood pressure was 180 mmHg. The intraocular haemorrhage has resorbed and the retina has reattached, but the retinal vessels are grossly abnormal and there is retinal degeneration. Both eyes were similarly affected and blindness is obviously permanent. The cat's general health was greatly improved.

alone because the vascular pathology is more advanced. Recurrent intraocular haemorrhage may result in complications such as glaucoma.

The effects on vision depend upon the acuteness of onset, the severity of the intraocular changes and, presumably, whether or not other complications such as cerebral oedema and cerebral haemorrhage are present.

The diagnosis is best confirmed by sequential measurement of blood pressure and assessment can now be carried out by indirect noninvasive methods using either an oscillometric sphygmomanometer or a Doppler-shift sphygmomanometer. The Doppler equipment measures only systolic blood pressure with any accuracy. The oscillometric monitor will record systolic, diastolic and mean arterial blood pressure. The range of normal values for the cat have not been established, although blood pressure measurements in awake, nonanxious, normal cats do not usually exceed 160/100 mmHg (Littman, 1994). Systolic values above 180 mmHg indicate the possibility of hypertension. Temperament, age and stress factors should be taken into account when making a series of readings.

Treatment of hypertension in cats is somewhat empirical as there is a paucity of information on the use and efficacy of antihypertensive agents in single or combination therapy. Treatment will be lifelong and dependent on the ability to monitor blood pressure and examine the eye. Medication should not just address the problem of elevated blood pressure, but should be tailored to the individual patient based on the presence of underlying disease and target organ involvement. Rational therapy is based on regimes which affect cardiac output and peripheral resistance because blood pressure is the product of these two parameters. Table 14.1 lists some possible regimes and these should be combined with cage rest initially and long-term monitoring of ocular appearance and blood pressure.

It is early cases with subtle fundus changes, including mild serous retinal detachment, that are most likely to respond favourably to therapy and retinal reattachment will occur with restoration of vision in some of these cases. Many cats, especially those with more serious retinal detachment and intraocular haemorrhage, will not regain any useful vision, despite retinal reattachment and resorption of intraocular haemorhage. Cats that remain blind cope well with their visual disability and may live for a considerable period of time after presentation. Treatment certainly improves the patient's quality of life and may control further target organ damage that results in some or all of cardiac failure, renal failure and cerebrovascular accidents.

Retinal degenerations

Taurine deficiency retinopathy

A feline central retinal degeneration (FCRD) was first reported in 1970 by Bellhorn and Fischer in pet cats in New York. The aetiology was unknown but it was not originally considered to be a nutritional retinopathy. However, a remarkably similar retinopathy was later recorded (Aguirre, 1978) in cats fed dog food and in 1973 Rabin *et al.* described a nutritionally induced retinal degeneration in cats resulting from taurine deficiency.

Taurine deficiency retinopathy, or FCRD, is a bilateral, usually symmetrical, progressive condition that occurs in both sexes. The retinal changes are typical, unusual and highly specific for this condition, particularly in the early stages. The first lesion appears at the area centralis, level with and temporal (lateral) to the optic disc in a region devoid of visible blood vessels. A zone of granularity (Fig. 14.53) has been described but the first obvious change is the presence of a horizontally oval, focal and well-demarcated millet-seed like spot of increased reflectivity (Fig. 14.54). Hyper-reflectivity in a tapetal region always indicates retinal thinning, i.e. retinal degeneration, whatever the cause. The affected area increases in size but remains clearly defined and horizontal and oval in shape (Figs. 14.55 and 14.57). Ophthalmoscopically, the appearance may suggest a pigmented border particularly along the upper and lower edges (Fig. 14.56). A second and similar area appears next on the nasal (medial) side of the disc. These two areas spread towards one another (Figs 14.58 and 14.59), meet, and fuse in a bridge

Table 14.1 Antihypertensive therapy

Regimes which affect cardiac output		
(a) By reducing extracellular fluid volume		
Sodium restriction	Low sodium diet	
Diuretics[+]	Frusemide	1–2 mg/kg each day per os (PO)
	Hydrochlorothiazide	1–2 mg/kg twice daily PO
(b) By reducing heart rate		
β-Adrenoceptor blocking drugs	Propranolol	0.1–0.2 mg/kg twice daily PO
Regimes which affect peripheral resistance		
α_1 Blocking drugs	Prazosin	0.25–1.0 mg twice or three times daily PO
Angiotensin-converting enzyme inhibitors	Benazepril*	0.25 mg/kg each day PO
	Enalapril maleate*	0.25–0.5 mg/kg every 12–24 h PO
Calcium-channel blockers	Amlodipine besylate*	0.625 mg every 24 h PO
	Diltiazem hydrochloride	1.75–2.4 mg/kg every 8–12 h PO

*Recommended drugs.
[+]Avoid in hypersensitive cats with renal disease.
Note: Benazepril and amlodipine besylate may be used together if the individual drugs do not reduce blood pressure significantly.

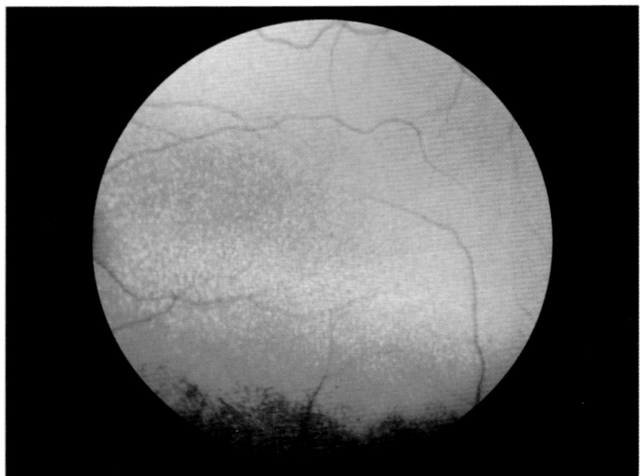

Fig. 14.53 *Zone of granularity at area centralis in early taurine deficiency.*

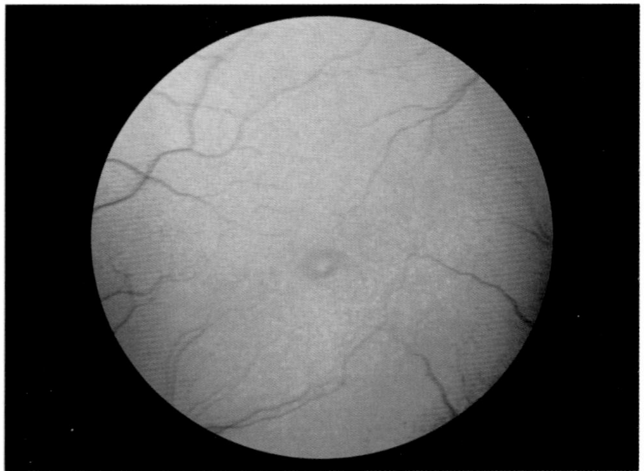

Fig. 14.54 *Small focal area of retinal degeneration at area centralis.*

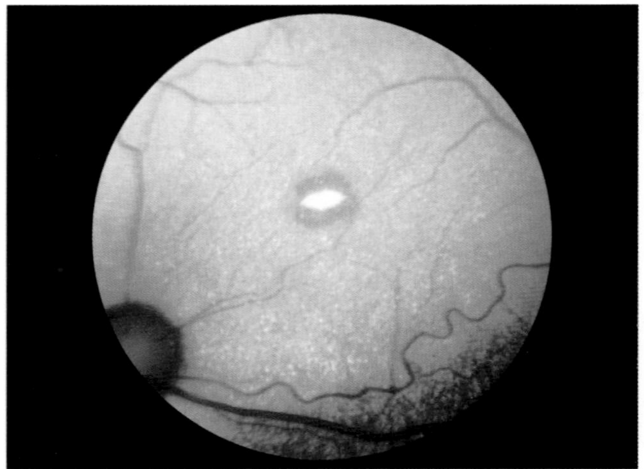

Fig. 14.55 *Slightly larger area of taurine deficiency retinopathy. Note that the area is slightly above the level of the optic disc.*

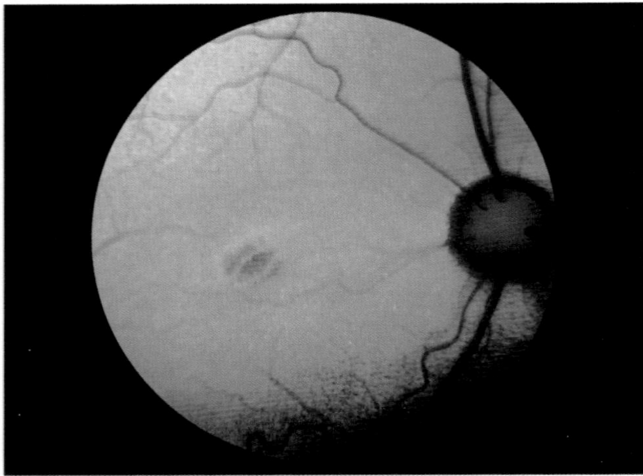

Fig. 14.56 *Similar sized area as Fig 14.55 but note the appearance of pigmentation ophthalmoscopically, simply owing to the angle of light and reflection.*

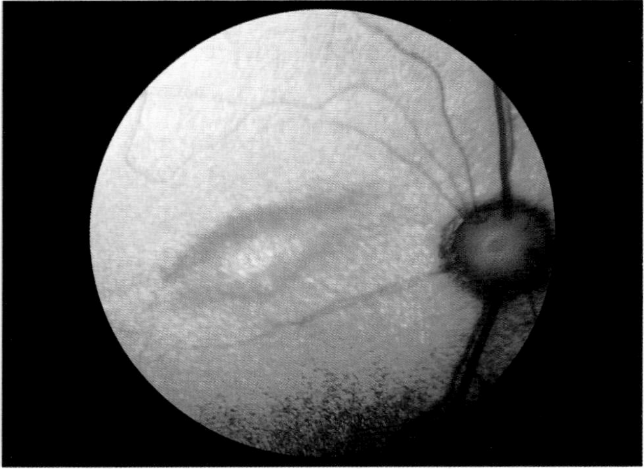

Fig. 14.57 *Increased size of area now approaching the optic disc.*

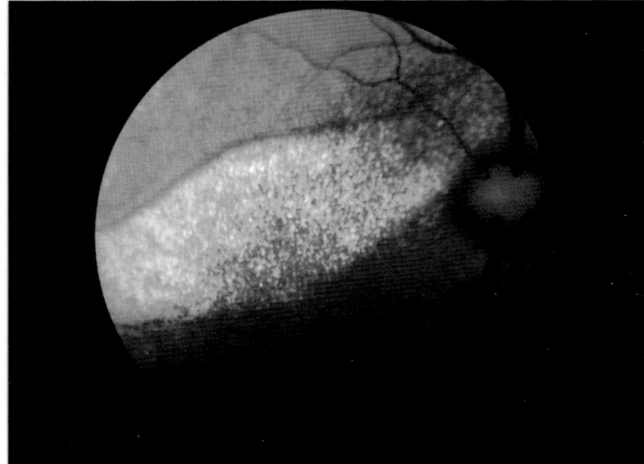

Fig. 14.58 *The degenerative area has now reached the optic disc.*

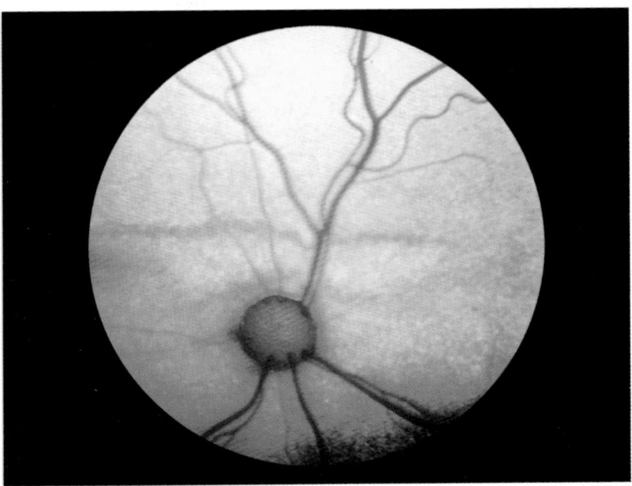

Fig. 14.59 *The two areas meet above the optic disc.*

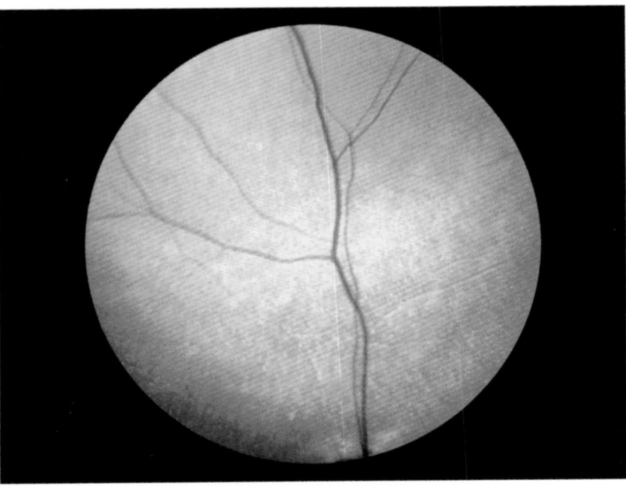

Fig. 14.61 *Generalized retinal degeneration with early attenuation of blood vessels.*

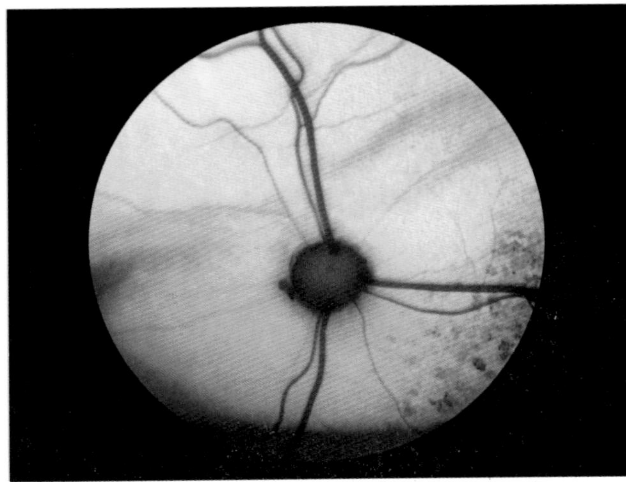

Fig. 14.60 *Bridge of taurine deficiency retinopathy superior to the optic disc.*

immediately superior to the optic disc (Fig. 14.60). Further progression occurs but until this time there has been no apparent loss of vision noticed clinically. The whole of the fundus is then affected with a generalized retinal degeneration which appears ophthalmoscopically as hyper-reflectivity in the tapetal region (Fig. 14.61); previously no change would have been noted except in the areas described above. Finally, attenuation of blood vessels and blindness ensues.

The highly distinctive ophthalmoscopic lesions illustrated in Figs 14.54 to 14.60 are similarly described by all authors and have been said to follow the lines of cone density. Histopathologically, there are no inflammatory changes; the outer retinal layers are most severely affected with loss of photoreceptors and associated nuclear layer and the inner layers remaining more normal; no changes by light microscopy have been described in the retinal pigment epithelium despite the apparently pigmented borders visible by ophthalmoscopy.

Feline retinopathy of dietary origin was first recorded by Greaves and Scott (1962) in cats fed a semipurified diet based on casein. In addition to the retinal degeneration other ocular signs were observed and a relationship with vitamin A was considered. Morris (1965) also produced a feline degenerative retinopathy with a synthetic diet based on casein but did not consider any involvement with vitamin A. It has been suggested (Rubin *et al.*, 1973) that all the nutritional retinopathies described in the cat are of similar origin but if this is the case then the typical ophthalmoscopic lesions of taurine deficiency retinopathy were not noted in the earlier reports. It is interesting that experimental cats fed a purified, amino acid, taurine-free diet (Burger and Barnett, 1979) developed the distinctive ophthalmoscopic progressive lesions of taurine deficiency but more slowly, and less advanced, than the reports on cats fed a semipurified, casein-based diet and these facts might indicate some anti-taurine factor in casein. The aminosulphonic acid taurine is now recognized as essential for the cat and approximately 10 mg per kg body weight has been shown to be the daily requirement for an adult cat (Burger and Barnett, 1982).

Figures 14.53 to 14.61 are retinal photographs of different cats fed a purified diet deficient in taurine in an investigation to study the development of this retinopathy. The study proved that cats require a dietary source of taurine. Pet food manufacturers are now aware of this fact and a sufficient supply of available taurine is present in proprietary cat foods. However, occasional cases of naturally occurring taurine deficiency retinopathy still occur in household cats which are sometimes kept indoors and fed unusual diets including entirely dog foods (dogs are able to synthesize their own taurine). Figure 14.62 depicts such a case.

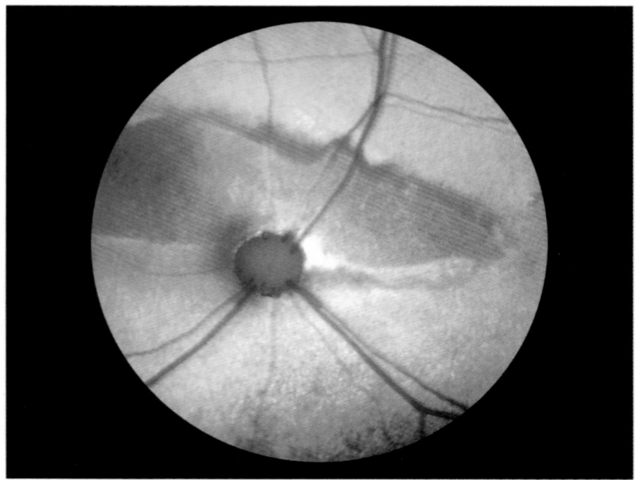

Fig. 14.62 *Typical taurine deficiency retinopathy. A naturally occurring case in a pet cat.*

Hereditary progressive retinal atrophy

Progressive retinal atrophy (PRA) is a well known and well recognized form of retinal degeneration due to inheritance in many breeds of dog throughout the world. In the UK 18 breeds of pedigree dogs are listed as having proven or suspected generalized PRA in the British Veterinary Association/Kennel Club/International Sheepdog Society scheme for the control of hereditary eye disease. The common mode of inheritance in all these breeds is a simple autosomal recessive gene. Generalized PRA, in contradistinction to central PRA or pigment epithelial dystrophy, has been divided into dysplasias and degenerations according to when the atrophy occurs. However, ophthalmoscopically these separate conditions are all identical, the only difference being the age at onset. It is remarkable that in the cat, to date, only one breed has proven hereditary progressive retinal atrophy and, furthermore, that breed, the Abyssinian, has two separate forms occurring at different ages, one caused by a dominant gene and the other by a recessive gene.

There are very few reports in the literature of feline PRA. Retinal degeneration with a suspected hereditary basis has been reported in the Siamese (Barnett, 1965) and further investigated (Carlisle, 1981). Possible hereditary retinal degeneration in two litters of Persian kittens was recorded in America (Rubin and Lipton, 1973) and abnormal photoreceptor development in two generations of mixed breed domestic cats (West-Hyde and Buyukmihci, 1982). However, none of these reports proved an hereditary cause. PRA in the Abyssinian cat was first described in Sweden and Finland by Narfstrom (1981) and in the United Kingdom by Barnett (1982) and several further reports have followed.

In the Abyssinian cat there are two distinctly separate forms of progressive retinal atrophy. Both are bilateral, symmetrical in the two eyes and progressive, and both have been proven to be hereditary. The first form affects young kittens and the first observable clinical sign is a dilated pupil, or

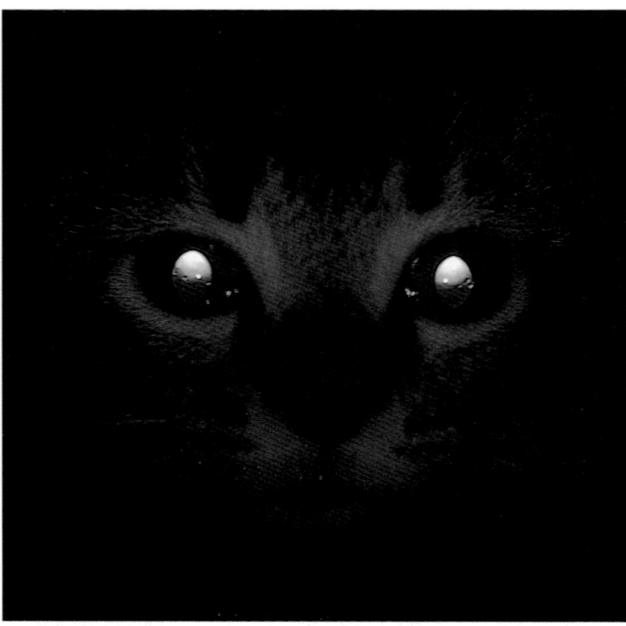

Fig. 14.63 *Pupils of an unaffected kitten.*

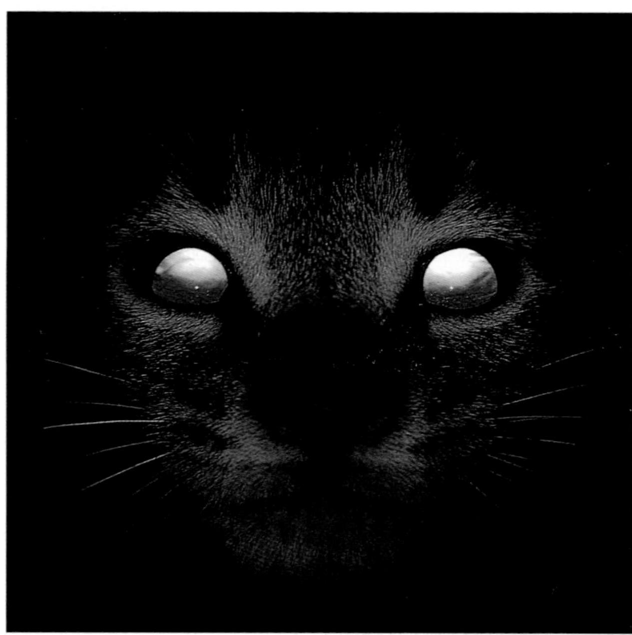

Fig. 14.64 *Mydriasis in an affected kitten; this was a littermate to the kitten in the previous figure.*

mydriasis, which is obvious in affected kittens when compared with their non-affected littermates at as early as 4 weeks old (Figs 14.63 and 14.64). The affected kittens also show nystagmus which is variable, intermittent and often rapid in its form. This form of PRA is a rod–cone dysplasia, degeneration of the photoreceptors occurring before maturation. The first observable ophthalmoscopic lesion is present at about 8 weeks old when affected kittens can be distinguished from non-affected littermates (Figs. 14.65 and 14.66). Progression is rapid and obvious differences ophthalmoscopically are present by 24 weeks old (Figs 14.67 and 14.68). Ophthalmoscopic signs are similar, as might be expected, to any dog with generalized PRA and consist of tapetal hyper-reflectivity and attenuation of the retinal blood vessels and loss of pigment in the nontapetal region (Fig. 14.69). With further progression loss of tapetal structure occurs several months later (Fig. 14.70), particularly in the area centralis region. Even in advanced cases, with ghost vessels visible ophthalmoscopically and tapetal degeneration evident, cats retain some pupillary light reflex in bright sunlight and there have been no cases of a secondary cataract, which is common with generalized PRA in the dog.

The rod–cone dysplasia in the Abyssinian cat described above has been shown to be due to an autosomal dominant gene by crossbreeding unrelated females of both mixed and pedigree breeding resulting in affected offspring in the first

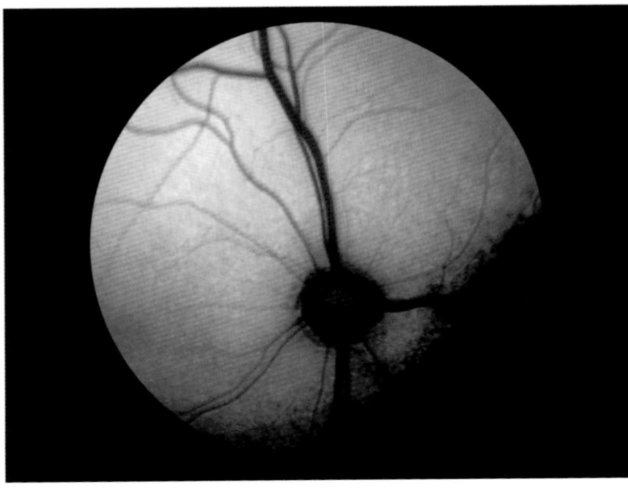

Fig. 14.67 *Fundus of normal kitten at 24 weeks old.*

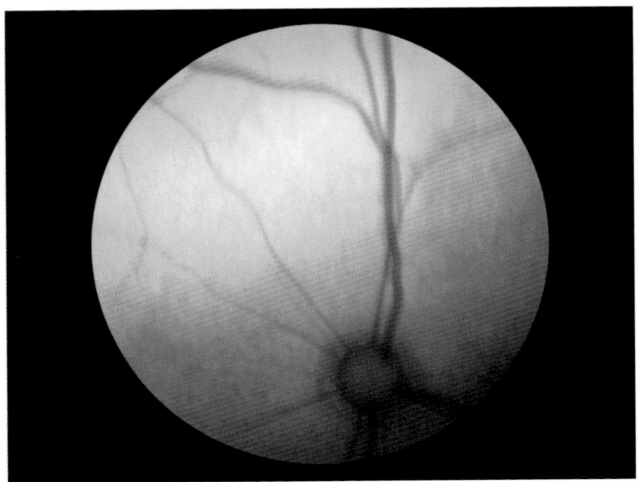

Fig. 14.65 *Fundus appearance of unaffected kitten at 8 weeks old.*

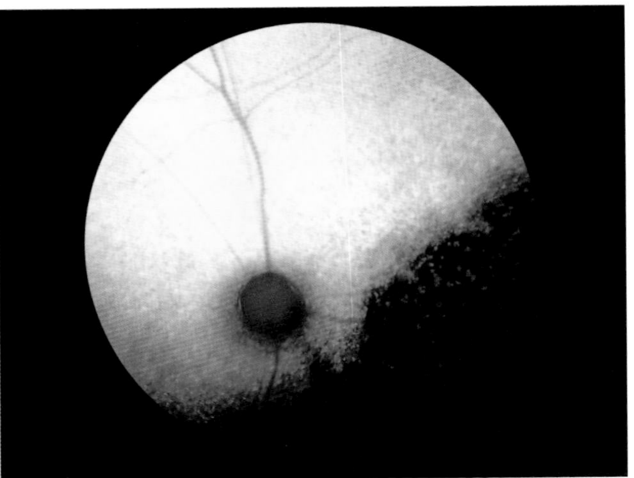

Fig. 14.68 *Fundus of affected kitten; this was a littermate to the kitten in the previous figure.*

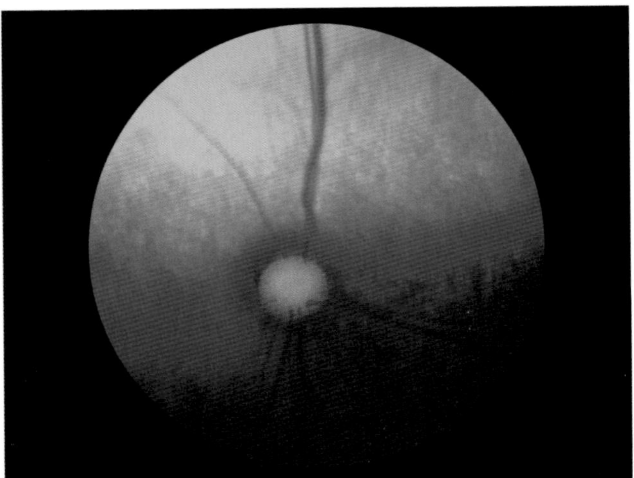

Fig. 14.66 *Fundus of affected kitten; this was a littermate to the kitten in the previous figure.*

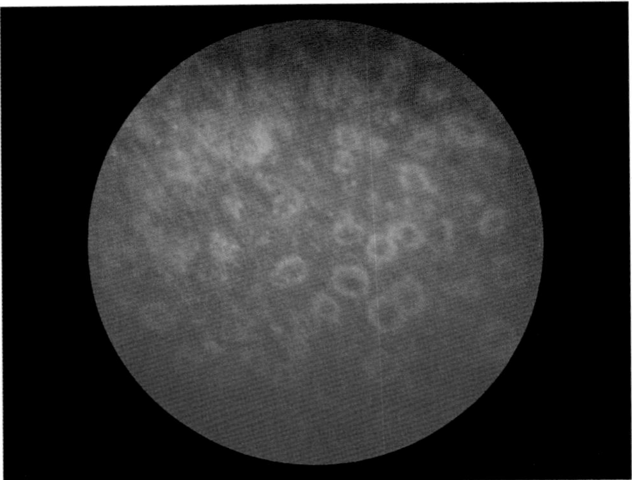

Fig. 14.69 *Loss of pigment from nontapetal fundus in affected kitten.*

generation; the proportion of affected and nonaffected parents being not significantly different from the ratio expected; and the production of normal kittens in litters born to parents both of whom were affected (Barnett and Curtis, 1985). The other form of progressive retinal atrophy in the Abyssinian cat occurs at a later age in young adults, the majority showing clinical signs by 1.5–2 years, occasionally 3–4 years of age (Narfstrom, 1983). This disease was also bilateral and progressive and advanced retinal atrophy varied from 3–6 years, with similar ophthalmoscopic signs to those described above (Figs 14.71 and 14.72). Interestingly, genetic analysis of these cases (Narfstrom, 1983) indicated an autosomal recessive mode of inheritance, evidence being that all offspring from two affected parents were themselves affected, affected offspring derived from matings between clinically unaffected (carrier) parents, and the expected proportion of normal and affected kittens born to matings between affected parents and carriers.

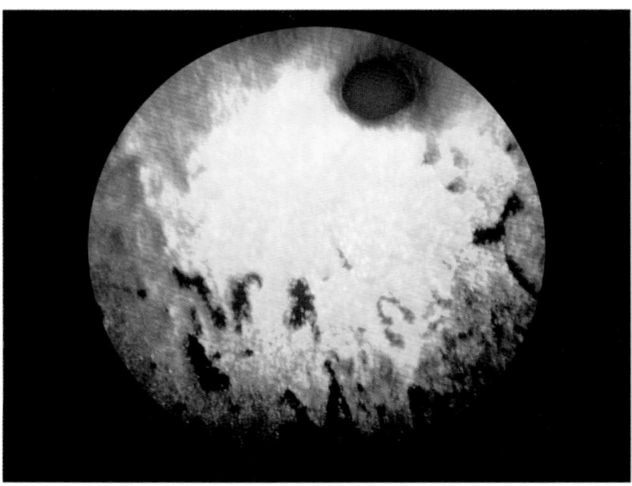

Fig. 14.70 *Loss of tapetal structure in a taurine deficient cat.*

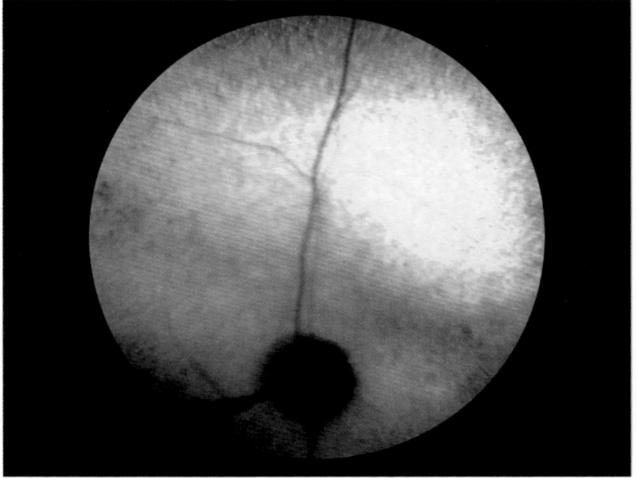

Fig. 14.71 *Generalized progressive retinal atrophy in an Abyssinian cat showing tapetal hyper-reflectivity and blood vessel attenuation (courtesy of K. Narfstrom).*

Inflammatory retinopathies

Active retinal inflammation may present with oedema, exudates, cellular infiltrates, granulomas and haemorrhage (see Chapter 12). Inactive, post-inflammatory retinopathies usually appear as hyper-reflective areas in the tapetal fundus and greyish areas in the nontapetal fundus. Pigmentary disturbance at the level of the retina, or choroid, or both, is a feature of both activity and inactivity, but is much more obvious in the latter.

Active viral, bacterial, parasitic and mycotic infections have been discussed and illustrated in Chapter 12 and are summarized below. Inactive chorioretinopathies, so common a finding in dogs, are much less common in cats (Fig. 14.73).

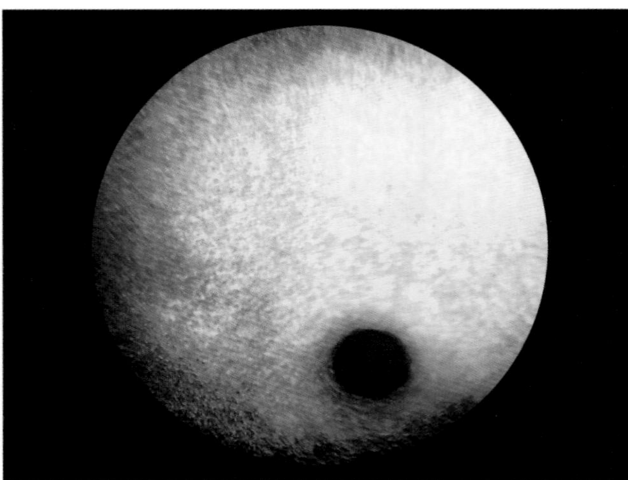

Fig. 14.72 *Generalized progressive retinal atrophy in an Abyssinian cat showing progression from previous figure (courtesy of K. Narfstrom).*

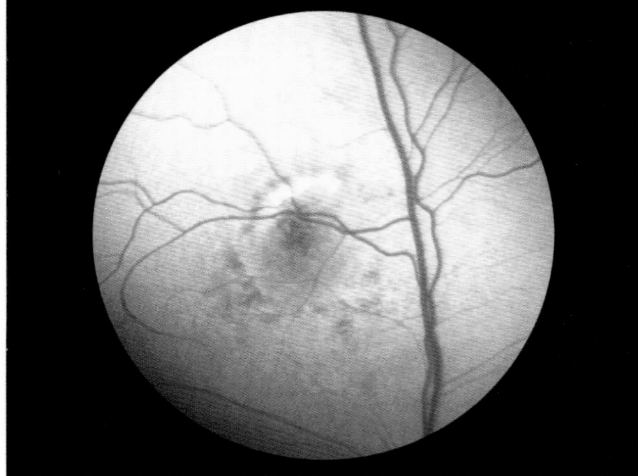

Fig. 14.73 *A 9-year-old Domestic shorthair. Inactive chorioretinopathy of unknown cause as an incidental finding on fundus examination.*

Viral

Feline infectious peritonitis is a classical cause of pyogranulomatous inflammation and intense vasculitis is often a prominent feature. Choroidal exudates (causing retinal separation and tapetal hyporeflectivity), retinal perivascular cellular exudates, retinal haemorrhage and retinal detachment are characteristic. Optic neuritis may be present. Hyperviscosity may also be apparent (see above) if plasma proteins are raised.

Feline leukaemia–lymphosarcoma complex is sometimes associated with posterior segment manifestations as a consequence of neoplastic cellular infiltration. Opthalmoscopic manifestations include pigmentary disturbance, chorioretinal infiltration, retinal detachment and optic neuritis.

Feline immunodeficiency virus is occasionally associated with posterior segment changes, which are assumed to be associated with immunosuppression, but also possibly reflect viral neuropathogenicity.

Bacterial

Choroiditis is the commonest ocular manifestation of mycobacterial infection.

Parasitic

Toxoplasmosis may be associated with retinitis and choroiditis as well as anterior uveitis and the clinical appearance has already been described.

Dipteran larvae are presumed to be the cause of ophthalmomyiasis interna posterior. The lesions are said to be pathognomonic and consist of linear and curvilinear criss-crossing 'tracks' which mark the route of parasite migration, although the parasite is rarely seen (Gwin *et al.*, 1984). The tracks have well-defined parallel edges and are present in both the tapetal and nontapetal fundus. Active migration is usually subretinal and may also be associated with haemorrhage. Considerable chorioretinal scarring may be a legacy of previous parasite activity.

No treatment is required if the eye is 'quiet' and systemic corticosteroids can be used when the eye is inflamed. The causal organism is rarely seen, so removal is not normally an option.

Mycotic

Opportunistic mycotic infections (e.g. cryptococcosis, histoplasmosis, blastomycosis, coccidiomycosis, candidiasis) typically produce granulomatous inflammation of the uveal tract. They usually gain entry by inhalation and reach the eye via the blood stream. Multiple focal pyogranulomatous lesions may be observed on fundus examination.

OPTIC NERVE

CONGENITAL PROBLEMS

Aplasia or hypoplasia of the optic nerve is uncommon, one or both eyes may be involved and other abnormalities (e.g. multiple ocular defects) may be present. Aplasia is associated with blindness, whereas the visual defect associated with hypoplasia will depend upon the extent of the defect. In the case of aplasia (Fig. 14.74) reported by Barnett and Grimes (1974) the retinal vasculature, nerve fibre layer and ganglion cell layer were missing, as were the optic nerves and optic tract. Optic nerve hypoplasia is associated with an optic disc which is smaller than normal and it is possible to demonstrate histologically that there are fewer retinal nerve fibres and ganglion cells.

Colobomatous defects involving the papillary and peripapillary region have already been described (Fig. 14.34).

ACQUIRED PROBLEMS

Papilloedema

Papilloedema is a swelling of the optic nerve head and is not commonly recognized in cats (see Chapter 15, Fig. 15.22). However, there are a number of situations in which papilloedema may be a feature of the clinical presentation in severe or advanced disease (e.g. hydrocephalus, hypertension, encephalitis, meningitis and neoplasia).

Optic Neuritis

Optic neuritis, which is inflammation of the optic nerve, is not unusual (Fig. 14.75) and is most commonly associated with inflammatory disease (intraocular, extraocular and as a consequence of extension from the central nervous system).

Glaucomatous Cupping

Glaucomatous cupping is a pathological recession of the optic nerve head and is a feature of chronic glaucoma (see Chapter 10). As there is indentation of the optic nerve head in normal cats, this is not as distinctive as in the dog (Fig. 14.76).

Optic Atrophy

This may be the end result of many ocular insults, these include traumatic proptosis, optic nerve avulsion and traction damage transmitted to the contralateral optic nerve as

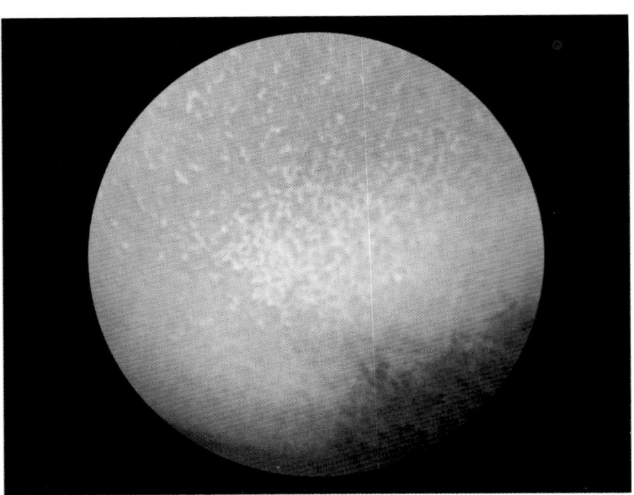

Fig. 14.74 *Domestic shorthair kitten with optic nerve aplasia.*

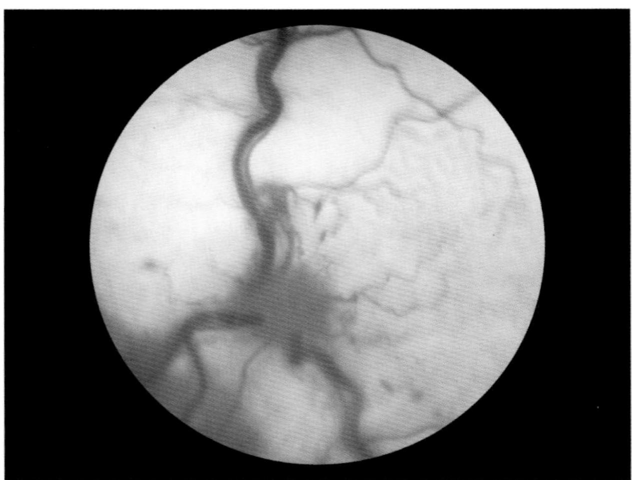

Fig. 14.75 *A 12-month-old Birman with acute onset of left-sided exophthalmos associated with orbital cellulitis (Pasteurella multocida cultured from the orbit). Optic neuritis apparent in the left eye. Orbital cellulitis subsequently developed on the other side. (Courtesy of P. W. Renwick.)*

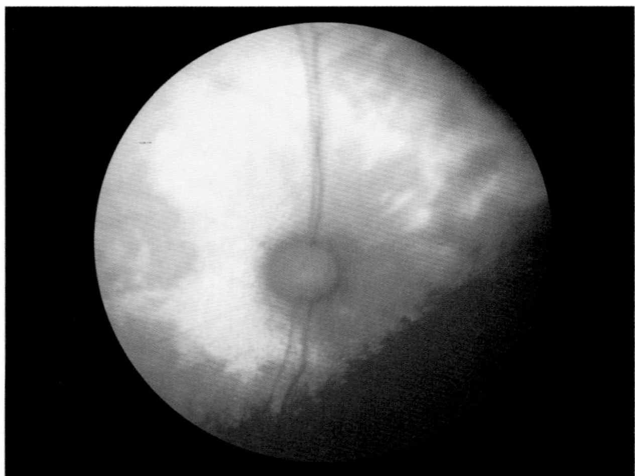

Fig. 14.76 *A 11-year-old Domestic shorthair. Obvious cupping of the optic disc and retinal degeneration secondary to chronic glaucoma.*

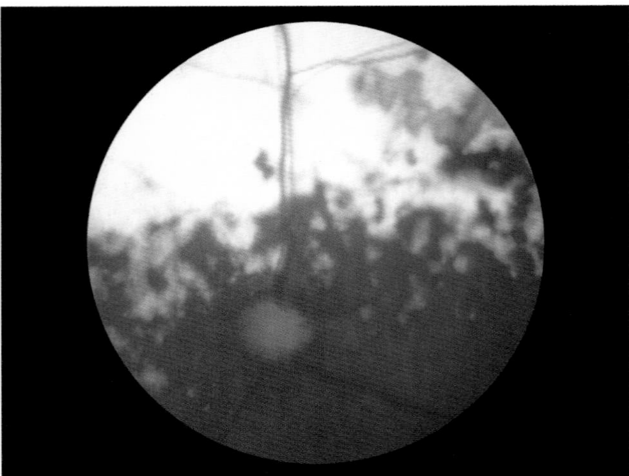

Fig. 14.77 *A 7-year-old Domestic shorthair neutered female. Blindness was apparent on recovery after uneventful enucleation of the fellow eye. The vision loss was unrelated to anaesthesia but occurred because of traction damage to the optic nerve transmitted via the optic chiasma. Some months later optic atrophy is obvious in the permanently blind eye.*

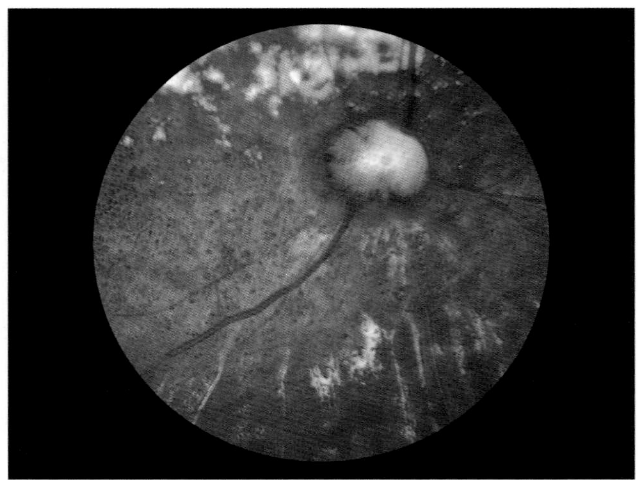

Fig. 14.78 *A 2-year-old Domestic shorthair. Optic atrophy with multiple neurological deficits including blindness and incontinence. Note the short section of grossly narrowed primary venule at '7 o'clock'.*

a complication of globe removal (Fig. 14.77). Optic atrophy may also occur as a sequel to chronic glaucoma, hypertension and degenerative conditions of the retina (Fig. 14.78).

Neoplasia of the ocular fundus

Retina and Choroid

Primary neoplasia is rare and often limited to single case reports; they include astrocytoma (Gross and Dubielzig, 1984), glioma (Jungherr and Wolf, 1939) and neuroblastoma (Grün, 1936).

Secondary neoplasia is more common (see also Chapters 4 and 12) and lymphosarcoma is the commonest neoplasm to involve the eye and orbit (Figs 14.79 – 14.81). Other tumours which may produce changes of fundus appearance (because of orbital involvement or direct infiltration) include squamous cell carcinoma, plasma cell myeloma, reticulosis, sarcomas (e.g. haemangiosarcoma) and carcinomas (e.g. adenocarcinoma). Iridal and ciliary body

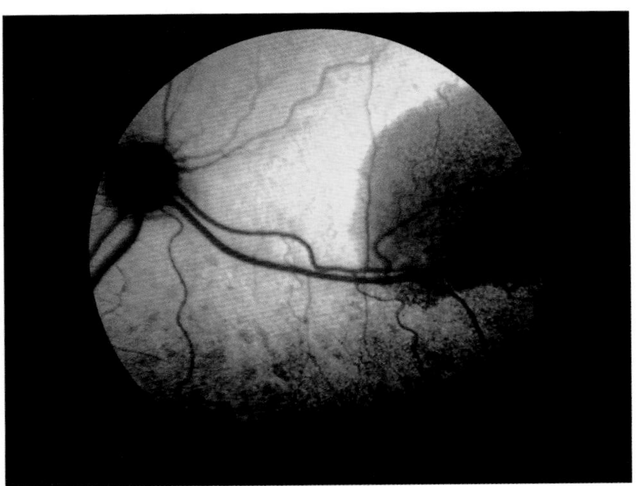

Fig. 14.79 A 3-year-old Domestic shorthair with generalized lymphosarcoma (see also Fig. 8.37 of the same cat).

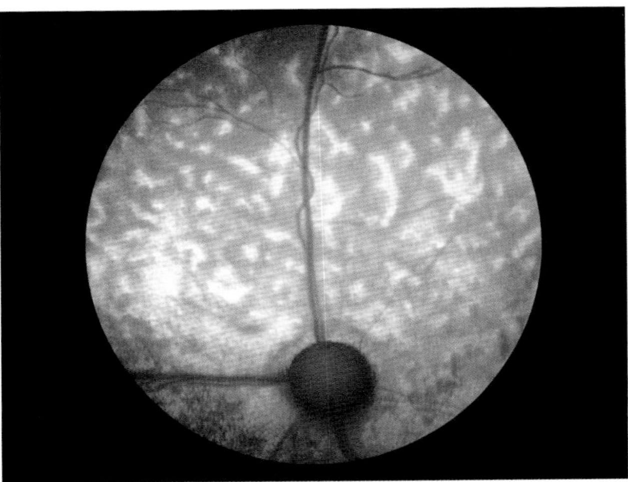

Fig. 14.81 A 13-year-old Domestic shorthair with generalized pigmentary disturbance, retinal degeneration and optic atrophy in a cat with ascites and suspected metastatic neoplasia.

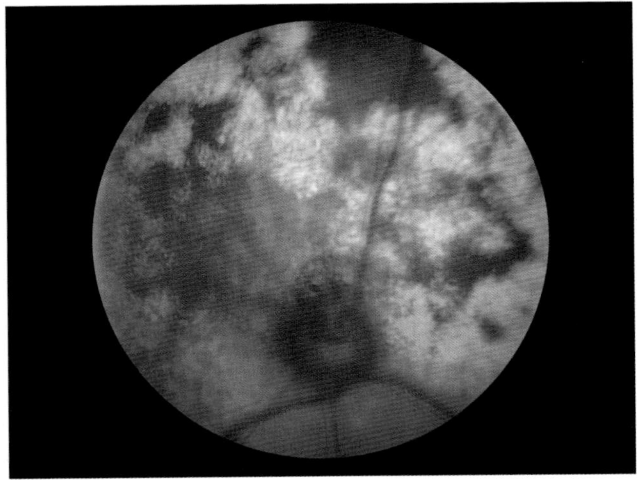

Fig. 14.80 A 7-year-old Domestic shorthair neutered male with generalized lymphosarcoma. This cat was presented because of poor condition. Investigations indicated a renal mass and generalized lymphadenopathy; lymphosarcoma was confirmed post mortem. Bilateral fundic changes were also present; the right eye is shown. In addition to increased retinal reflectivity and bizarre pigmentation there is also intraretinal haemorrhage. Note the attenuation of the retinal vessels and optic atrophy.

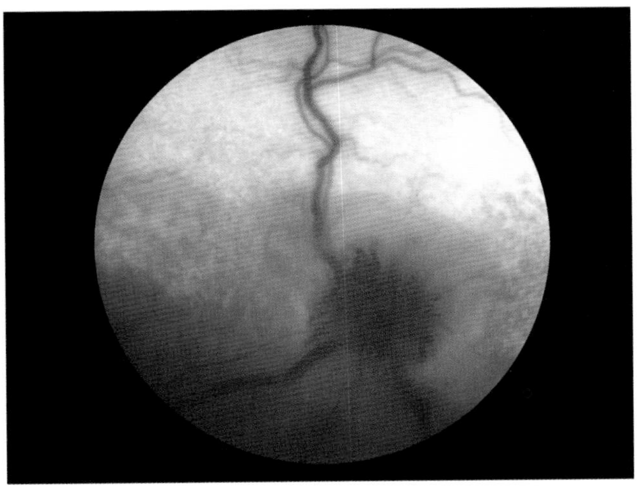

Fig. 14.82 A 10-year-old Domestic shorthair neutered male. Optic nerve meningioma with neovascularization of the optic papilla.

melanomas occasionally extend into the peripheral choroid.

Optic nerve and meninges

Of primary tumours, meningioma is the most likely to be identified and is the commonest intracranial neoplasm of cats (Fig. 14.82), other tumours are rare, they include glioma and astrocytoma. Secondary neoplasia is as described above for the retina and choroid.

References

Aguirre GD (1978) retinal degeneration associated with the feeding of dog foods to cats. *Journal of the American Veterinary Medical Association* **172**: 791–796.

Albert DM, Lahav M, Colby ED, Shadduck JA, Sang DN (1977) Retinal neoplasia and dysplasia. I. Induction by feline leukaemia virus. *Investigative Ophthalmology and Visual Science* **16**: 325–337.

Barclay SM, Riis RC (1979) Retinal detachment and reattachment associated with ethylene glycol intoxication in a cat. *Journal of the American Animal Hospital Association* **15**: 719–724.

Barnett KC (1965) Retinal atrophy. *Veterinary Record* **77**: 1543–1560.

Barnett KC (1982) Progressive retinal atrophy in the Abyssinian cat. *Journal of Small Animal Practice* **23**: 763–766.

Barnett KC, Curtis R (1985) Autosomal dominant progressive retinal atrophy in Abyssinian cats *J. Hered.* 76: 168–170.

Barnett KC, Grimes TD (1974) Bilateral aplasia of the optic nerve in a cat. *British Journal of Ophthalmology* **58**: 663–667.

Bellhorn RW, Fischer CA (1970) Feline central retinal degeneration. *Journal of the American Veterinary Medical Association* **157**: 842–849.

Bellhorn RW, Barnett KC, Henkind P (1971) Ocular colobomas in domestic cats. *Journal of the American Veterinary Medical Association* **159**: 1015–1021.

Blakemore WF (1986) A case of mannosidosis in the cat: Clinical and histopathological findings. *Journal of Small Animal Practice* 27: 447–455.

Boldy K (1983) Clinical and histological findings of systemic hypertension in dogs and cats. *Transactions of the American College of Veterinary Ophthalmologists* **14**: 14.

Burger IH, Barnett KC (1979) *Essentiality of Taurine for the Cat.* Kal Kan Symposium for the treatment of dog and cat diseases, September 1979, pp. 64–70. Kal Kan Foods Inc. Vernon, California, USA.

Burger IH, Barnett KC (1982) The taurine requirement of the adult cat. Waltham Symposium No. 4, *Recent Advances in Feline Nutrition*, pp. 533–537.

Carlisle JL (1981) Feline retinal atrophy *Veterinary Record* **108**: 311.

Christmas R, Guthrie B (1989) Bullous retinal detachment in a cat. *Canadian Veterinary Journal* 30: 430–431.

Crispin SM (1993) Ocular manifestations of hyperlipoproteinaemia. *Journal of Small Animal Practice* **34**: 500–506.

Dukes J (1992) Hypertension: A review of the mechanisms, manifestations and management. *Journal of Small Animal Practice* **33**: 119–129.

Dziezyc J, Millichamp NJ (1993) The feline fundus. In Petersen-Jones SM and Crispin SM (eds) *Manual of Small Animal Ophthalmology*, pp. 259–265. BSAVA Publications.

Ginzinger DG, Lewis MES, Ma Y, Jones BR, Liu G, Jones SD, Hayden MR (1996) A mutation in the lipoprotein lipase gene is the molecular basis of chylomicronemia in a colony of domestic cats. *Journal of Clinical Investigation* 97: 1257–1266.

Greaves JP, Scott PP (1962) feline retinopathy of dietary organ. *Veterinary Record* 74: 904–905.

Gross SL, Dubielzig RR (1984) Ocular astrocytomas in a dog and cat. *Proceedings of the American College of Veterinary Ophthalmologists* 15: 243.

Grün K (1936) Die Geschwülste des Zentralnervensystems und seiner Hüllen bei unseren Haustieren. Dissertation, Berlin.

Gunn-Moore DA, Watson TDG, Dodkin SJ, Blaxter AC, Crispin SM, Gruffydd-Jones TJ (1997) Transient hyperlipidaemia and associated anaemia in kittens. *Veterinary Record* **140**: 355–359.

Gwin RM, Merideth R, Martin C, Kaswan R (1984) Ophthalmomyiasis interna posterior in two cats and a dog. *Journal of the American Animal Hospital Association* **20**: 481–486.

Haskins ME, Jezyk PF, Patterson DF (1979) Mucopolysaccharide storage disease in three families of cats with arylsulfatase B deficiency: Leukocyte studies and carrier identification. *Paediatric Research* **13**: 1203–1210.

Hubler M, Haskins ME, Arnold S, Kaser-Hotz B, Bosshard NU, Briner J, Spycher MA, Gizelmann R, Sommerlade H-J, von Figura K (1996) Mucolipidosis type II in a domestic shorthair cat. *Journal of Small Animal Practice* 37: 435–441.

Jungherr E, Wolf A (1939) Gliomas in animals. *American Journal of Cancer* 37: 493–500.

Kobayashi DL, Peterson ME, Graves TK, Lesser M, Nichols CE (1990) Hypertension in cats with chronic renal failure or hyperthyroidism. *Journal of Veterinary Internal Medicine* **4**: 58–62.

Labato MA, Ross LA (1991) Diagnosis and management of hypertension. In August JR (ed.) *Consultations in Feline Internal Medicine*, pp. 301–308. WB Saunders, Philadelphia.

Littman MP (1994) Spontaneous systemic hypertension in 24 cats. *Journal of Veterinary Internal Medicine* **8**: 79–86.

Morgan RV (1986) Systemic hypertension in four cats: Ocular and medical findings. *Journal of the American Animal Hospital Association* **22**: 615–621.

Morris ML (1965) Feline degenerative retinopathy. *Cornell Veterinarian* **50**: 295–308.

Mould JRB (1993) Ophthalmic pathology of systemic hypertension in the dog and cat. Dissertation, Royal College of Veterinary Surgeons Diploma in Veterinary Ophthalmology.

Murray JA, Blakemore WF, Barnett KC (1977) Ocular lesions in cats with GM_1-gangliosidosis with visceral involvement. *Journal of Small Animal Practice* **18**: 1–10.

Narfstrom K (1981) Progressive retinal atrophy in Abyssinian cats. *Svensk Veterinartidning* 33(6): 147–150.

Narfstrom K (1983) Hereditary progressive retinal atrophy in the Abyssinian cat. *J. Hered* **74**: 273–276.

Percy DH, Scott FW, Albert DM (1975) Retinal dysplasia due to feline panleukopenia virus infection. *Journal of the American Veterinary Medical Association* **167**: 935–937.

Rabin AR, Hayes KC, Berson EL (1973) Cone and rod responses in nutritionally induced retinal degeneration in the cat. *Investigative Ophthamology* **12**: 694–704.

Rubin LF (1974) *Atlas of Veterinary Ophthalmoscopy*, p. 249. Lea & Febiger, Philadelphia.

Rubin LF, Lipton DE (1973) Retinal degeneration in kittens. *Journal of the American Veterinary Association* **162**: 467–469.

Sansom J, Barnett KC, Dunn KA, Smith KC, Dennis R (1994) Ocular disease associated with hypertension in 16 cats. *Journal of Small Animal Practice* **35**: 604–611.

Stiles J, Polzin DJ, Bistner SI (1994) The prevalence of retinopathy in cats with systemic hypertension and chronic renal failure or hyperthyroidism. *Journal of the American Animal Hospital Association* **30**: 564–572.

Szymanski C (1987) Holzworth J. (ed.) *Diseases of the cat.* WB Saunders Co, Philadelphia.

Tilley L, King JN, Humbert-Droz E, Maurer M (1996) Benezepril activity in cats: inhibition of plasma ACE and efficacy in the treatment of hypertension. *Proceedings of the 14th American College of Internal Medicine Forum*, p. 745.

Turner JL, Brogdon JD, Lees GE, Greco DS (1990) Idiopathic hypertension in a cat with secondary hypertensive retinopathy associated with a high salt diet. *Journal of the American Veterinary Medical Association* **26**: 647–651.

West-Hyde L, Buyukmihci N (1982) Photoreceptor degeneration in a family of cats. *Journal of the American Veterinary Association* **181**: 243–247.

15 NEURO-OPHTHALMOLOGY

INTRODUCTION

The cat is a successful predator with excellent special senses; the sense of smell is not as well-developed as that of dogs, but hearing is acute and tactile vibrissae allow the cat to manoeuvre with confidence under conditions of darkness. Cats are very hesitant in the dark if they lack tactile vibrissae and their presence helps to explain the uncanny abilities of cats to cope with severe visual disability and blindness.

The cat has an arrythmic eye, which permits activity in a range of lighting conditions, but is particularly effective under conditions of low illumination because of a combination of optics, the presence of a tapetum cellulosum and a rod-dominated retina. Both a rod and cone electroretinogram can be demonstrated in the cat, green and blue absorbing photoreceptors are present and colour vision is somewhat rudimentary. The eyes are frontally placed and some 35% of retinal nerve fibres remain uncrossed – a prerequisite for binocular vision, stereopsis and conjugate eye movement.

NEUROLOGICAL EXAMINATION OF THE CAT WITH OCULAR DISEASE

A complete neurological examination is an essential, but challenging, part of the investigation of any cat with suspected neuro-ophthalmological disease. The aims of the neurological examination are:

(1) Confirmation of neurological abnormalities: objective information is obtained to confirm or rule out the presence of neurological disease
(2) Localization of neurological disease: a single, focal site of disease within the central or peripheral nervous system should be sought that could account for the neurological abnormalities detected. If this is not possible, then a multifocal or diffuse disease may be present
(3) An assessment of the severity of the disease: based partly on historical features, and partly on the neurological examination. Because cats adapt well to gradual visual loss, the history may be crucial, particularly the owner's observations in relation to the cat in familiar and unfamiliar environments
(4) Differential diagnoses: the findings of the neurological examination, together with the ophthalmic examination, history and background details will allow appropriate differential diagnoses to be considered, and therefore facilitate a rational approach to the subsequent diagnostic investigations.

The value of repeat neurological examinations (a few hours, or a day later) to demonstrate whether findings are genuine or artifactual should not be underestimated. This is particularly helpful when the initial findings suggest the presence of mild neurological deficits.

Observation of the cat (even if just for a few minutes) is important prior to commencement of the neurological examination to assess mental status, posture and gait. A full neurological examination incorporates careful assessment of cranial nerves, postural reactions, spinal reflexes, and nociception. Aspects of the neurological examination relating specifically to ocular disease (cranial nerve examination and visual placing reactions) are outlined below, followed by some examples of neurological diseases with ocular manifestations. Standard neurology texts should be consulted for detailed neurological examination, particularly of the head and eyes and for a more comprehensive guide to neurological diseases with ocular manifestations (De Lahunta, 1983; Oliver *et al.*, 1987; Scagliotti, 1990; Chrisman, 1991; Moreau and Wheeler, 1995; Petersen-Jones, 1995).

CRANIAL NERVE ASSESSMENT

CRANIAL NERVE II (OPTIC)

The optic nerve (CN II) is actually a tract of the central nervous system which acts as the afferent pathway for vision (for abnormalities of the central visual pathways see below) and the pupillary light reflex (for abnormalities of the pupils see below). The visual pathway consists of the neurosensory retina, the optic nerve, the optic chiasm, the optic tract, the lateral geniculate nucleus, the optic radiation and the visual cortex (Fig. 15.1). A normal ophthalmic examination and intact pupillary light responses do not necessarily imply intact vision.

Assessment of Vision

The obstacle test This assesses the cat's ability to avoid obstacles while wandering round the room. Normal cats are often reluctant to move around in strange surroundings, so an obstacle course may be of limited value in this species.

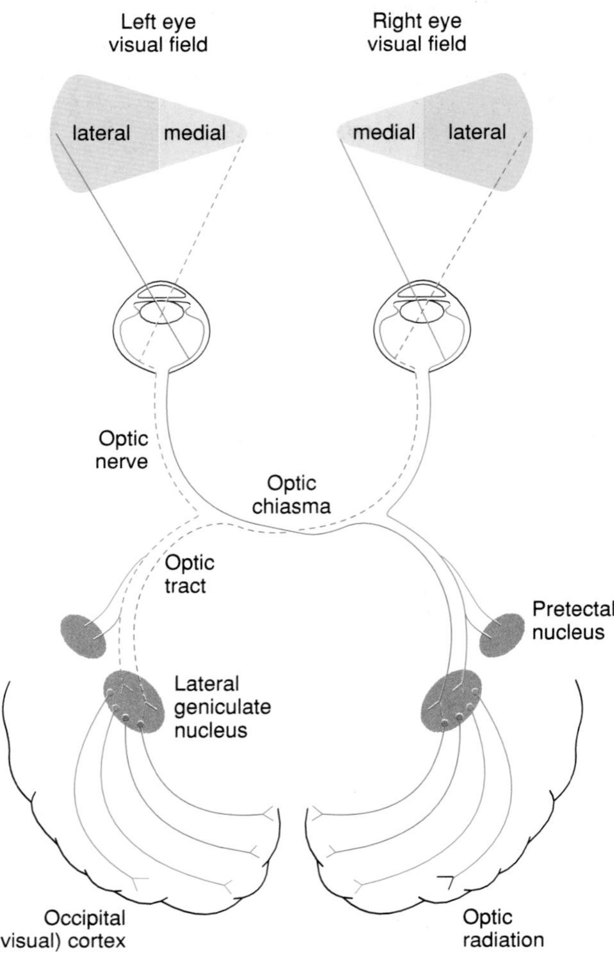

Fig. 15.1 *The central visual pathway. Reproduced with permission of BSAVA, Manual of Small Animal Neurology.*

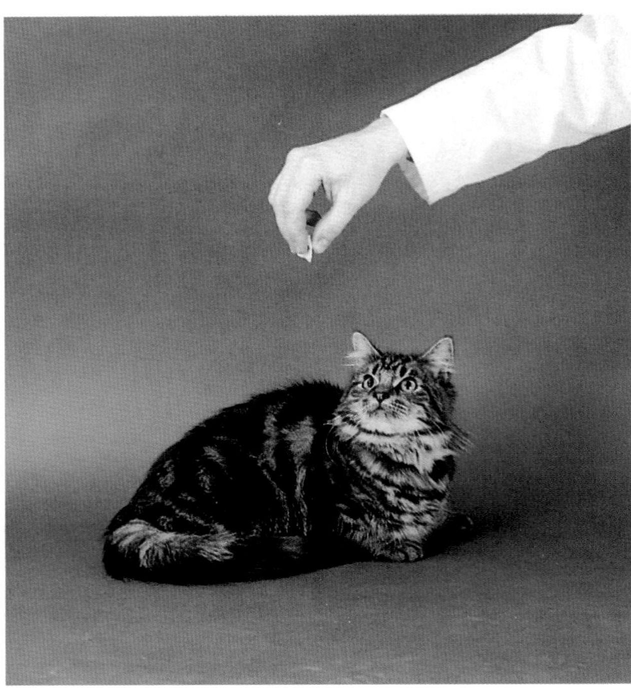

Fig. 15.2 *The following response, prior to dropping the cotton wool.*

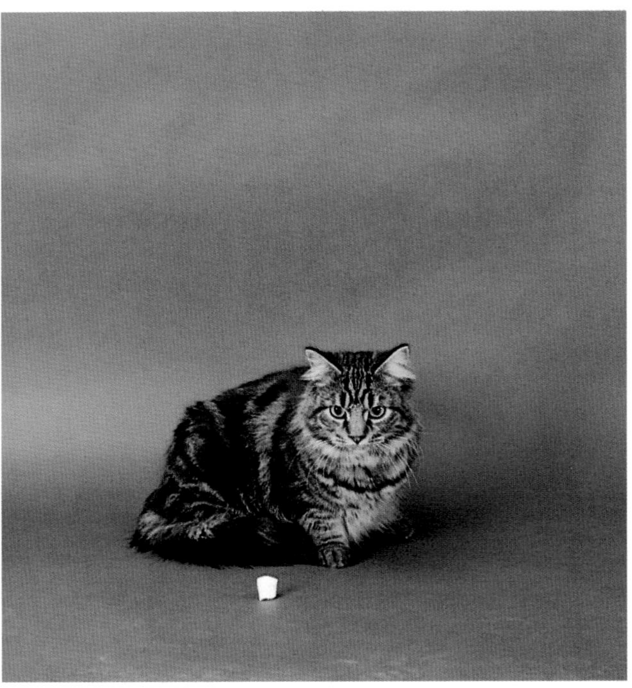

Fig. 15.3 *The following response, after the cotton wool has been dropped.*

The following response This is the ability to follow a cotton wool ball which is dropped or tossed in the air (Figs 15.2 and 15.3) under normal conditions of room lighting. Central vision is tested when the cotton wool ball is dropped in front of the animal and peripheral vision when the cotton wool ball is dropped from each side. In addition, a bright light can be shone from a variety of angles in a darkened room. Unfortunately, many normal cats show no inclination to participate in tests of this type, so results should be interpreted with caution.

The menace response Blinking in response to a hand or object moved slowly and steadily towards the eye. In addition to the afferent sensory pathway (CN II), a motor pathway via the facial nerve (CN VII) is involved. It is important not to stimulate the cornea (CN V) during performance of the menace response.

The retinal light (dazzle) reflex This is a subcortical reflex which initiates a bilateral partial eyelid closure when a bright light is shone into the eye

Visual placing response This involves moving the cat towards the edge of a table and observing for appropriate extension and placing of the thoracic limbs on the table.

Cranial nerve III (oculomotor)

The oculomotor nerve (CN III) is responsible for pupillary constriction (via parasympathetic innervation), innervation of extra-ocular muscles (dorsal, medial and ventral rectus, and the ventral oblique) and partial innervation of the upper eyelid (levator palpebrae superioris).

Assessment

CN III is assessed by observation of pupil size (symmetry, direct and indirect pupillary light response, eye position and eye movements). Deficits of CN III produce mydriasis, an inability to contract the pupil in response to light, ventrolateral strabismus with no movement of the globe except laterally, and ptosis.

Cranial nerves IV (trochlear) and VI (abducens)

These nerves supply motor function to extra-ocular muscles. The trochlear (CN IV) innervates the dorsal oblique, and the abducens (CN VI) innervates the lateral rectus and retractor oculi muscles.

Assessment

A deficit of the trochlear (CN IV) causes mild rotation of the globe with the dorsal aspect turned laterally (dorso-lateral rotation); the abnormal direction is easiest to discern by examination of the accompanying pupil rotation.

A deficit of the abducens (CN VI) causes medial strabismus and a lack of globe retraction in response to touching the cornea (corneal reflex, tested in conjunction with CN V which provides the sensory input).

Cranial nerve V (trigeminal)

The trigeminal nerve (CN V) is responsible for sensory input from the entire face and also provides motor function to the muscles of mastication.

Assessment

A deficit of motor function results in an inability to close the mouth and reduced tone (± atrophy) of the masticatory muscles.

Sensory function can be assessed in the three main branches of the nerve (ophthalmic, maxillary and mandibular), but only the ophthalmic branch is considered here as it is this branch which conveys afferent sensory stimulation from the eye. The ophthalmic branch is tested by the palpebral (blink) reflex (elicited by touching the medial canthus, tested in conjunction with CN VII which provides the motor input for the blink) and the corneal (blink) reflex (see CN IV). Stimulation of afferent fibres of the ophthalmic branch will also stimulate tear secretion. Sensory deficits of the cornea result in an exposure keratopathy which particularly affects the exposed area of cornea in the palpebral aperture.

Cranial nerve VII (facial)

The facial nerve (CN VII) provides motor innervation to the muscles of facial expression and parasympathetic fibres supply the lacrimal glands (see below). The facial nerve becomes closely associated with the vestibulocochlear nerve once it has left the brain stem and they enter the internal auditory meatus together; a single lesion may involve both nerves.

Assessment

Abnormality causes facial paralysis and there may be reduced tear production. Unilateral deficits may be observed as asymmetry of the ears, eyelids, lips and nose. Specific tests include the palpebral reflex (see CN V), the menace response (see CN II), the Schirmer tear test and observation of normal ear and facial movements. When the cat attempts to blink, the globe is retracted and the third eyelid sweeps across the cornea, but there is no movement of the upper and lower eyelids.

Cranial nerve VIII (vestibulocochlear)

The cochlear portion of the eighth cranial nerve (CN VIII) is responsible for hearing, and the vestibular portion is responsible for equilibrium of posture and gait and coordination of eye movements (see below).

Assessment

Cochlear deficits result in deafness while vestibular deficits may manifest as nystagmus. If spontaneous horizontal nystagmus is present, the fast phase moves away from the side of the lesion. Nystagmus can be horizontal, vertical or rotatory, but if it is vertical this implies that the disease may be central in origin (i.e. a disease affecting the vestibular nucleus). The other two forms of nystagmus can occur with either central or peripheral (vestibular nerve or vestibular apparatus) disease. Positional nystagmus may also be detectable, with nystagmus occurring or changing as the position of the head is altered (e.g. lying the cat on its side or back).

Note that an hereditary horizontal nystagmus is seen in some Siamese cats, without other signs of vestibular disease (see below).

Unilateral vestibular disease will also result in a head tilt and circling to the side of the lesion, with ataxia. The head tilt, if mild or inapparent, may be exaggerated by suspending the cat from its pelvis. Normally the thoracic limbs reach towards the ground and the head is held at approximately 45° to the ground. A marked head tilt will be seen in unilateral vestibular disease, and in bilateral disease the head becomes hyperflexed with the chin tucked onto the sternum.

Postural reactions

Postural reactions include wheelbarrowing, the extensor postural thrust, hemi-standing and hemi-walking, hopping, proprioception and placing responses. The visual placing response is the only one of these that specifically includes an assessment of vision (see above).

Light reflex pathway

Pupil size is controlled by the iris sphincter muscle (under cholinergic parasympathetic control) and the iris dilator muscle (under adrenergic sympathetic control, see below) and the balance between the two systems is in a constant state of flux. The light reflex, also known as the pupillary light response (PLR), originates in the retina following stimulation of receptors (probably the photoreceptors) by bright light and the afferent pathway begins in the ganglion cell layer. A proportion of the second-order neurones in the optic nerve carrying impulses derived from stimulation of receptor cells are pupillomotor fibres, which exit the optic tract to enter the midbrain where they synapse with third-order neurones in the pretectal nucleus, which in turn synapse with the parasympathetic component of the oculomotor nucleus (known as the Edinger–Westphal nucleus in man). There is extensive crossover of both second-order neurones at the optic chiasm, and third-order neurones at the caudal commissure (between the pretectal and oculomotor nuclei) allowing a bilateral pupillary response to stimulation with light. Efferent parasympathetic fibres from the oculomotor nucleus are contained in the oculomotor nerve (CN III), they enter through the orbital fissure to synapse at the ciliary ganglion lateral to the optic nerve, with post-ganglionic fibres passing in two short ciliary nerves (nasal or medial and malar or lateral) to innervate the iris musculature (Fig. 15.4).

Oculosympathetic pathway

Sympathetic innervation to the iris originates in the hypothalamus. Upper motor neurones synapse with lower motor neurones at the T1–T3 level of the spinal cord, and their axons exit and travel in the thoracic and vago-sympathetic trunk to synapse in the cranial cervical ganglion close to the tympanic bulla. Postganglionic fibres pass through the middle ear and join the ophthalmic branch of the trigeminal (CN V) nerve to innervate the iris dilator muscle and the smooth muscle of the periorbital muscles and eyelid (Fig. 15.5).

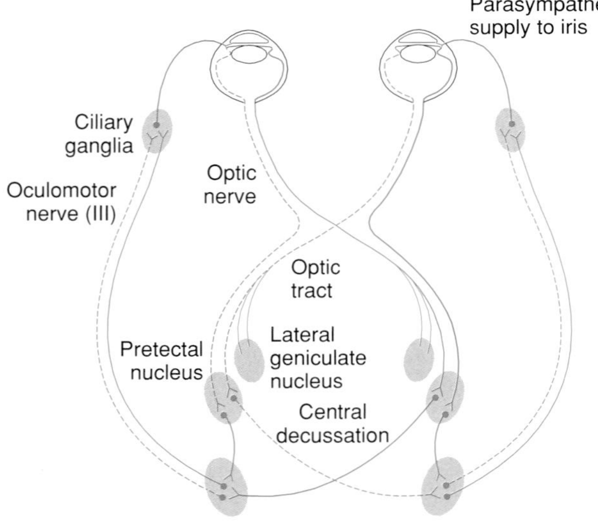

Fig. 15.4 *The light reflex pathway. Reproduced with permission of BSAVA, Manual of Small Animal Neurology.*

Assessment of pupillary response

Pupillary assessment under a range of lighting conditions is a standard feature of neuro-ophthalmological examination. The shape, size and position of the pupils under normal conditions of illumination are examined first, then the examination is repeated with the lights dimmed – a technique which helps in the differentiation of sympathetic and parasympathetic defects. In bright light miosis caused by sympathetic dysfunction may be difficult to detect because of the dominance of the parasympathetic system. In dim light, however, such a defect is obvious as the anisocoria becomes more marked, with the smaller pupil being on the affected side. Conversely, the mydriasis found in parasympathetic paralysis (e.g. traumatic damage to the ciliary ganglion), may be obvious in bright light, but difficult to detect in dim light.

The direct (ipsilateral) and consensual (indirect or contralateral) response to bright light is assessed next and this test is best performed in conditions of near darkness. Partial decussation of the optic nerve fibres at the optic chiasm and caudal commissure of the midbrain ensures that the normal pupil response to a bright light directed into one eye will be more intense miosis in the stimulated eye (dynamic contraction anisocoria). If the light is swung to stimulate the other eye then the pupil of this eye will, in turn, become more miotic and if the light is swung from one eye to the other, the miosis will alternate (alternating contraction anisocoria). This is the basis of the swinging flashlight test which can be used to detect the presence of a relative afferent pupillary defect (Marcus Gunn phenomenon). With a prechiasmal lesion, for example, when the light is swung to stimulate the other eye, the miotic pupil of this eye suddenly dilates while receiving direct illumination (a positive swinging flashlight test).

Ocular manifestations of neurological disease

Pupil abnormalities with normal vision

Pharmacological Mydriasis and Miosis

Mydriatic and cycloplegic drugs (e.g. atropine, tropicamide) will dilate the pupil, miotic drugs (e.g. pilocarpine) will constrict the pupil. Anaesthetic agents such as ketamine also produce mydriasis. In assessment of pupillary abnormalities it is important to determine whether drugs of this type have

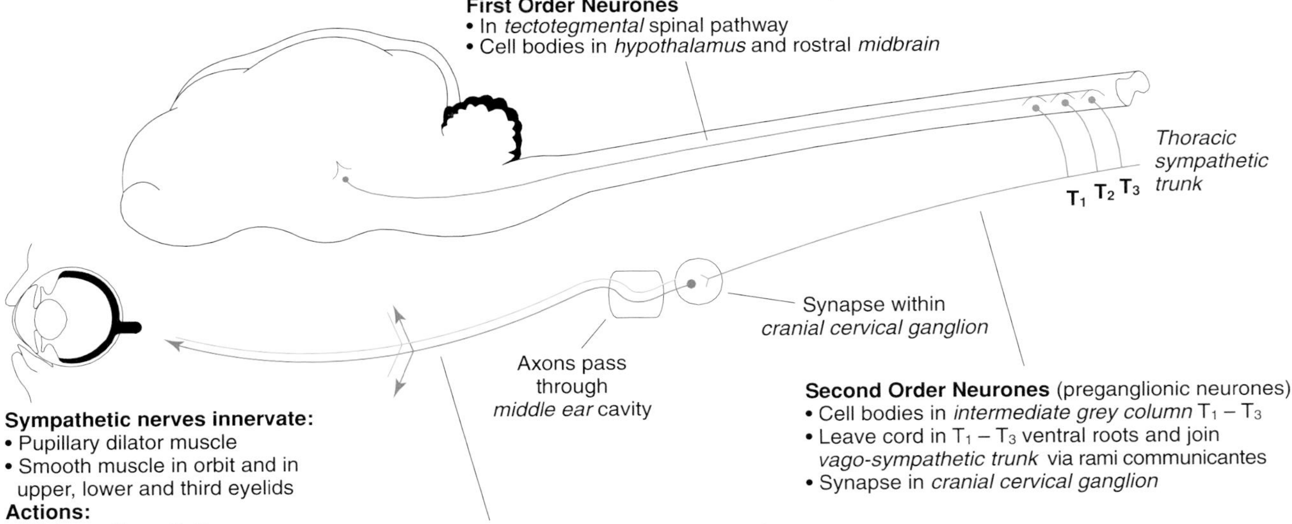

Fig. 15.5 *The oculosympathetic pathway. Reproduced with permission of BSAVA, Manual of Small Animal Neurology.*

been given, particularly in referral cases. It is also sensible to check the recent anaesthetic history.

Pharmacological testing can be useful in the differentiation of preganglionic and postganglionic lesions of the sympathetic and parasympathetic nervous system and is based on the principle of denervation hypersensitivity. The denervated muscle cells become hypersensitive to exogenously applied 'neurotransmitter' so that the pupillary response of the denervated eye occurs sooner, is more extensive and persists for a longer period of time when compared with that of the normal eye (Collins and O'Brien, 1990).

Anisocoria

Anisocoria (inequality of pupil size) may arise as a result of abnormalities of the eye, the oculosympathetic system, the light reflex pathway, the midbrain or the cerebellum (Figs 15.6–15.10). The underlying cause is not always obvious (Fig. 15.7), particularly in relation to inflammatory disorders and detailed investigations may be required (Neer and Carter, 1987; Collins and O'Brien, 1990; Bercovitch *et al.*, 1995). It is important to detect which eye is abnormal when anisocoria is present, and this may require careful observation of direct and consensual pupillary light reflexes and pupillary dilation in response to low lighting conditions. Other causes of anisocoria (Fig. 15.6) such as congenital or acquired iris problems (e.g. iris hypoplasia, iris atrophy and iritis), glaucoma and fundus abnormalities are discussed elsewhere (see Chapters 10, 12 and 14).

Idiopathic anisocoria Mild inequality of pupil size is quite common in cats and is assumed to be caused by differences in basal sympathetic or parasympathetic tone to the two eyes. The origin of this type of anisocoria may be

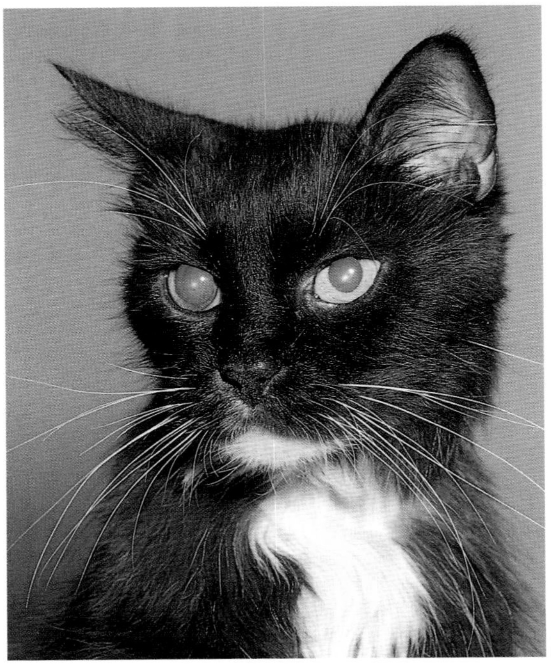

Fig. 15.6 *An 11-year-old Domestic shorthair with anisocoria as consequence of right-sided uveitis complicated by glaucoma secondary to idiopathic uveitis. Note the keratic precipitates, change of iris colour and dilated pupil.*

'central' in so far as it relates to asymmetries of supranuclear inhibitory control of the parasympathetic nuclei of the oculomotor nerves.

Unilateral miosis – Horner's syndrome Anisocoria is the single most common sign of Horner's syndrome, which usually presents as miosis, ptosis, enophthalmos and third eyelid protrusion on the affected side (Fig. 15.8). In some cases anisocoria is the only presenting ocular sign (Fig. 15.9). Horner's syndrome arises from damage to the sympathetic innervation on the affected side (Neer, 1984; van den Broek, 1987; Morgan and Zanotti, 1989; Kern *et al.*, 1989) and although damage may occur to the sympathetic fibres within the brain or spinal cord, it is more common for the lesion to occur outside the cord.

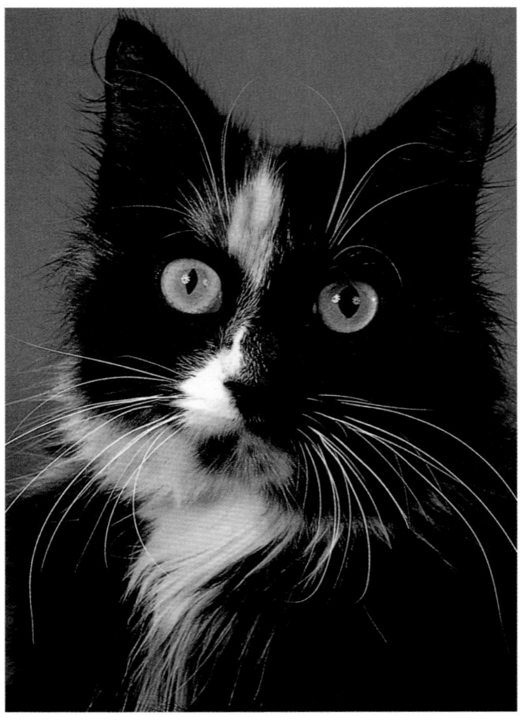

Fig. 15.7 *A 3-year-old Domestic longhair neutered female. Anisocoria, left eye affected; sparse, discrete focal opacities were present in the ocular fundi of both eyes. Diffuse inflammation of the central nervous system with progressive neurological deficits.*

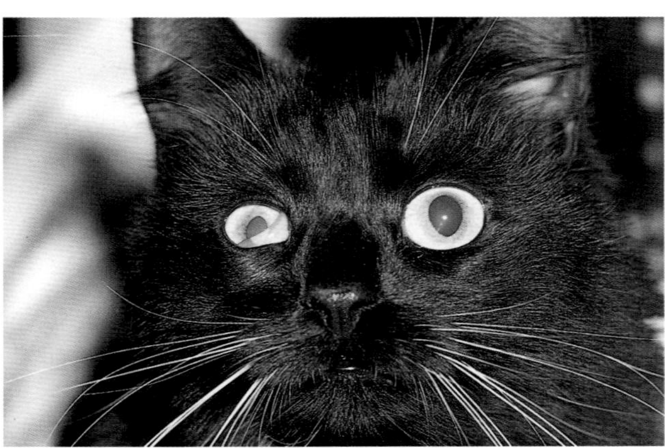

Fig. 15.8 *A 7-month-old Domestic longhair with unilateral Horner's syndrome (right side affected) which developed after the ears had been cleaned with a detergent solution. Note the ptosis, miosis, enophthalmos and prominence of the third eyelid which is present.*

Horner's syndrome can be classified according to the site of involvement: as central (first order), preganglionic (second order) and postganglionic lesions (third order). Pharmacological testing for lesion localization, based on the principle of denervation hypersensitivity, is possible using a directly acting agent such as topical 1% phenylephrine (10% phenylephrine diluted 1:10 with saline); the results obtained will vary according to the time after the insult, the completeness of the lesion and its distance from the iris. The normal eye will not respond to the weak concentration of the drug. If the lesion is postganglionic the pupil dilates within 20 min, whereas if the lesion is preganglionic the pupil will take 30–40 min to dilate. An indirectly acting agent such as hydroxyamphetamine can also be used, but the tests must be performed on different days. Further details of pharmacological testing can be obtained from Collins and O'Brien (1990).

In some cases of Horner's syndrome the aetiology cannot be identified, but common identifiable causes include head or neck trauma (damage to the vagosympathetic trunk),

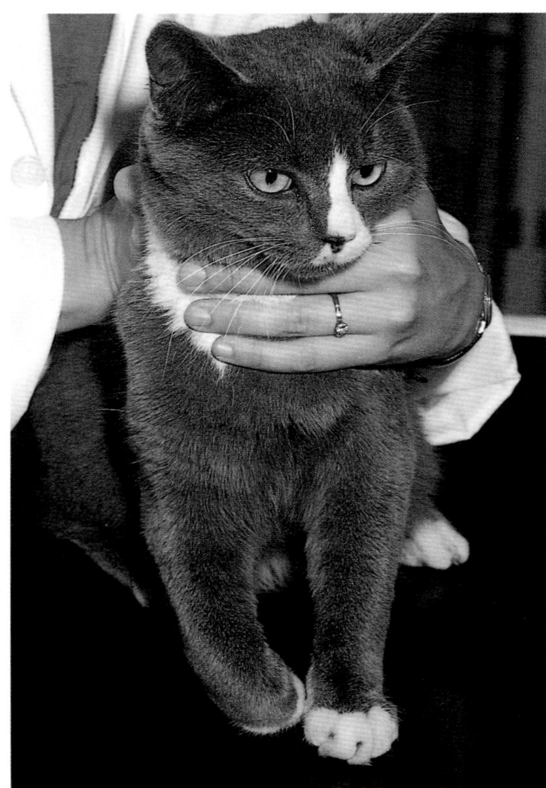

Fig. 15.9 *A 10-month-old Domestic shorthair. Unilateral Horner's syndrome (right side affected) which developed after a road traffic accident (avulsion of the brachial plexus). Note the anisocoria with a more constricted pupil on the right, although the third eyelid is not noticably prominent. Radial nerve paralysis is also present on the right side.*

anterior mediastinal disease (e.g. anterior mediastinal lymphosarcoma), brachial plexus and chest trauma, middle/inner ear disease (may be concurrent vestibular syndrome) and iatrogenic damage (during surgery of the neck or tympanic bulla). In cats, second-order Horner's syndrome may present with concurrent ipsilateral laryngeal hemiplegia (Holland, 1996).

Unilateral mydriasis Lesions affecting the afferent arm of the light reflex pathway (Fig. 15.10), the parasympathetic component of the oculomotor nerve (CN III) or the oculomotor nucleus, may result in unilateral mydriasis. Oculomotor dysfunction is uncommon, but underlying causes include trauma and neoplasia. If paralysis is complete, the pupil will be widely dilated and unresponsive to bright light, but vision is unaffected. Unless the damage is restricted to the parasympathetic part of the nerve/nucleus, other signs of oculomotor damage should be seen (i.e. ventrolateral strabismus with or without ptosis). The term 'internal ophthalmoplegia' is applied to paralysis of the intraocular muscles (i.e. iris sphincter and ciliary body muscles).

Unilateral mydriasis may sometimes be seen with lateralized cerebellar disease (there is contralateral pupillary dilation). The anisocoria will be accompanied by primary signs of cerebellar disease.

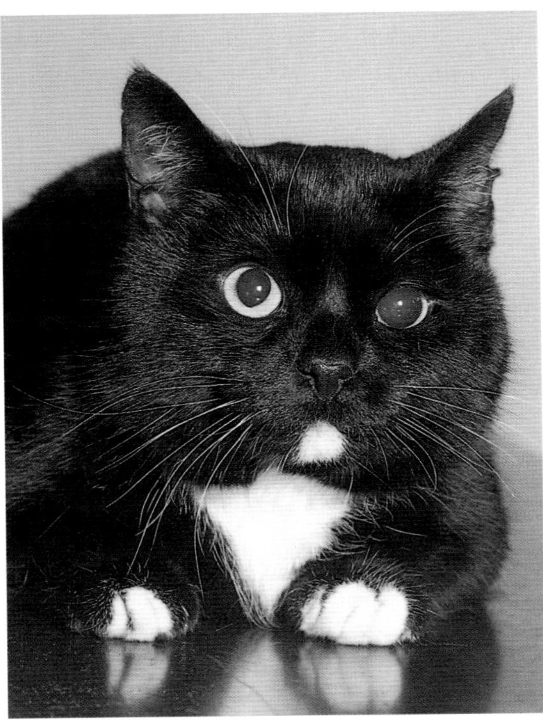

Fig. 15.10 *An 8-year-old Domestic shorthair. Anisocoria with the affected eye (dilated pupil) on the left. The left eye was blind as a consequence of previous traumatic proptosis, permanent facial nerve (VII) damage was also present. Retraction of the globe and rapid protrusion of the third eyelid provided an effective alternative to normal blinking and tear replacement therapy provided ocular surface lubrication. The right eye of this cat is illustrated in Fig. 14.42.*

Static anisocoria (Spastic pupil syndrome) Partial bilateral miosis with mild anisocoria which remains partially or completely unchanged during dark adaptation (static anisocoria) has been reported in association with FeLV-infection, possibly as a direct result of viral infection of the short ciliary nerves or ciliary ganglia. Vision is unaffected. The severity of the changes may alter and signs may even be intermittent early in the disease. Occasionally, affected animals present with bilateral partial mydriasis, rather than miosis. Static anisocoria may also be associated with other viruses such as feline immunodeficiency virus (Fig. 15.11).

Hemidilated pupil (partial internal ophthalmoplegia, 'D-shaped' pupil) This refers to the condition where only one of the two ciliary nerves supplying the iris constrictor muscle is paralysed, which results in a 'D-shaped' or 'reverse D-shaped' pupil, depending on which of the two nerves is affected (Figs 15.12 and 15.13). If, for example, the lateral (malar) nerve is damaged, a D-shaped pupil will be observed if the left eye is affected and a reverse D if the right eye is affected. Conversely, damage to the medial

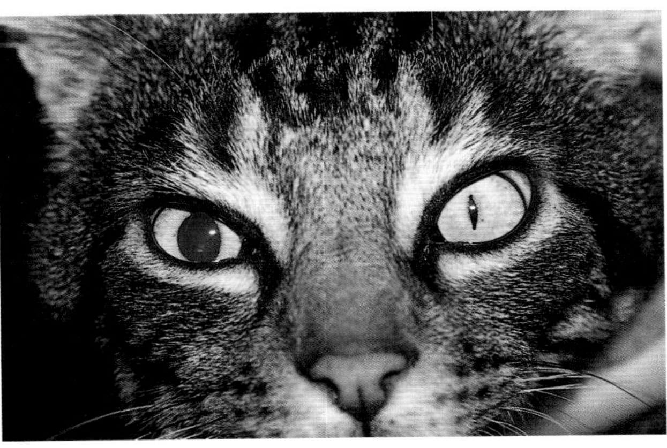

Fig. 15.11 *A 3-year-old Domestic shorthair. Static anisocoria ('spastic pupil syndrome') associated with FIV.*

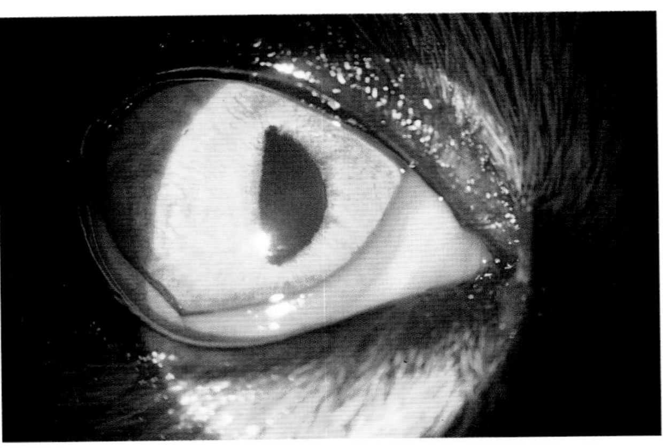

Fig. 15.12 *A 10-year-old Domestic shorthair with damage to the nasal ciliary nerve of the right eye resulting in a 'D'-shaped pupil. The cat also had bilateral posterior uveitis and was FIV positive.*

(nasal) short ciliary nerve will produce a D-shaped pupil if the right eye is affected and a reverse D if the left eye is affected. This type of ophthalmoplegia may be seen, for example, in FeLV-associated lymphosarcoma infiltration of one ciliary nerve.

Bilateral Mydriasis

Bilateral mydriasis with intact vision has been associated with a variety of neurological conditions.

Dysautonomia Although not as common in the UK now as when originally reported (Key and Gaskell, 1982) cases of feline dysautonomia still occur in Europe and, less commonly, the USA. The sympathetic and parasympathetic systems are both affected. Bilateral, dilated, unresponsive pupils, often accompanied by third eyelid protrusion (Fig. 15.14), reduced tear production and photophobia, are common ocular signs. Other evidence of generalized dysautonomia is usually evident (for example, depression, anorexia, weight loss, dry mucous membranes, intermittent regurgitation, megoesophagus, ileus, constipation, urinary retention, bradycardia), but in some cases classical clinical signs may be absent or less prominent. Degeneration of autonomic nerves and ganglia is seen on post-mortem examination.

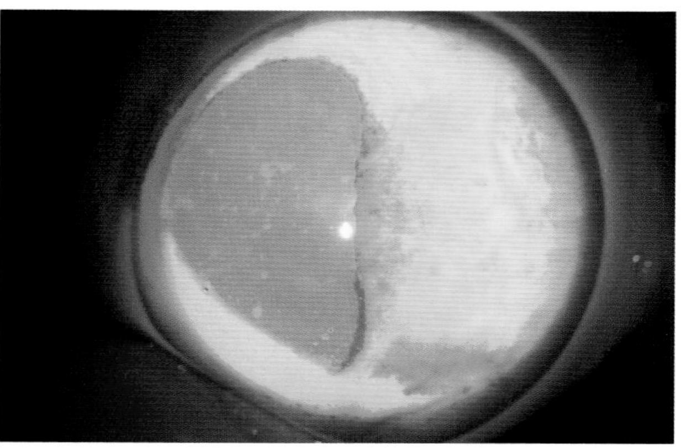

Fig. 15.13 *Adult Domestic shorthair with damage to the nasal ciliary nerve of the left eye resulting in a reverse 'D' pupil. This was associated with lymphosarcoma.*

Application of one drop of 0.1% pilocarpine to the eye of an affected cat may produce miosis and third eyelid retraction within minutes (Fig. 15.15) as a result of denervation hypersensitivity in established cases, whereas topical application of 0.25% physostigmine sulphate should have no effect (Guilford *et al.*, 1988). If both drugs are used the indirectly acting physostigmine should be given first, followed by the directly acting pilocarpine the next day. However, pharmacological testing can be stressful and the disadvantages may outweigh the advantages in sick cats. These agents should not be used as a form of therapy.

The management of dysautonomia cases requires good nursing care, with parenteral feeding or feeding via a pharyngostomy tube during the acute phase and moist food thereafter, until the mucous membranes are no longer dry. Tear replacement therapy (e.g. 0.2% polyacrylic acid, Viscotears CIBA Vision; 0.2% w/w Carbomer 940, GelTears, Chauvin) is also necessary until tear production has returned to normal. The prognosis is guarded in severely incapacitated cats and nursing care is required for months, even in successfully treated cases. Recovery may be partial in some cats and stress may trigger apparent relapses in others.

Hepatic encephalopathy During encephalopathic episodes, some cats will exhibit bilateral mydriasis. This is invariably accompanied by other neurological signs such as ataxia, altered behaviour and hypersalivation.

Feline spongiform encephalopathy (FSE) Bilateral mydriasis and blindness have been a feature of some cats with FSE. The pupillary light response may be poor or absent. Other ocular abnormalities are usually absent (Fig. 15.16). A range of neurological signs such as persistent and progressive ataxia, altered behaviour (e.g. extreme apprehension) and ptyalism are also present. The diagnosis is confirmed by brain histopathology (Gruffydd-Jones *et al.*, 1991).

Thiamine deficiency Clinical signs of thiamine (vitamin B_1) deficiency in cats are characteristic and include anorexia, cerebellar-type ataxia, ventroflexion of the neck and bilateral

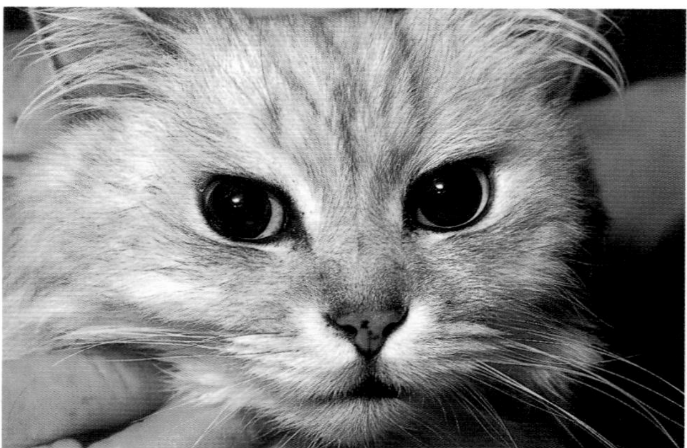

Fig. 15.14 *A 6-year-old Persian neutered male. Dysautonomia with bilateral dilation of the pupils.*

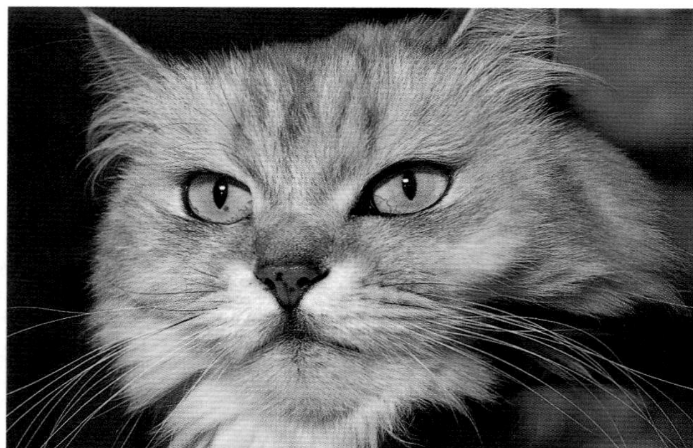

Fig. 15.15 *The same cat as illustrated in Figure 15.12, 20 min after the application of 0.1% pilocarpine.*

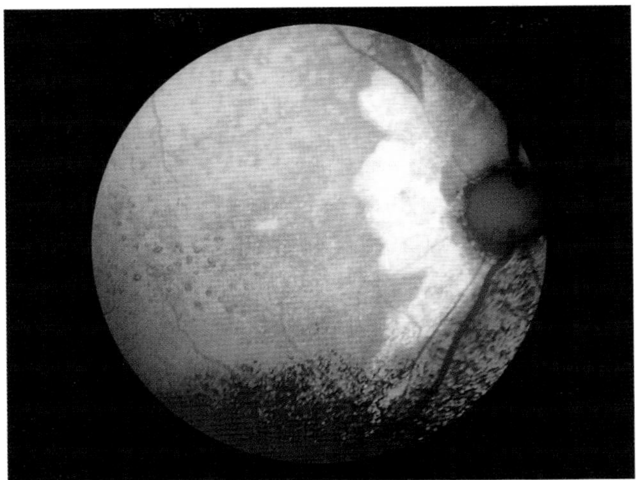

Fig. 15.16 A 4-year-old Siamese cross neutered male. Unusual fundus appearance in a cat with feline spongiform encephalopathy.

mydriasis. Fundus examination may reveal peripapillary oedema and papillary neovascularization (Fig. 14.41), but these are not specific for thiamine deficiency as inflammatory and neoplastic conditions may produce similar changes (see Chapter 14). Treatment includes systemic corticosteroids to reduce the oedema in addition to thiamine to correct the deficit; both may be given intravenously initially.

Acute brain disease Mydriasis may accompany acute generalized diseases of the midbrain such as swelling or compression. If the mydriasis is bilateral it carries a grave prognosis. The potential clinical signs of central nervous system trauma and its management are beyond the scope of this book, but further details may be found elsewhere (Griffiths, 1987; Hopkins, 1995).

Cavernous Sinus Syndrome

The cavernous sinus is a venous sinus on either side of the pituitary fossa, but also contains fibres of all the cranial nerves, except the optic nerve, that innervate the globe. Many disease processes can affect the cavernous sinus; for example, neoplasia, inflammatory diseases and vascular disorders can affect this site and cause unilateral or bilateral fixed (slightly mydriatic) pupils and loss of ocular motility. There may also be ptosis and third eyelid prominence and, occasionally, strabismus will be present depending upon specific or multiple cranial nerve palsies (Fig. 15.17). Cavernous sinus syndrome is the commonest reason for complete ophthalmoplegia (paralysis of extraocular and intraocular muscles).

Bilateral Miosis

Organophosphate poisoning Profound miosis (Fig. 15.18) is one of the characteristics of organophosphate poisoning, and is accompanied by other neurological signs such as ptyalism, vomiting and diarrhoea, abdominal cramps, muscle twitching, fasciculations and even convulsions (Wheeler, 1993).

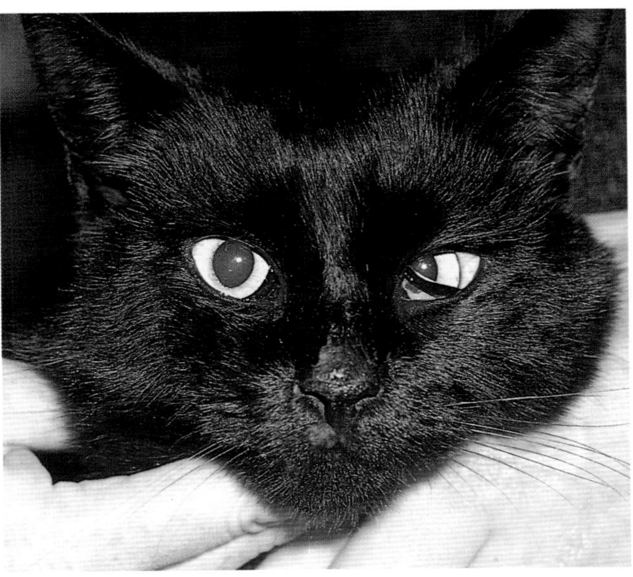

Fig. 15.17 Domestic shorthair with mild ptosis, mydriasis and obvious esotropia (medial squint) associated with the cavernous sinus syndrome.

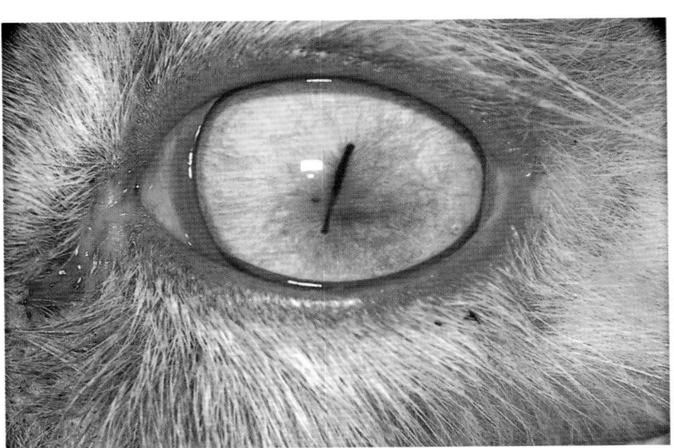

Fig. 15.18 A 2-year-old Birman with bilateral miosis associated with organophosphate poisoning; the left eye is illustrated.

Acute brain disease As with mydriasis, miosis can be a feature of severe midbrain disease (Fig. 15.19), possibly as a result of loss of inhibition from higher centres (e.g. because of severe midbrain compression associated with tentorial herniation). The prognosis is grave when pupils progress from miotic to mydriatic.

VISUAL DEFICITS ASSOCIATED WITH THE CENTRAL VISUAL PATHWAY

Those abnormalities which can affect vision and which are routinely detectable by ophthalmoscopy have been described earlier (see Chapters 12 and 14) and include congenital abnormalities such as optic nerve aplasia, optic nerve hypoplasia and optic nerve colobomas and acquired prob-

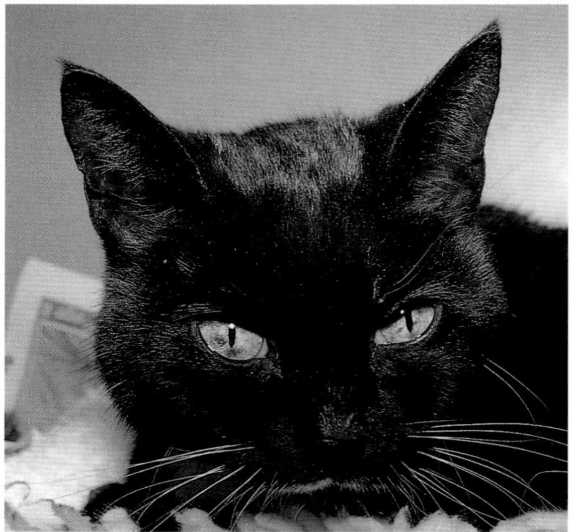

Fig. 15.19 *Domestic shorthair with bilateral miosis associated with a brain tumour.*

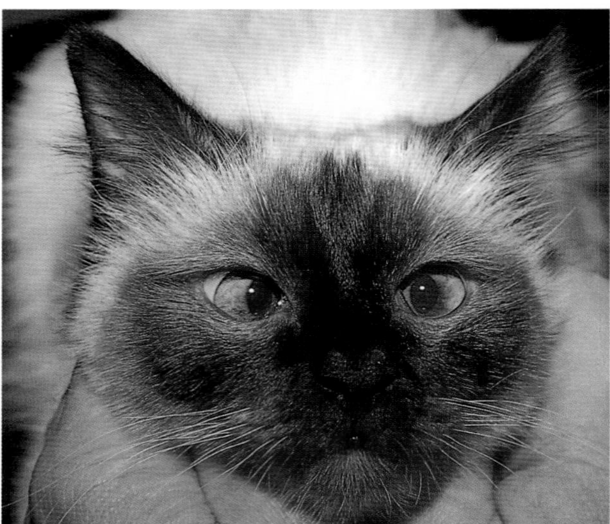

Fig. 15.20 *Birman cat with early onset convergent strabismus.*

lems such as optic neuritis and optic atrophy. This section describes some of the conditions which may affect the central visual pathway from the optic nerve to the occipital cortex of the cerebral cortex.

Visual deficits may be difficult to detect and partial deficits often go unnoticed by all but the most observant owner. They are equally difficult to demonstrate on clinical examination, but occasionally the configuration may be so distinctive as to allow precise localization of the lesion and this, in turn, may lead to an understanding of its cause. Undoubtedly, it is much more difficult to reach a precise diagnosis in cats compared with humans, but improved imaging techniques, in particular the introduction of magnetic resonance imaging, have opened up exciting possibilities for the future.

It is customary to place the lesions of the central visual pathway in four categories and these are summarised in Table 15.1. Some examples of neurological disorders which affect the central visual pathway follow.

Abnormal Visual Pathways

Convergent strabismus (Fig. 15.20) and nystagmus are common abnormalities in imperfect albinos such as Siamese and Himalayan cats in which pigment production is deficient (Creel, 1971; Johnson, 1991). Other breeds (e.g. Birman) may also be affected on occasions. Melanin, an essential regulator of axonal growth, is deficient in the retinal pigment epithelium of these breeds and this leads to misdirected axonal projections from the eye to the brain, so that central visual pathways do not develop properly. The misrouting of the central visual fibres results in reduced visual acuity and absence of binocular vision. The convergent strabismus (esotropia) which develops at about 3 months in some cats is probably a consequence of abnormal visual perception and attempts by the brain to create a complete visual field. The mechanism underlying the nystagmus which is present in most affected cats, is less well understood, but may result from contradictory information perceived at the level of the mesencephalon.

Hydrocephalus

Hydrocephalus denotes, in general terms, an increase in the volume of cerebrospinal fluid (CSF). Hydrocephalus in cats is likely to be either a congenital problem because of malformation and hypoplasia of brain tissue or acquired because of ischaemic encephalopathy, neoplasia or severe meningitis and ependymitis (e.g. feline infectious peritonitis).

Congenital hydrocephalus is associated with abnormal skull shape, including an enlarged calvaria with open sutures (Fig. 15.21). The bony orbits are also enlarged and the globes are displaced ventrolaterally, probably as a consequence of the orbital malformation rather than neuropraxia. Teratogenic damage from drugs such as griseofulvin or infection with the feline panleukopenia virus may induce congenital hydrocephalus.

Hydrocephalus occurring as a result of ischaemic encephalopathy is caused by a compensatory increase of CSF volume which fills the space resulting from tissue destruction. Neoplasia and severe inflammation usually produce hydrocephalus because of obstruction to the flow of CSF, or interference with its absorption.

The clinical signs are variable, although affected animals invariably demonstrate behavioural changes such as lethargy. Bilateral visual deficits with a normal pupillary light response is the most common and consistent sign observed in affected cats (De Lahunta, 1983). Depending on the cause, and whether or not CSF pressure is raised, other neuro-ophthalmological changes may be present (Fig. 15.22). The management of hydrocephalus depends upon establishing the cause and specialist neurological advice will be needed; many cases are not amenable to treatment.

Table 15.1 Lesions of the Central Visual Pathway

Pre-chiasmal lesions	
Vision	Visual deficit: either partial or total blindness results. One or both eyes can be affected
PLR	Unilateral lesions: static anisocoria in normal light with pupil of affected eye slightly more dilated. Both pupils evenly dilated in darkness. An abnormal swinging flashlight test is demonstrable. The direct and consensual PLR from the affected eye are absent Bilateral lesions: fixed, dilated pupils
Aetiology	Retrobulbar optic neuritis, neoplasia, trauma and optic nerve compression
Chiasmal lesions	
Vision	Total lesions cause total blindness in both eyes. Incomplete lesions may lead to partial bilateral deficits (e.g. loss of lateral visual fields – bitemporal hemianopsia)
PLR	Complete lesions lead to bilateral fixed dilated pupils. Partial lesions produce variable effects
Aetiology	Cerebral vascular infarction (resulting in ischaemic necrosis of the optic chiasm), neoplasia (rare), inflammation and abscessation
Optic tract lesions	
Vision	Vision is not always affected and it may be difficult to demonstrate visual defects in other cases. Bilateral involvement is rare Unilateral lesions: loss of medial visual field in eye ipsilateral to lesion, loss of lateral field in contralateral eye (incongruous homonymous hemianopsia). Field loss is greatest in the eye contralateral to the tract lesion Hemisensory and hemimotor defects affecting the side of the body contralateral to the lesion may also be present
PLR	Proximal (rostral) two-thirds: unilateral lesions, static anisocoria in normal light. An afferent pupillary defect may be seen in the eye contralateral to the tract lesion Distal (caudal) one-third: The afferent pupillary fibres leave the optic tract some two-thirds of the way along the optic tract, so lesions of the distal one-third produce no defect of PLR
Aetiology	Space-occupying lesions, inflammation and abscessation, vascular infarction and ischaemia. Most cases are unilateral but severe inflammation may produce bilateral involvement
Lesions of the lateral geniculate nucleus, optic radiation and occipital cortex	
Vision	Homonomous hemianopsia as described for unilateral optic tract lesions
PLR	Unaffected, as described for unilateral optic tract lesions affecting the distal one-third of the tract
Aetiology	Unilateral lesions: space-occupying lesions (e.g. neoplasia, haemorrhage), inflammation (encephalitis, meningoencephalomyelitis) and abscessation, trauma, vascular infarction Bilateral lesions: space-occupying lesions, inflammation (encephalitis) and abscessation, trauma, toxins (e.g. lead poisoning, hepatoencephalopathy)

Lysosomal Storage Diseases

A number of recessively inherited neurometabolic storage diseases have been described in the cat and others await description (see also Chapters 9 and 14). Although neurological signs are common to many of these diseases, their characterization is neither complete nor precise. Blindness is usually the result of central neuropathy and can occur for example in the gangliosidoses (Fig. 15.23) and sphingomyelinosis. Mucopolysaccharidosis I has also been associated with meningiomas and hydrocephalus (Haskins and McGrath, 1983).

Anoxia, Hypoxia and Ischaemia

See Chapter 3.

Vascular Infarction

Cerebral infarction may occur in a variety of sites. For example, those in the region of the optic chiasm result in bilateral blindness with bilateral dilated pupils, whereas those which involve the occipital (visual) cortex and optic radiation result in unilateral visual impairment and a normal pupillary light response.

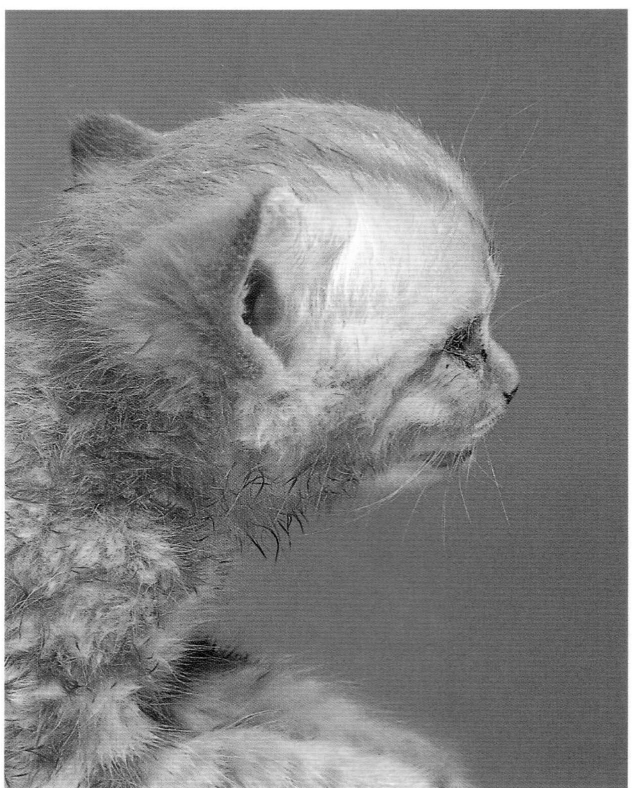

Fig. 15.21 *Domestic shorthair kitten with congenital hydrocephalus. Note the obviously domed skull. (Courtesy of D. A. Gunn-Moore.)*

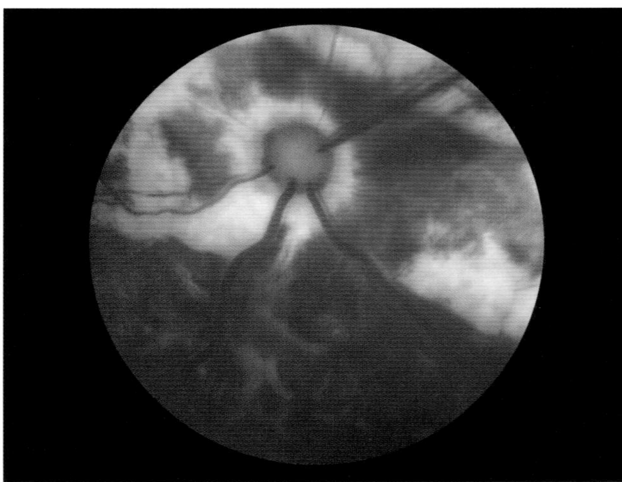

Fig. 15.22 *A 1-year-old Domestic shorthair. Acquired hydrocephalus associated with feline infectious peritonitis. Note the extensive haemorrhage and papilloedema. Intracranial pressure and cerebro-spinal fluid pressure were raised.*

Others

A number of infectious and inflammatory diseases may be associated with central visual deficits and blindness,

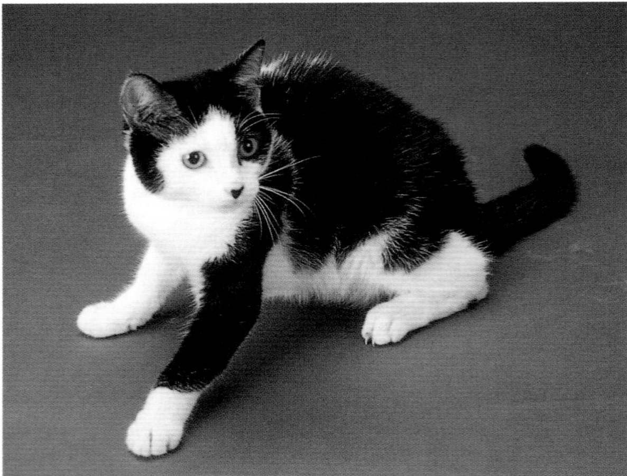

Fig. 15.23 *Domestic shorthair kitten. GM_1 gangliosidosis. Mild diffuse corneal clouding, discrete focal retinal opacities and defective vision were present. Note the wide-based stance; the kitten was also ataxic.*

although it is often the case that no visual abnormalities are detected. Most of these conditions have been described in Chapters 12 and 14. Those which have been associated with defective vision include feline infectious peritonitis, the feline leukaemia–lymphosarcoma complex, feline immunodeficiency virus, toxoplasmosis and mycotic infections.

Neurological abnormalities of eye position and movement

The quality of the visual image is dependent on two principal types of eye movement: those that keep images steady on the retina via the vestibular and optokinetic systems and those that change the line of sight, mainly via the saccadic system (Scagliotti, 1990). Assessment of abnormal eye position and movement is complex and beyond the scope of this book; a comprehensive overview of neuro-ophthalmology is provided by Scagliotti (1990).

The vestibulo-ocular reflex (VOR) acts to steady retinal images during head movement by producing eye movement which is equal and opposite. Sensory cells within the semicircular canals detect the motion, the vestibular nerve transmits the signal and the motor control is effected via CN III, IV and VI.

Saccadic eye movements are the most rapid of eye movements; they enable the eye to redirect the line of sight so that the subject of interest will be focused on that part of the retina with the best visual acuity (the area centralis under normal lighting conditions). Saccadic eye movements include voluntary and involuntary changes of fixation and the quick phases of vestibular and optokinetic nystagmus.

Strabismus is the term used to describe ocular misalignment. Inborn defects are usually the result of benign misrouting of the central visual fibres, as already outlined for the Siamese and Himalayan cat. Acquired abnormalities (Fig. 15.17) are usually peripheral as a consequence of damage to the extraocular muscles or their nerve supply (see also under cranial nerve assessment and cavernous sinus syndrome) and the term external ophthalmoplegia describes the paralysis of the extraocular muscles which may result.

Nystagmus is an involuntary rhythmical movement of the eyes with a slow and a fast phase. Congenital nystagmus is most commonly associated with the abnormal visual pathways of the Siamese and Himalayan cat. Acquired nystagmus is most likely to be seen in association with early vision loss (e.g. early-onset generalized progressive retinal atrophy) and vestibular disease (both central and peripheral).

Neurological abnormalities affecting the adnexa

Disorders of Eyelid Closure

Closure of the eyelids is performed by the orbicularis oculi muscle under the influence of the palpebral branch of the facial nerve (CN VII). Damage to this efferent nerve will lead to inability to close the eyelids and the menace response will also be negative. Because the optic and trigeminal nerves mediate the afferent arm of eyelid closure it is important to separate the various nerve components during assessment of any one of them.

A peripheral cause of facial nerve dysfunction is trauma to the nerve as it crosses the temporal region of the zygomatic arch. Despite defective eyelid closure the cornea can appear clinically normal; this is because lesions at this location spare the innervation to the lacrimal gland, hence tear production is unaffected, futhermore, third eyelid function is intact, so that the distribution of the tear film remains normal.

More central lesions may lead to facial asymmetry, drooping of the lip, drooling of saliva, deviation of the nasal philtrum and reduced tear production (Fig. 15.24). This can occur because of trauma, otitis media, neoplasia and as a complication, albeit temporary, of aural surgery, especially bulla osteotomy (Fig. 15.25). Corneal devitalization is more common in these animals because of the concurrent tear film abnormality. One drop of 1% pilocarpine added to the food twice daily may stimulate tear production in these cases, but cats object both to the adulterated food and the side-effects of the drug, so tear replacement therapy may be a more practical alternative. Tarsorrhaphy, a third eyelid flap, or a conjunctival graft is occasionally indicated.

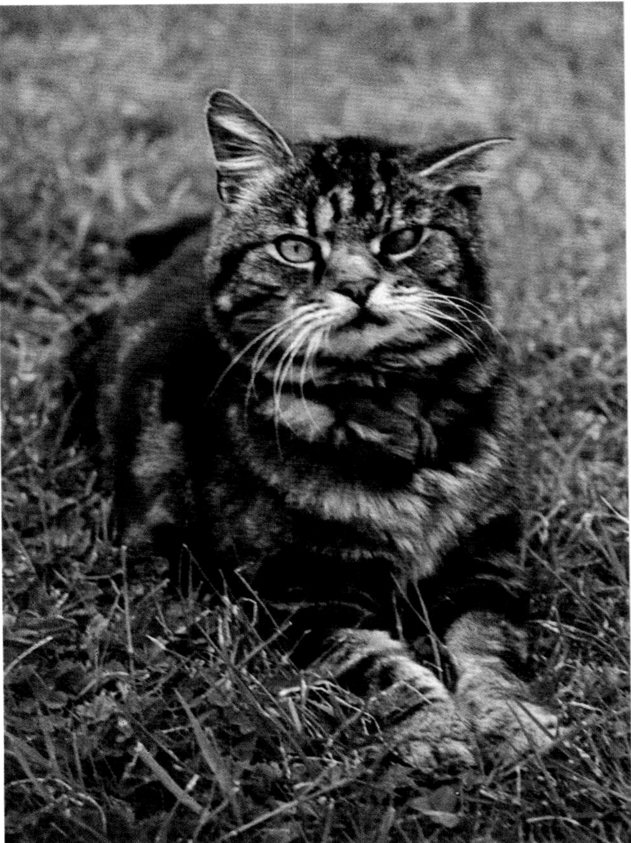

Fig. 15.24 *A 14-year-old Domestic shorthair with permanent facial nerve paralysis (left side) following head injury in a road traffic accident. Note facial asymmetry and keratitis resulting from reduced tear production and inability to close the eye.*

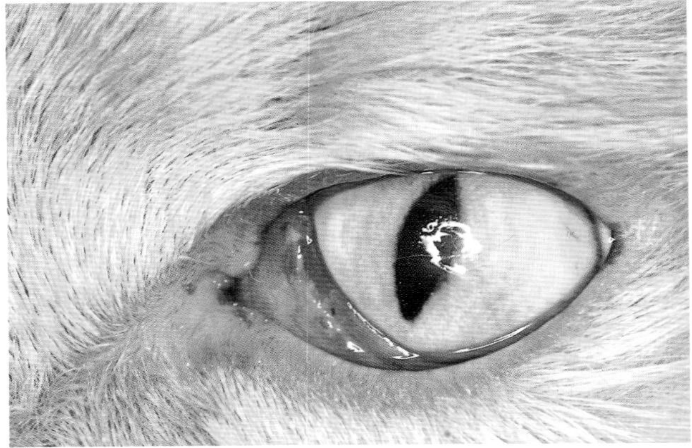

Fig. 15.25 *Domestic shorthair with temporary facial nerve paresis and Horner's syndrome after a left-sided bulla osteotomy. Note the mild exposure keratopathy.*

Disorders of Eyelid Opening

Ptosis, or drooping of the upper lid, can occur because of damage to the oculomotor nerve at any level, or less commonly, because of direct damage to the levator palpebrae superioris muscle. The oculomotor nerve innervates most of the extraocular muscles and parasympathetic fibres supply the iris sphincter muscle, so it is sometimes possible to localize the site of damage with reasonable precision.

Ptosis is also a feature of Horner's syndrome (see above) as a consequence of damage to the efferent sympathetic pathway. In Horner's syndrome the upper eyelid droops and the lower eyelid is slightly elevated so that the palpebral fissure is narrowed (Fig. 15.8). The other features of the syndrome (third eyelid prominence, miosis and enophthalmos) should simplify diagnosis.

Disorders of the Third Eyelid

The third eyelid has both smooth muscle (supplied by sympathetic nerves) and skeletal muscle (an extension of the lateral rectus innervated by the abducens nerve CN VI). The normal state of retraction of the third eyelid is due to sympathetic tone in the third eyelid smooth muscle and orbital smooth muscle; loss of sympathetic tone (Horner's syndrome) thus leads to third eyelid prominence (Fig. 15.8) which has been described earlier. Damage to the abducens nerve or its nucleus may also result in third eyelid prominence (Fig. 15.17).

Chronic diarrhoea is sometimes associated with bilateral prominence of the third eyelid (see Chapter 6).

Tetanus is an occasional disease of the cat and is usually a result of wound contamination (Fig. 15.26). In addition to the usual hypersensitivity to sound and touch, and the rigidity and stiffness which typify the condition, affected animals may exhibit brief and rapid bilateral protrusion of the third eyelids.

Disorders of Lacrimation

Three different types of lacrimation can be distinguished (see also Chapter 7). Reflex tear production results from exposure to wind, cold, light, chemicals and foreign bodies for example, and is mediated via free sensory nerve endings of the trigeminal nerve (afferent pathway) and parasympathetic fibres in the facial nerve (efferent pathway). Basal (i.e. continuous) tear production in the cat is by accessory lacrimal glands, including the seromucous superficial gland of the third eyelid, and this also is under the control of the parasympathetic nervous system (Fig. 15.10). The third type of lacrimation (induced tear production) is initiated by a variety of drugs, notably those agents which act by causing direct irritation or allergic reaction, as well as those such as pilocarpine which induce tearing by their direct parasympathomimetic action on the secretory cells of the lacrimal gland (Scagliotti, 1990).

Assessment The Schirmer I and Schirmer II tear tests are used to provide a quantitative assessment of combined basal and reflex production and basal production alone respectively. Further details of tear film assessment and tear film disorders are given in Chapters 1 and 7 respectively.

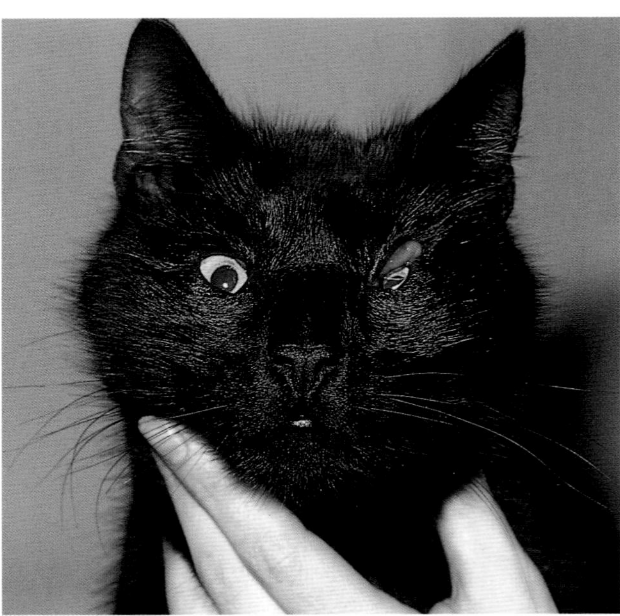

Fig. 15.26 *Young adult Domestic shorthair. Tetanus developed following a puncture wound penetrating the skull as well as the overlying skin and muscle. The cat made a full recovery after treatment.*

References

Bercovitch M, Krohne S, Lindley D (1995) A diagnostic approach to anisocoria. *The Compendium on Continuing Education for the Practicing Veterinarian* **17**: 661–673.

Chrisman CL (1991) *Problems in Small Animal Neurology*, 2nd edn. Philadelphia, Lea and Febiger.

Collins BK, O'Brien DP (1990) Autonomic dysfunction of the eye. *Seminars in Veterinary Medicine and Surgery* **5**: 24–36.

Creel DJ (1971) Visual anomaly associated with albinism in the cat. *Nature* **231**: 465–466.

De Lahunta A (1983) *Veterinary Neuroanatomy and Clinical Neurology*, 2nd edn. WB Saunders, Philadelphia.

Griffiths IR (1987) Central nervous system trauma. In Oliver JE, Hoerlein BF, Mayhew IG (eds) *Veterinary Neurology*, pp. 303–320. WB Saunders Co, Philadelphia.

Gruffydd-Jones TJ, Galloway PE, Pearson GR (1991) Feline spongiform encephalopathy. *Journal of Small Animal Practice* **33**: 471–476.

Guilford WG, O'Brien DP, Aller A, Ermeling HM (1988) Diagnosis of dysautonomia in a cat by autonomic nervous system function testing. *Journal of the American Veterinary Medical Association* **193**: 823–828.

Haskins ME, McGrath JT (1983) Meningiomas in young cats with mucopolysaccharidosis I. *Journal of Neuropathology and Experimental Neurology* **42**: 664–670.

Holland CT (1996) Horner's syndrome and ipselateral laryngeal hemiplegia in three cats. *Journal of Small Animal Practice* **37**: 442–446.

Hopkins AL (1995) Special neurology of the cat. *In* Wheeler SJ (ed) *Manual of Small Animal Neurology*, 2nd edn, pp. 219–232. BSAVA Publications.

Johnson BW (1991) Congenitally abnormal visual pathways of Siamese cats. *The Compendium on Continuing Education for the Practicing Veterinarian* **13**: 374–377.

Kern TJ, Aramondo MC, Erb HN (1989) Horner's syndrome in cats and dogs: 100 cases (1975–1985). *Journal of the American Veterinary Medical Association* **195**: 369–373.

Key T, Gaskell CJ (1982) Puzzling syndrome in cats associated with pupillary dilation (correspondence). *Veterinary Record* **110**: 160.

Moreau PM, Wheeler SJ (1995) Examination of the head. In Wheeler SJ (ed) *Manual of Small Animal Neurology*, 2nd edn, BSAVA Publications. pp. 13–26.

Morgan RV, Zanotti SW (1989) Horner's syndrome in dogs and cats: 49 cases (1980–1986). *Journal of the American Veterinary Medical Association* **194**: 1096–1099.

Neer TM (1984) Horner's syndrome: Anatomy, diagnosis and causes. *The Compendium on Continuing Education for the Practicing Veterinarian* **6**: 740–746.

Neer TM, Carter JD (1987) Anisocoria in dogs and cats: ocular and neurologic causes. *Compendium on Continuing Education for the Practicing Veterinarian* **9**: 817–823.

Oliver JE, Hoerlein BF, Mayhew IG (eds) (1987) *Veterinary Neurology*. WB Saunders Co, Philadelphia.

Petersen-Jones SM (1995) Abnormalities of Eyes and Vision. In Wheeler SJ (ed) *Manual of Small Animal Neurology*, 2nd edn, BSAVA Publications. pp. 125–142.

Scagliotti RH (1990) Neuro-ophthalmology. *Progress in Veterinary Neurology* **1**: 157–170.

van den Broek AHM (1987) Horner's syndrome in cats and dogs: A review. *Journal of Small Animal Practice* **28**: 929–940.

Wheeler SJ (1993) Disorders of the Nervous System. In Wills J, Wolf A (eds) *Handbook of Feline Medicine*. Pergamon, Oxford. pp. 267–282.

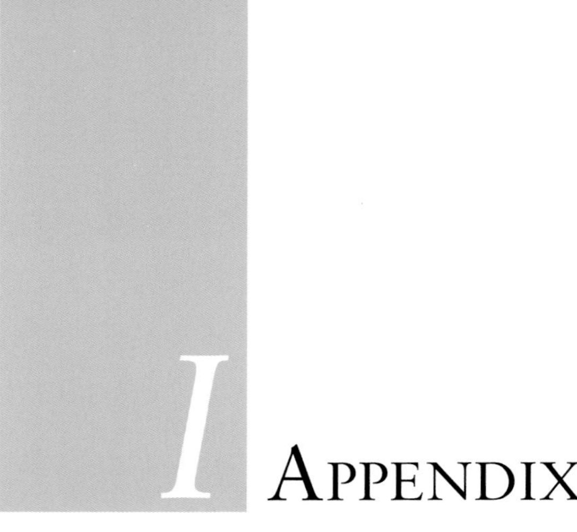

I Appendix

Equipment

Basic Instruments

Condensing lens (e.g. Heine, Nikon, Volk or Welch Allyn)
Direct ophthalmoscope (e.g. Heine, Keeler or Welch Allyn)
Magnifying loupe (e.g. Heine or Keeler)
Otoscope (e.g. Heine, Keeler or Welch Allyn)
Pen-light (e.g. Heine, Keeler or Welch Allyn)

Additional Instruments

Aesthesiometer
Binocular indirect ophthalmoscope (e.g. Clement Clarke, Heine, Keeler, Welch Allyn)
Finoff transilluminator (e.g. Heine, Keeler or Welch Allyn)
Hand-held fundus camera (Kowa Genesis; Keeler)
Monocular indirect ophthalmoscope (American Optical Company; Reichert Ophthalmic Instruments)
Portable slit lamp biomicroscope (e.g. Kowa SL 14; Keeler, Haag-Streit 904, Clement Clarke)
Tonometer (Schiøtz tonometer or some form of electronic applanation tonometer)

Disposables

Cotton wool
Lacrimal cannulae (metal or plastic)
Mydriatic (1% tropicamide, Mydriacyl; Alcon)
Ophthalmic stains (1% fluorescein sodium, Minims Fluorescein Sodium and 1% Rose Bengal, Minims Rose Bengal, both preparations manufactured by Smith and Nephew)
Routine culture media (e.g. blood agar, Sabouraud's agar)
Schirmer tear test papers (Sno Strips; Smith and Nephew)
Spatula and glass slides for cytology
Swabs for bacteriological culture and viral isolation
Topical local anaesthetic (0.5% proxymetacaine hydrochloride, Ophthaine; Squibb)
Viral and chlamydial transport medium

II Appendix

Congenital and early onset anomalies

Chapter 4: Globe and orbit

Anophthalmos
Buphthalmos
Cyclopia
Microphthalmos
Nystagmus
Ophthalmia neonatorum
Strabismus

Chapter 5: Upper and lower eyelids

Agenesis and coloboma
Ankyloblepharon
Dermoid
Incomplete development of canthus
Ophthalmia neonatorum

Chapter 7: lacrimal system

Atresia and hypoplasia of the naso-lacrimal system

Chapter 8: Conjunctiva, limbus, episclera and sclera

Anterior segment dysgenesis
Dermoid
Symblepharon

Chapter 9: Cornea

Dermoid
Microcornea/megalocornea

Chapter 10: Aqueous and glaucoma

Buphthalmos

Chapter 11: Lens

Aphakia
Cataract
Coloboma
Lenticonus
Microphakia

Chapter 12: Uveal tract

Abnormal pupil shape
Albinism
Coloboma
Heterochromia
Hypoplasia
Persistent pupillary membrane

Chapter 13: Vitreous

Persistent hyaloid artery

Chapter 14: Fundus

Aplasia/hypoplasia optic nerve
Coloboma retina/optic nerve
Retinal dysplasia

Chapter 15: Neuro-ophthalmology

Hydrocephalus
Nystagmus
Strabismus

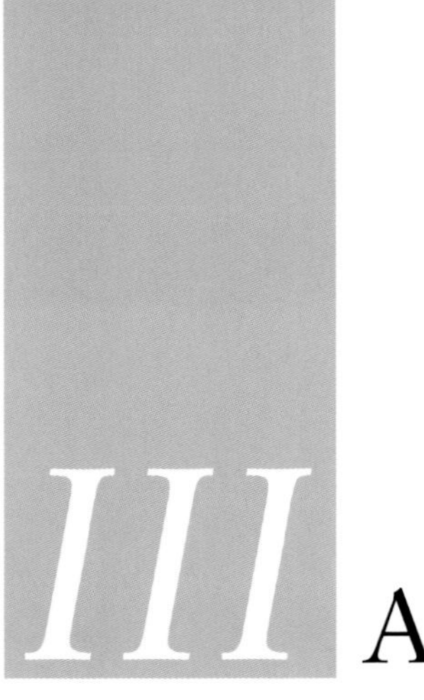

III Appendix

Hereditary eye disease

Chapter 4: Globe and orbit

Nystagmus (Siamese)
Strabismus (Siamese and Himalayan)

Chapter 5: Upper and lower eyelids

Ankyloblepharon (Persian)
Dermoid (Burmese and Birman)
Entropion (Persian)
Incomplete development of canthus (Burmese)

Chapter 8: Conjunctiva, limbus, episclera and sclera

Dermoid (Birman)

Chapter 9: Cornea

Corneal sequestrum (Birman, Burmese, Colourpoint, Himalayan, Persian, Siamese)
Dermoid (Birman)
Endothelial corneal dystrophy (Domestic shorthair)
Lysosomal storage disease (Domestic shorthair)
Stromal corneal dystrophy (Manx)

Chapter 11: Lens

Cataract (Persian, British shorthair)
Chédiak-Higashi syndrome (Blue-smoke Persian)

Chapter 12: Uveal tract

Chédiak-Higashi Syndrome (Blue-smoke Persian)

Chapter 14: Fundus

Chylomicronemia
Lysosomal storage disease (Domestic shorthair)
Progressive retinal atrophy – recessive (Abyssinian)
Rod-cone dysplasia – dominant (Abyssinian)

Chapter 15: Neuro-ophthalmology

Nystagmus (Siamese)
Strabismus (Siamese and Himalayan)

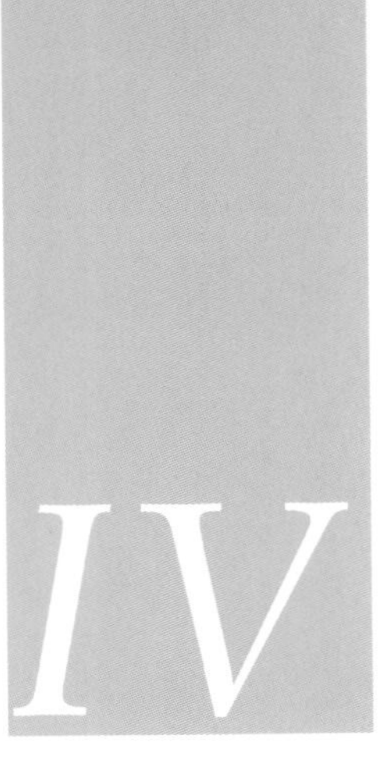

Appendix

Neoplasia

*Denotes most common neoplasm(s) at the specified site

Chapter 3: Emergencies and trauma

(see under lens for poorly differentiated sarcoma)

Chapter 4: Globe and orbit

Adenocarcinoma
Ameloblastoma
Carcinoma
Chondroma
Fibrosarcoma
Haemangiosarcoma
Lymphosarcoma
Melanoma
Meningioma
Osteoma
Osteosarcoma
Rhabdomyosarcoma
Sarcoma
Squamous cell carcinoma

Chapter 5: Upper and lower eyelids

Adenoma
Adenocarcinoma
Basal cell carcinoma
Fibroma
Fibrosarcoma
Haemangioma
Haemangiosarcoma
Mast cell tumour
Melanoma
Neurofibroma
Neurofibrosarcoma
Papilloma
Sarcoma (feline sarcoma virus)
Squamous cell carcinoma*
Undifferentiated carcinoma

Chapter 6: Third eyelid

Adenocarcinoma
Fibrosarcoma
Lymphosarcoma
Mast cell tumour
Squamous cell carcinoma
Undifferentiated carcinoma

Chapter 7: Lacrimal system

Adenocarcinoma
Lymphosarcoma
Squamous cell carcinoma

Chapter 8: Conjunctiva, limbus, episclera and sclera

Adenocarcinoma
Fibrosarcoma
Lymphosarcoma
Melanoma
Squamous cell carcinoma*

Chapter 9: Cornea

Primary neoplasia not recorded.
Secondary involvement:-

Fibrosarcoma
Lymphosarcoma
Scleral shelf melanoma

Chapter 10: Aqueous and glaucoma

Glaucoma may be secondary to invasive neoplasia.

Adenocarcinoma
Haemangiosarcoma
Lymphosarcoma
Melanoma

Chapter 11: Lens

Possible lens epithelium-derived tumour may follow trauma to the globe and lens (recorded in the literature as poorly differentiated sarcoma).

Chapter 12: Uveal tract

Adenoma
Adenocarcinoma
Fibrosarcoma
Haemangiosarcoma
Leiomyoma
Leiomyosarcoma
Lymphosarcoma
Melanoma*
Plasma cell myeloma
Squamous cell carcinoma

Chapter 13: Vitreous

No primary neoplasia recorded. Secondary involvement because of extension from neighbouring structures, usually the uveal tract.

Chapter 14: Fundus

Retina

Adenocarcinoma
Astrocytoma
Carcinoma
Glioma
Haemangiosarcoma
Lymphosarcoma
Neuroblastoma
Plasma cell myeloma
Reticulosis
Sarcoma

Optic nerve

Astrocytoma
Glioma
Lymphosarcoma
Meningioma*
Squamous cell carcinoma

Chapter 15: Neuro-ophthalmology

Ocular manifestations may be associated with a number of tumours, of which meningioma is the most common primary tumour and lymphosarcoma the most common secondary tumour. Other possible tumours are also listed.

Ependymoma
Lymphosarcoma*
Medulloblastoma
Meningioma*
Pituitary tumours
Reticulosis

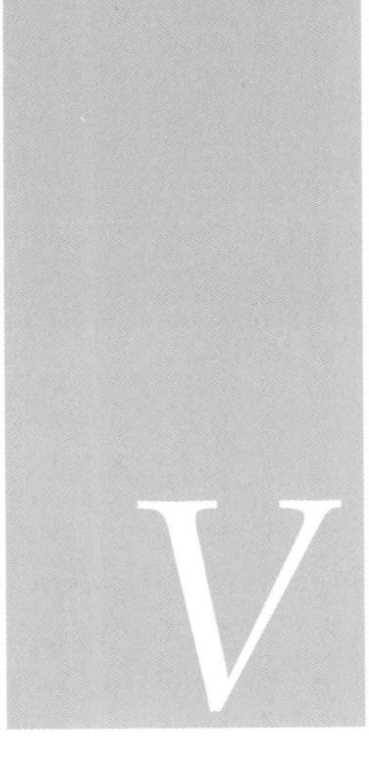

Appendix

Systemic disease

Generalized (metastatic) neoplasia is listed in Appendix IV

Chapter 3: Ocular emergencies and trauma

Brain tumours (see Appendix IV)
Generalized inflammatory disease
Hypertension

Chapter 4: Globe and orbit

Congenital hydrocephalus is associated with enlargement of the calvaria and bony orbits and the globes are deviated ventrolaterally
Disseminated infection, e.g. *Penicillium* sp.
Nutritional pansteatitis
Orbital extension may also be a complication of e.g. dental disease and sinusitis
Parasitic disease: within orbit (e.g. *Thelazia californiensis* and cuterebra larvae)
within eye (e.g. nematodes and dipteran larvae)

Chapter 5: Upper and lower eyelids

Allergic blepharitis, e.g. food allergies
Immune-mediated, e.g. Pemphigus erythematosus, Pemphigus foliaceus, systemic lupus erythematosus.
Mycotic, e.g. *Microsporum canis*
Parasitic, e.g. *Notoedres cati*, cuterebra larvae

Chapter 6: Third eyelid

Chronic diarrhoea associated with possible viral disease (bilateral prominence)
Disseminated infection and orbital cellulitis (unilateral or bilateral prominence)
Dysautonomia (bilateral prominence)
Horner's syndrome (unilateral, rarely bilateral prominence), see under neuro-ophthalmology, Chapter 15)
Tetanus (*Clostridium tetani*) (bilateral prominence)

Chapter 7: Lacrimal system

Dacryoadenitis (e.g. mycobacterial infection)
Dacryocystitis (e.g. as a complication of chronic rhinitis)
KCS associated with dysautonomia

Chapter 8: Conjunctiva, limbus, episclera and sclera

Extension from neighbouring tissues (e.g. sinusitis, orbital cellulitis and abscess)
Parasitic (e.g. thelaziasis)
Respiratory tract viruses (e.g. feline herpesvirus 1, feline calicivirus)

Chapter 9: Cornea

Bacterial: *Mycobacterium* sp.
Diabetes mellitus increases susceptibility to corneal infection
Immune-mediated (e.g. relapsing polychondritis) and note the influence of immunosuppression (e.g. FeLV and FIV) on corneal disease
Lipid deposition associated with dyslipoproteinaemia is rare
Metabolic: inborn errors of metabolism (e.g. GM_1 and GM_2 gangliosidosis, mucopolysaccharidosis I, VI, VII, mannosidosis)
Mycotic: *Candida albicans, Aspergillus fumigatus, Drechslera spicifera, Rhinosporidium* spp.
Parasitic: *Microsporidium* spp.
Viral: feline herpesvirus 1

Chapter 10: Aqueous and glaucoma

Hyphaema (e.g. hypertension, blood dyscrasias)
Lipaemic aqueous (e.g. hypertriglyceridaemia, hyperchylomicronaemia)

Chapter 11: Lens

Cataract associated with metabolic disease (e.g. diabetes mellitus, hypoparathyroidism), nutritional (e.g. arginine deficiency), drug-induced (e.g. associated with chronic use of anticholinesterases)

Chapter 12: Uveal tract

Mycotic: cryptococcosis, histoplasmosis, blastomycosis, coccidiomycosis
Parasitic: *Toxoplasma gondii*, cuterebra larvae, *Dirofilaria immitis*
Viral: feline infectious peritonitis virus, feline leukaemia virus, feline immunodeficiency virus

Chapter 13: Vitreous

Haemorrhage (e.g. secondary to hypertensive retinopathy)
Infectious diseases as for Chapter 11, Uvea, and Chapter 14, Fundus, vitreal involvement is secondary

Chapter 14: Fundus

Retina and Choroid

Chédiak–Higashi syndrome (colour dilution)
Congenital retinal dysplasia as a result of in utero feline panleukopenia infection (with or without cerebellar hypoplasia). Panleukopenia infection may also be associated with chorioretinitis in older cats (see below)
Detachment: hypertension, toxins (e.g. ethylene glycol), infectious causes as listed above, neoplasia
Haemorrhage: hypertension, thiamine deficiency, *Haemobartonella felis* infection, parasitic migration
Inborn errors of metabolism: GM_1 gangliosidosis, mucopolysaccharidosis VI, alphamannosidosis, mucolipidosis type II
Nutritional: taurine deficiency, thiamine deficiency
Mycotic: cryptococcosis, histoplasmosis, blastomycosis, coccidiomycosis, candidiasis
Parasitic: *Toxoplasma gondii*, migrating nematode and dipteran larvae
Vessel changes: Lipid – lipaemia retinalis due to hyperchylomicronaemia
Hyperviscosity – polycythaemia (e.g. congenital heart disease)
Anaemia (e.g. aplastic, autoimmune haemolytic, related to neoplasia)
Hyperproteinaemia (e.g. myeloma, feline infectious peritonitis)
Hypertension – primary and secondary
Viral: feline infectious peritonitis virus, feline leukaemia virus, feline immunodeficiency virus, feline panleukopenia virus

Optic Nerve

Optic neuritis–feline infectious peritonitis, feline leukaemia–lymphosarcoma complex

Chapter 15: Neuro-ophthalmology

Pupil Abnormalities

Dysautonomia
Hepatic encephalopathy
Horner's syndrome (e.g. due to cervical insult, mediastinal space-occupying lesion, brachial plexus damage, middle ear infection or polyp, iatrogenic – following, for example, bulla osteotomy)
Neoplasia (e.g. feline leukaemia–lymphosarcoma complex)
Organophosphate poisoning
Thiamine deficiency

Blindness

Chronic taurine deficiency
Consequence of anoxia, hypoxia, ischaemia
Optic neuritis (see above)
Lysosomal storage disease (e.g. sphingomyelinosis, gangliosidoses)
Vascular infarction

Further reading

Acland G (1979) Intraocular tumours in dogs and cats. *Compendium on Continuing Education for the Practicing Veterinarian* **1**: 558–565.

Aguirre GD, Gross SL (1980) Ocular manifestations of selected systemic disease. *Compendium on Continuing Education for the Practicing Veterinarian* **2**: 144–153.

American Society of Veterinary Ophthalmology (1965) *Canine and Feline Ocular Fundus*. American Animal Hospital Association.

American Society of Veterinary Ophthalmology (1970) *Diseases of the Canine and Feline Conjunctiva and Cornea*. American Animal Hospital Association.

Barnett KC (1990) *A Colour Atlas of Veterinary Ophthalmology*. Wolfe Publishing Ltd, London.

Barnett KC, Ricketts JD (1985) The Eye. In: *Feline Medicine and Therapeutics* (EA Chandler, ADR Hilbery, CJ Gaskell, eds) pp. 176–197. Blackwell Scientific Publications, Oxford.

Bjorab MJ (ed.) (1990) *Current Techniques in Small Animal Surgery*, 3rd edn. Lea and Febiger, Philadelphia.

Bonagura JD (ed.) (1995) *Kirk's Current Veterinary Therapy XII Small Animal Practice*. W.B. Saunders, Philadelphia.

Catcott EJ (ed.) (1975) *Feline Medicine and Surgery*, 2nd edn. American Veterinary Publications Inc., Santa Barbara.

Chrisman CL (1991) *Problems in Small Animal Neurology*, 2nd edn. Lea and Febiger, Philadelphia.

Crouch JE (1969) *Text-Atlas of Cat Anatomy*. Lea and Febiger, Philadelphia.

Collin JRO (1989) *A Manual of Systematic Eyelid Surgery*, 2nd edn. Churchill Livingstone, Edinburgh.

De Lahunta A (1983) *Veterinary Neuroanatomy and Clinical Neurology*, 2nd edn. W.B. Saunders, Philadelphia.

Gelatt KN (1979) Feline Ophthalmology. *Compendium on Continuing Education for the Practicing Veterinarian* **1**(8): 576–583.

Gelatt KN (ed.) (1981) *Veterinary Ophthalmology*. Lea and Febiger, Philadelphia.

Gelatt KN (ed.)(1991) *Veterinary Ophthalmology*, 2nd edn. Lea and Febiger, Philadelphia.

Gelatt KN, Gelatt JP (1994) *Handbook of Small Animal Ophthalmic Surgery*, Vols I and II. Pergamon, Oxford.

Glaze MB (1995) The Retina and Optic Nerve. In: *Veterinary Pediatrics – Dogs and Cats from Birth to Six Months* (JD Hoskins ed.) pp. 325–336. W.B. Saunders, Philadelphia.

Glaze MB (ed.) (1996) *Ophthalmology in Small Animal Practice. The Compendium Collection*. Veterinary Learning Systems, Trenton, New Jersey.

Goldston RT, Hoskins JD (eds) (1995) *Geriatrics and Gerontology of the Dog and Cat*. W.B. Saunders, Philadelphia.

Ketring KL, Glaze MB (1994) *Atlas of Feline Ophthalmology*. Veterinary Learning Systems Co., Inc., Trenton, New Jersey.

Kirk RW, Bonagura JD (eds) (1992) *Kirk's Current Veterinary Therapy XI Small Animal Practice*. W.B. Saunders, Philadelphia.

Millichamp NJ, Dziezyc J (eds) (1990) *Veterinary Clinics of North America: Small Animal Practice* **20**(3). W.B. Saunders, Philadelphia.

Mustardé JC (ed.) (1991) *Repair and Reconstruction in the Orbital Region*. 3rd Edn. Churchill Livingstone, Edinburgh.

Nasisse MP (1991) Feline Ophthalmology. In: *Veterinary Ophthalmology*, 2nd edn (KN Gelatt, ed.) pp. 529–575. Lea and Febiger, Philadelphia.

Oliver JE, Hoerlein BF, Mayhew IG (eds) (1987) *Veterinary Neurology*. W.B. Saunders, Philadelphia.

Patraik AK, Mooney S (1988) Feline melanoma: A comparative study of ocular, oral and dermal neoplasms. *Veterinary Pathology* **25**: 105.

Peiffer RL (1981) Feline Ophthalmology In: *Veterinary Ophthalmology* (KN Gelatt, ed.) pp. 521–568. Lea and Febiger, Philadelphia.

Peiffer RL (ed.) (1989) *Small Animal Ophthalmology: a Problem-oriented Approach*. W.B. Saunders, London.

Peiffer RL (ed.) (1990) *Veterinary Clinics of North America: Small Animal Practice*. **10**(2). W.B. Saunders, Philadelphia.

Peiffer RL & Petersen-Jones SM (eds) (1997) *Small Animal Ophthalmology: A Problem-oriented Approach*, 2nd edn. W.B. Saunders, London.

Petersen-Jones SM, Crispin SM (eds) (1993) *Manual of Small Animal Ophthalmology*. British Small Animal Veterinary Association Publications, Cheltenham.

Phillipson AT, Hall LW, Pritchard WR (eds) (1980) Scientific Foundations of Veterinary Medicine. William Heinemann Medical Books Ltd, London.

Pratt PW (ed.) (1983) *Feline Medicine*. American Veterinary Publications Inc, Santa Barbara.

Prince JH, Diesem CD, Eglitis I, Ruskell GL (1960) *Anatomy and Histology of the Eye and Orbit in Domestic Animals*. Charles C Thomas, Springfield, Illinois.

Rose M (ed.) (1992) Ophthalmologie du Chat. *Pratique Médicale et Chirurgicale* **27**: Supplement No. 3.

Rubin LF (1974) *Atlas of Veterinary Ophthalmoscopy*. Lea and Febiger, Philadelphia.

Sansom J (1994) The Eye. In: *Feline Medicine and Therapeutics*, 2nd edn. (EA Chandler, CJ Gaskell, RM Gaskell, eds) pp. 322–359. Blackwell Scientific Publications, Oxford.

Slatter D (1990) *Fundamentals of Veterinary Ophthalmology*, 2nd edn. W.B. Saunders, Philadelphia.

Slatter D (ed.) (1993) *Textbook of Small Animal Surgery*, 2nd edn. W.B. Saunders, Phildelphia.

Szymanski C (1987) The Eye. In: *Diseases of the Cat* (Holzworth J, ed.) pp. 676–723. WB Saunders Co, Philadelphia.

Walde I, Schäffer EH, Kostlin RG (1990) *Atlas of Ophthalmology in Dogs and Cats*. B.C. Decker Inc., Toronto, Philadelphia.

Walde I, Schäffer EH, Kostlin RG (1997) *Atlas der Augenerkrankungen bei Hund und Katz*, 2nd edn. Schattauer Stuttgart, New York.

Wheeler SJ (ed.) (1995) *Manual of Small Animal Neurology*. British Small Animal Veterinary Association Publications, Cheltenham.

Whitley RD, Moore CP (1984) Advances in feline ophthalmology. *Veterinary Clinics of North America: Small Animal Practice* (JR August, AS Loar, eds) **14**: 1271–1288.

Whitley RD, Hamilton HL, Weigand CM (1993) Glaucoma and disorders of the uvea, lens, and retina in cats. *Veterinary Medicine* **88**: 1164–1173.

Whitley RD, Gilger BC, Whitley EM, McLaughlin SA (1993) Diseases of the orbit, globe, eyelids and lacrimal system in the cat. *Veterinary Medicine* **88**: 1150–1162.

Whitley RD, Whitley EM, McLaughlin SA (1993) Diagnosing and treating disorders of the feline conjunctiva and cornea. *Veterinary Medicine* **88**: 1138–1149.

Wilkie DA (1994) Diseases and Surgery of the Eye. In: *The Cat: Diseases and Clinical Management, Volume II*, 2nd edn. (RG Sherding, ed.) pp. 2011–2046. Churchill Livingstone, New York.

Wills J, Wolf A (eds) (1993) *Handbook of Feline Medicine*. Pergamon, Oxford.

Wyman M (1986) *Manual of Small Animal Ophthalmology*. Churchill Livingstone, New York.

Index